Recent Advances in Noncoding RNAs
http://dx.doi.org/10.5772/intechopen.98151
Edited by Lütfi Tutar

Contributors
Mashooq Ahmad Ahmad Dar, Ishteyaq Majeed Shah, Kaiser Ahmad Bhat, Tashook Ahmad Dar, Fayaz Ahmad, Syed Mudasir Ahmad, Lütfi Tutar, Hussein Al-Dahmoshi, Noor Salman Al-Khafaji, Moaed E. Al-Gazally, Maha F. Smaism, Zena Abdul Ameer Mahdi, Suhad Y. Abed, Thanh Thi Ngoc Nguyen, Thu Huynh Ngoc Nguyen, Luan Huu Huynh, Hoang Ngo Phan, Hue Thi Nguyen, Mohsin Munawar, Irfana Liaqat, Shaukat Ali, Neetu Singh, Shahzad Irfan, Farhat Jabeen, Haseeb Anwar, Patricia Silveyra, Maksat Babayev, Tomomi Fujii, Tomoko Uchiyama, Maiko Takeda, Manoel Teixeira Souza Junior, Fernanda Salgado, Priscila Grynberg

First published in London, United Kingdom, 2022 by IntechOpen
IntechOpen is the global imprint of INTECHOPEN LIMITED, registered in England and Wales, registration number: 11086078, 5 Princes Gate Court, London, SW7 2QJ, United Kingdom

British Library Cataloguing-in-Publication Data
A catalogue record for this book is available from the British Library

Additional hard and PDF copies can be obtained from orders@intechopen.com

Recent Advances in Noncoding RNAs
Edited by Lütfi Tutar
p. cm.
Print ISBN 978-1-80356-014-4
Online ISBN 978-1-80356-015-1
eBook (PDF) ISBN 978-1-80356-016-8

For EU product safety concerns:
IN TECH d.o.o., Prolaz Marije Krucifikse Kozulić 3, 51000 Rijeka, Croatia,
info@intechopen.com or visit our website at intechopen.com.

Meet the editor

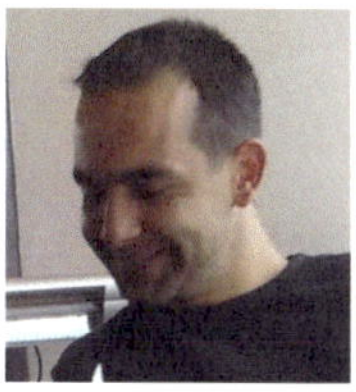

Dr. Lütfi Tutar is currently an assistant professor in the Department of Molecular Biology and Genetics, Faculty of Art and Sciences, Kırşehir Ahi Evran University, Turkey. His interdisciplinary research focuses on bioinformatics analysis of high-throughput data, microRNAs, small RNAs, and heat shock proteins (HSPs) in human diseases and other multicellular organisms.

Contents

Preface

Noncoding RNAs (ncRNAs), which play important roles in regulating gene expression in animals, plants, and various human diseases, have had a huge impact on RNA biology. This book provides an overview of current ncRNA research dealing with miRNA- and ncRNA-related human diseases and molecular diagnosis, plant ncRNAs, and the role of lncRNAs in cancer.

The introductory chapter provides an overview of ncRNAs, and the subsequent chapters constitute an essential resource for researchers in the field of ncRNAs, miRNAs and lncRNAs. Chapter 2 discusses the origin of lncRNAs, their biogenesis, their mechanism of action and their role in many biological and pathological processes such as epigenetics, genome imprinting, several cancers and autoimmune diseases. Chapter 3 examines the advantage of noncoding RNA in molecular diagnosis and looks in detail at the roles of miRNAs in various cancers. The processes leading to the identification of their target molecules are described, and the latest diagnostic strategies using miRNAs are discussed with specific examples. Chapter 4 focuses on the role of ncRNAs in lung cancer pathogenesis as well as their potential use as biomarkers or therapies against lung cancer. Chapters 5 and 6 describe the roles of miRNAs in pancreatic ß cell functional modulation and breast cancer. Chapter 5 discusses the multiple effects of different types of microRNAs on ß cell physiology in the context of maintenance and function in type 2 diabetes. Chapter 6 describes the SNP prediction in mature miRNAs dysregulated in breast cancer. Chapter 7 describes the roles and molecular mechanisms of lncRNAs in neural stem cell self-renewal, neurogenesis, gliogenesis and synaptogenesis over the course of neural development. Chapter 8 describes lncRNA and miRNA interactions in digestive system tumors and the vital role played by ncRNAs (both miRNA and lncRNA) in some digestive system tumors, either as oncogene promoting cancer viability, invasiveness, proliferation, and metastasis or as tumor suppressor inhibiting tumorigenicity or inducing apoptosis. Chapter 9 looks at the miRNA-mediated regulatory mechanism related to male infertility. The final chapter summarizes current knowledge on miRNA involvement in oil palm plant response to abiotic stress and suggests possible miRNA-based strategies for the genetic improvement of oil palm salinity and drought stress tolerance. Overall, this book provides a unique perspective for scientists in the field of ncRNA biology.

Lütfi Tutar
Kırşehir Ahi Evran University,
Kırşehir, Turkey

Chapter 1

Introductory Chapter: Noncoding RNAs–A Brief Introduction

Lütfi Tutar

1. Introduction

The discovery of ribosomal RNAs (rRNAs) and transfer RNAs (tRNAs) in 1960s led to first steps of noncoding RNA (ncRNA) research [1–3]. In 1980, 90–220 nucleotides long small nuclear RNAs (snRNAs) were involved in splicing reported by Lerner *et al.* [4]. When microRNAs (miRNAs) were discovered in the late 1990s, the noncoding RNA research gained a momentum [5, 6]. Furthermore, development of the next-generation sequencing technologies and advanced bioinformatics opens a new era for noncoding RNAs (ncRNAs).

Ubiquitously, ncRNAs are present in all three domains of life and less than 2% of the human genome code for proteins. Generally, ncRNAs do not code for proteins, but there is some exceptions coding for small bioactive peptides [7, 8]. The two major groups of ncRNAs may be separated from each other by having less or more 200 nucleotides (nts): small noncoding RNAs (sncRNAs) are shorter than 200 nts, and long noncoding RNAs (lncRNAs) are longer than 200 nts.

Noncoding RNAs may be grouped into some categories; tRNA (transfer RNA), rRNA (ribosomal RNA), snRNA (small nuclear RNA), snoRNA (small nucleolar RNA), Telomerase RNA, tRF (transfer RNA-derived RNA fragments), and tiRNA (tRNA-derived stress-induced RNAs) are all "housekeeping" RNAs. "Regulatory" RNAs are miRNA (microRNA), siRNA (small interfering RNA), piRNA (P-element-induced wimpy testis (PIWI) interacting RNA), eRNA (enhancer RNA), lncRNA (long noncoding RNA), circRNA (circular RNA), YRNA, crasiRNA (centromere repeat associated short interacting RNA), and TelsRNA (telomere-specific small RNA). Based on structure, LincRNA (long intergenic noncoding RNA), TUCRNA (transcribed ultraconserved RNA), eRNA, and NAT (natural antisense transcript) are "linear" RNAs while ciRNA, ecircRNA (exonic circular RNA), and elciRNA (exon–intron circRNA) are "circular" RNAs. Based on the location, RNAs may be grouped as sense, antisense, intronic, intergenic, and bidirectional RNAs. Some of the ncRNA families are briefly reviewed below. Rfam is a public online database, which provides information for all RNA families, each represented by multiple sequence alignments, consensus secondary structures, and covariance models (https://rfam.xfam.org/) [9].

2. miRNAs (microRNAs)

miRNAs are ~20 nts long molecules that generally regulate gene expression by inducing mRNA degradation or translational repression. miRNAs originated from pri-miRNA and mature miRNAs regulate protein coding genes. Understanding the regulation of gene expression is changed after the discovery of first miRNA called lin-4 on *Caenorhabditis elegans* in 1993 [5]. Furthermore, miRNAs are potential biomarkers for several human diseases since they are responsible for many biological processes in the cell such as cell differentiation, cell proliferation, cell death, and development by inducing mRNA degradation or translational repression. Especially, oncomirs such as mir-21 are generally upregulated in cancer patients, and miRNAs attract researchers because of their potential as diagnostic and prognostic biomarkers. miRNA gene sequences are publicly deposited on miRBase catalogs (https://www.mirbase.org/) [10].

3. siRNAs (small interfering RNAs)

siRNAs are about 20–22 nts in size and evolved from double-stranded RNAs. They perform silent transcription of genes via inducing mRNA degradation. siRNAs are very attractive for therapeutic applications in cancer and other diseases [11]. Especially, siRNAs target genes within the tumor cells to inhibit expansions of tumors by RNAi (RNA interference) technology [12]. Moreover, RNAi is a powerful tool in agriculture for crop improvement, including development against biotic or abiotic stress, seedless fruit development, improvement of nutritional quality, and induction of male sterility [13]. Furthermore, a database of siRNA sequences called siRNAdb located on http://sirna.cgb.ki.se/ provides information for siRNAs [14].

4. piRNAs (P-element-induced wimpy testis (PIWI) interacting RNAs)

piRNAs are small noncoding RNAs, which originated from long single chain precursor transcripts. These RNAs are about 21–35 nts long and interact with PIWI proteins to form the piRNA silencing complex (piRISC). piRNAs play key roles in transposon repression, DNA methylation, silencing transposable elements, regulating gene expression, and fighting with viral infections. Since their abnormal expression is reported for many cancer types, they have potential to be diagnostic tools, prognostic markers, and therapeutic targets for cancer [15]. There are two important databases for piRNAs on the web, piRNAdb and piRNABank. piRNAdb is a piwi-interacting RNA sequences storage and search system, providing some other relevant information such as alignments, clusters, datasets, and targets of these piRNAs on its URL (https://www.pirnadb.org/index). piRNABank provides comprehensive information on piRNAs in the three widely studied mammals, namely Human, Mouse, Rat and one fruit fly, Drosophila on the http://pirnabank.ibab.ac.in/ web address [16].

5. lncRNAs (long noncoding RNAs)

lncRNAs with longer than 200 nts are not translated into functional proteins and evolved from multiple ways and mainly transcribed by RNA polymerase II (and also by other RNA polymerases). lncRNAs regulate gene expressions in multiple ways including chromatin structure modulation, regulation of function and the transcription of neighboring and distant genes, and alteration of RNA splicing, stability and translation by interacting with DNA, RNA, and proteins. Moreover, lncRNAs can play roles in the formation and regulation of organelles [17]. Furthermore, they take roles in chromatin remodeling, cancer cell invasion and metastasis, and cell differentiation by acting as cis- or trans-regulators in biological processes [18]. lncRNAs are linked to some human diseases including hepatocellular carcinoma, Alzheimer's disease, and diabetes [19]. Owing to their key roles in diseases, lncRNAs have a potential to be therapeutic targets. Recently, antisense oligonucleotides (ASOs) technology is used to perform therapeutic lncRNA targeting [20, 21]. However, since lncRNAs lack of functional open reading frames, targeting them with CRISPR–Cas system is more difficult compared with targeting protein-coding genes [22]. There are too many lncRNA databases on the internet, but most comprehensive lncRNA database is RNAcentral located at https://rnacentral.org/ on the World Wide Web [23]. RNAcentral offers integrated access to a comprehensive and up-to-date set of ncRNA sequences.

6. Future perspectives

Mounting data, evidence, and recent discoveries of novel short and long regulatory noncoding RNAs have changed the understanding of genome and transcriptome in the cell. Advanced bioinformatics, public databases, and sequencing technologies led to fast understanding of biogenesis and function of ncRNA types and families. ncRNAs are potential biomarkers to perform therapeutic applications for diseases and to improve crops for agriculture. Further illumination of function, biogenesis, and interactions of ncRNAs will empower our understanding of natural dogma with the aid of developing bioinformatics, sequencing, and biochemical techniques.

Author details

Lütfi Tutar
Faculty of Arts and Sciences, Department of Molecular Biology and Genetics, Kırşehir Ahi Evran University, Kırşehir, Turkey

*Address all correspondence to: lutfitutar@gmail.com

References

[1] Crick FHC. The origin of the genetic code. Journal of Molecular Biology. 1968;**38**(3):367-379

[2] Crick FHC, Barnett L, Brenner S, Watts-Tobin RJ. General nature of the genetic code for proteins. Nature. 1961;**192**(4809):1227-1232

[3] Nirenberg M, Leder P. RNA codewords and protein synthesis. Science (80-.). 1964;**145**(3639):1399-1407

[4] Lerner MR, Boyle JA, Mount SM, Wolin SL, Steitz JA. Are snRNPs involved in splicing? Nature. 1980;**283**(5743):220-224

[5] Lee RC, Feinbaum RL, Ambros V. The C. elegans heterochronic gene lin-4 encodes small RNAs with antisense complementarity to lin-14. Cell. 1993;**75**(5):843-854

[6] Tutar L, Tutar E, Tutar Y. MicroRNAs and cancer; an overview. Current Pharmaceutical Biotechnology. 2014;**15**(5):430-437

[7] Anderson DM et al. A micropeptide encoded by a putative long noncoding RNA regulates muscle performance. Cell. 2015;**160**(4):595-606

[8] Kondo T et al. Small peptides switch the transcriptional activity of Shavenbaby during Drosophila embryogenesis. Science. 2010;**329**(5989):336-339

[9] Kalvari I et al. Non-coding RNA analysis using the Rfam database. Current Protocols in Bioinformatics. 2018;**62**(1):e51

[10] Kozomara A, Birgaoanu M, Griffiths-Jones S. miRBase: From microRNA sequences to function. Nucleic Acids Research. 2019;**47**(D1):D155-D162

[11] Nam N-H, Parang K. Current targets for anticancer drug discovery. Current Drug Targets. 2003;**4**(2):159-179

[12] Senapati D et al. Promising approaches of small interfering RNAs (siRNAs) mediated cancer gene therapy. Gene. 2019;**719**:144071

[13] Rajam MV. RNA silencing technology: A boon for crop improvement. Journal of Biosciences. 2020;**45**(1):118

[14] Chalk AM. siRNAdb: A database of siRNA sequences. Nucleic Acids Research. 2004;**33**(Database issue):D131-D134

[15] Guo B, Li D, Du L, Zhu X. piRNAs: Biogenesis and their potential roles in cancer. Cancer Metastasis Reviews. 2020;**39**(2):567-575

[16] Sai Lakshmi S, Agrawal S. piRNABank: A web resource on classified and clustered Piwi-interacting RNAs. Nucleic Acids Research. 2008;**36**(suppl_1):D173-D177

[17] Statello L, Guo C-J, Chen L-L, Huarte M. Gene regulation by long non-coding RNAs and its biological functions. Nature Reviews. Molecular Cell Biology. 2021;**22**(2):96-118

[18] Dhanoa JK, Sethi RS, Verma R, Arora JS, Mukhopadhyay CS. Long non-coding RNA: Its evolutionary relics and biological implications in mammals: A review. Journal of Animal Science and Technology. 2018;**60**:25

[19] DiStefano JK. "The emerging role of long noncoding RNAs in human disease". 2018:91-110

[20] Lee J-S, Mendell JT. Antisense-mediated transcript knockdown triggers premature transcription termination. Molecular Cell. 2020;**77**(5):1044-1054.e3

[21] Lai F, Damle SS, Ling KK, Rigo F. Directed RNase H cleavage of nascent transcripts causes transcription termination. Molecular Cell. 2020;**77**(5):1032-1043.e4

[22] Esposito R, Bosch N, Lanzós A, Polidori T, Pulido-Quetglas C, Johnson R. Hacking the cancer genome: Profiling therapeutically actionable long non-coding RNAs using CRISPR-Cas9 screening. Cancer Cell. 2019;**35**(4):545-557

[23] Petrov AI et al. RNAcentral: A comprehensive database of non-coding RNA sequences. Nucleic Acids Research. 2017;**45**(D1):D128-D134

Chapter 2

Long Non-Coding RNAs: Biogenesis, Mechanism of Action and Role in Different Biological and Pathological Processes

Ishteyaq Majeed Shah, Mashooq Ahmad Dar, Kaiser Ahmad Bhat, Tashook Ahmad Dar, Fayaz Ahmad and Syed Mudasir Ahmad

Abstract

RNA or ribonucleic acid constitutes of nucleotides, which are ribose sugars coupled to nitrogenous bases and phosphate groups. Nitrogenous bases include adenine, guanine, cytosine and uracil. Messenger RNA, ribosomal RNA and Transfer RNA are three main types of RNA that are involved in protein synthesis. Apart from its primary role in synthesis of protein, RNA comes in variety of forms like snRNA, miRNA, siRNA, antisense RNA, LncRNA etc., that are involved in DNA replication, post-transcriptional modification, and gene regulation etc. LncRNAs regulate gene expression by various ways including at, transcriptional, post-transcriptional, translational, post-translational and epigenetic levels by interacting principally with mRNA, DNA, protein, and miRNA. Among other biological functions, they are involved in chromatin remodelling, transcriptional interference, transcriptional activation, mRNA translation and RNA processing. In this chapter we shall be discussing the origin of lncRNAs, their biogenesis, their mechanism of action and their role in many biological and pathological processes like epigenetics, genome imprinting, several cancers and autoimmune diseases.

Keywords: long non-coding RNAs, epigenetics, chromatin remodelling, gene expression regulation, cancer, autoimmune diseases

1. Introduction

The genome of higher organisms contains less than 3% of protein coding genes while rest of genome is known as junk/or non-coding. With recent advances in science and technology we are learning more about the complexity of organisms, which has led to the discovery of the remarkable complexity of RNA. Large-scale projects such as ENCODE and FANTOM, for the systematic annotation and functional depiction of genes have pointed that 80% of genomic DNA of mammals are effectively transcribed and intricately controlled with majority belonging to noncoding RNA genes [1]. The figure of ncRNA genes varies by species. Frequency of ncRNA genes but not protein-coding genes, is strongly linked with the complexity of an organism emphasising the growing relevance of ncRNAs [2]. On the basis of molecular size ncRNAs can be classified into two groups. One group includes short RNAs that are less than 200 nucleotides in length such as microRNAs (20–25 nucleotides Length), piwi-interacting RNAs etc. The other group includes Long-non coding RNAs of around 200 nucleotides or more in length. Among the ncRNAs, long non coding RNAs represent a greater portion. Regulatory non coding RNAs with length $\geq$ 200 nucleotides belong to long non coding RNAs (lncRNAs). Due to their low expression levels, lncRNAs in the beginning were considered to be transcription noise. According to HUMAN GENCODE statistics, there are around 16,000 lncRNA genes, although some estimates put the number at over 100,000 [3, 4]. RNA polymerase II is primarily responsible for lncRNA transcription, but other RNA polymerases are also involved. The resultant lncRNAs are frequently capped at their 5′ ends with 7-methyl guanosine (m7G), polyadenylated at their 3′ ends, and spliced similarly to mRNAs. lncRNAs, in contrast, have a median turnover of 3.5 h, while it is 5.1 h for mRNAs. After transcription, the widely held lncRNAs stay in the nucleus [5]. LncRNAs regulate gene expression at different domains including the ones at epigenetic, transcriptional, post-transcriptional, translational, and post-translational levels by interacting principally with DNA, mRNA, protein, and miRNA [5]. LncRNAs regulate gene transcription by promoting or inhibiting the formation of transcription loops and recruiting or blocking regulators. LncRNAs also operate as precursors to other ncRNAs, such as microRNAs (miRNAs), and influence mRNA splicing [6]. They are involved in RNA processing, transcriptional interference, chromatin remodelling, transcriptional activation, and mRNA translation, among other biological processes. Besides these roles they also act as oncogenes or tumour suppressors by regulating different signalling cascades [7]. Based on their functions lncRNAs are classified into three types: non-functional lncRNAs, these are products of transcriptional noise; lncRNAs for which the act of transcription is adequate for their activity but the transcript itself is not required and functional lncRNAs that act in both cis and trans ways [8]. In recent years, lncRNAs which account for the immense majority of non-coding RNAs (ncRNAs), have become a hot topic in disease diagnostics and target therapeutics in recent years.

2. Biogenesis of lncRNAs

Understanding the biosynthesis of these lncRNAs is not only crucial but also ineluctable in order to decipher their functional value, relevance, and differentiation from other forms of RNAs. LncRNA biogenesis is both cell type and stage specific, regulated by stage and cell specific stimuli [9]. Enhancers, promoters, and intergenic regions are among the DNA components in eukaryotic genomes that transcribe diverse types of lncRNAs [10]. LncRNA biogenesis involve ribonuclease P for cleavage to create mature ends, the production of protein (snoRNP) complex caps at their ends, small nucleolar RNA, and the development of circular structures [11, 12]. During specific lncRNAs biogenesis, "paraspeckles" (sub-nuclear structures) have been discovered [13]. The identity of 4 paraspeckle proteins (PSPs) required for paraspeckle formation was made possible by RNAi analyses of 40 paraspeckle proteins [14]. Overall, the biology dealing with regulation, synthesis of various lncRNAs is still unknown.

3. Origin of LncRNAs

Compared to protein-coding genes, very less information regarding origins and evolution of lncRNAs is available. They reveal that among mammals, sequence conservation is poor and evolution is fast [15]. For the origin of lncRNAs, various evolutionary assumptions have been considered. The first idea is that the protein-coding gene undergoes transformation as a result of a gene-duplication process [16, 17]. Throughout evolution, one copy of a protein-coding gene acquires mutations and loses its capacity to code for proteins. Then, among other coding fractions, a new functional lncRNA gene is generated with polyadenylation sequences, splicing signals, regulatory elements and exon sequences [16, 18].

X inactive-specific transcript (XIST), meant for dosage compensation in mammals is assumed to have arisen from the chicken protein-coding Lnx3 gene [16, 17, 19], was classified as a pseudo gene [18]. The 5-UTR of Lnx3 exons 1 and 2 were used to create the XIST promoter region. Lnx3 exons 4 and 11 were also used to create exons 4 and 5 of the XIST gene of humans [20]. Other lncRNA genes, such as short and long non-coding RNAs, can duplicate segments or whole genes to generate lncRNAs. According to genomic research large homologous protein-coding gene families, protein coding gene duplication is ubiquitous; yet apart from protein coding genes, there is minimal proof for the entire duplication of lncRNAs. This might be owing to the fast sequence divergence of lncRNAs. The duplicated lncRNA mouse nuclear-enriched abundant transcript 2 is paralogous to non exonic sequences in the mouse genome [18]. The generation of lncRNAs appears to be aided by segmental gene duplication within antisense non-coding RNAs (ancRNAs).

De novo creation is another option for lncRNA origins. Examples include genome changes viz. chromosomal rearrangement, creation of (proto-) splice sites and (proto-) promoters transformed non-functional genomic stretches into functional lncRNAs [16]. Genesis of lncRNAs via insertion of transposable elements is the most recent and final hypothesis [17, 18, 21]. The bulk of human lncRNAs have TE segments as related to other genes such as pseudo genes, tiny lncRNAs, and protein-coding genes. Internal exons, transcription start sites, polyadenylation (polyA) sites, or a mix of these components can all include TEs. According to this research at least 75% of human lncRNAs contain at least one exon containing partial TE origin.

4. Mechanism of action of LncRNAs

4.1 LncRNAs as chromatin regulators

The figure of lncRNAs with known roles is gradually increasing, and the majority of the studies focus on their controlling potential. Histone modifications, DNA methylation, and chromatin remodelling are all functional steps where lncRNAs regulate chromatin structure.

LncRNAs are frequently used as important regulators (modulators) of protein coding gene expression by acting in cis and trans ways [22]. Binding of lncRNAs to histone modification complexes like PRC1 and PRC2 [in-specific] causes methylation of lysine 27 on histone 3, a histone signature connected to suppressed transcriptional state. Xist, a lncRNA abundantly generated from inactive X chromosomes in females (Xi), enhances PRC2 recruitment to the Xi to mute gene expression, according to studies on mammalian X chromosome inactivation [23, 24]. Other example includes HOTAIR lncRNA, synthesised from the HoxC gene cluster but targets histone H3K4me1/2 demethylase LSD1 and PRC2 complex to induce transcriptional gene suppression at the HoxD locus in trans [25]. Some well-studied lncRNAs, including ANRIL and KCNQ1OT1, bring epigenetic modifiers to particular loci, allowing for chromatin remodelling. For example, KCNQ1OT1, binds to PRC2 as well as the methyl-transferase G9A, whereas ANRIL binds to both polycomb repressive complexes [26]. Many different lncRNAs act as scaffolds and work by leading restrictive histone modifying complexes to particular loci [26]. By forming complexes with the trithorax group (TrxG) and the polycomb repressive complex 2, lncRNA steroid receptor RNA activator also plays a role in transcriptional control [27].

Examples of lncRNA that interact with PRC1 complex include FAL1 RNA (focally amplified lncRNA on chromosome 1). BMI1, a PRC1 subunit, interacts with FAL1. FAL1 controls not only the stability of BMI1, but also its connection with target promoter regions, altering target gene expression [28].

4.2 Transcriptional regulation

At gene promoters transcription is thought to be regulated by the interaction of transcription factors and chromatin modifying factors. LncRNAs regulate gene expression by interacting with other molecules such as Proteins, RNA and DNA near their target genes promoters or enhancers. LncRNAs have a number of ways for controlling transcription.

I. Enhancer RNAs: Enhancer RNAs (eRNAs) are a sort of long noncoding RNA (lncRNA) derived from gene enhancer regions that act along with DNA to upregulate gene transcription via two mechanisms: transcriptional machinery tracking and enhancer-promoter looping [29]. Kim et al. found a 2 kb eRNA transcribed bidirectional from active enhancers. The function of enhancer region was correlated with the expression of this eRNA, suggesting that eRNAs play a task in enhancer function and influence gene transcription [30, 31].

II. Activating ncRNAs: Class of lncRNAs that acts as a transcriptional activator and is produced from independent loci instead of enhancers. In an RNA-dependent way, activating ncRNAs need the activation of the coding gene promoter and exclusively trigger the transcription of neighbouring coding genes. The mediator complex has been connected to a variety of activating ncRNAs, and attenuation of such complex prevents looping between the activating ncRNAs locus and its target gene.

III. By recruitment of chromatin modifiers: LncRNAs can modulate target genes by triggering epigenetic alteration viz. DNA methylation, histone modification, and by bringing chromatin remodelling complexes to specific genomic loci, typically promoter regions. LncRNAs might have two purposes. Firstly, by attaching to a protein or protein complex, lncRNAs act as a bridge scaffold for chromatin conformational changes [32]. Second, lncRNAs lead chromatin modifying enzymes to particular DNA patterns by acting as a tethered scaffold. For instance, the lncRNA HOTAIR serves as an epigenetic protein scaffold with several binding domains for various proteins. HOTAIR aids in the demethylation of H3K4 by interacting with LSD1 (lysine-specific histone demethylase 1A), REST (restriction element 1-silencing transcription) factor & REST corepressor1 at the 3′ end. HOTAIR (At the 5′ end) is a transcriptional gene silencing factor derived from the HOXC locus that leads to transcriptional gene silencing in trans across 40 kb of the HOXD locus by inducing a repressive chromatin state, recruiting PRC2, & reinforcing H3K27 methylation [33].

Long non-coding RNAs also function as cofactors, influencing the activity of transcription factors. For example, the ncRNA Evf2 is produced from a conserved distal enhancer and attracts DlX2 (TF) to the same enhancer, causing neighbouring protein-coding genes to be expressed.

4.3 Regulation after transcription

Because ncRNAs can recognise complementary sequences, they can affect how mRNAs are processed after transcription, including capping, splicing, editing, transport, translation, destruction, and stability. LncRNAs compete with microRNAs to impact mRNA levels by changing mRNA stability, degradation, and translation [34].

I. **Regulation of mRNA splicing by LncRNAs**: Alternative splicing can be aided by lncRNAs in a number of ways. LncRNAs interact with splicing factors most of the time to regulate gene splicing. MALAT1, a notable lncRNA is involved in pre-mRNA splicing. MALAT1 is needed for the precise localization of SRSF1 and numerous other splicing factors to nuclear speckles. Deletion of MALAT1 is associated with the change in the alternative splicing of a group of transcripts [35]. Other lncRNA like Gomafu/MIAT, restricted to a nuclear domain and expresses neuronally, may influence mRNA splicing and obstruct spliceosome formation by sequestering splicing factor1 [36]. Chromatin-mediated splicing control is the other way through these ncRNAs can modulate alternative splicing. For instance, nuclear antisense lncRNA generated from FGFR2 locus promotes FGFR2 epithelial-specific alternative splicing. The lncRNA establishes a chromatin environment that precludes the binding of a restrictive chromatin-splicing adaptor complex required for mesenchymal-specific splicing by attracting Polycomb-group proteins and KDM2a (Histone demethylase) [37].

II. **Regulation of mRNA stability**: Because of interactions between their 3′-UTR and RBPs (RNA Binding Proteins), many genes have a limited mRNA half-life. Because lncRNAs can interact with RBPs, this type of interaction is expected to alter not just the number of RBPs in the pool, but also the functioning of lncRNAs that share binding sites with other genes, both coding and noncoding. By this way, mRNA molecules are either stabilised or destabilised. RBPs of different kinds may have a function in mRNA stability and, as a result, mRNA level. HuR is destabilised when the lncRNA OCC-1 binds with it and recruits the ubiquitin E3 ligase-TrCP1 to it [38]. HuR works as a stabilising factor for a wide number of mRNAs, causing HuR-targeted mRNAs to be down regulated. Linc-RoR interacts with hnRNP I (stabilising factor) and AUF1 (destabilising factor) in the opposite way that it interacts with c-Myc mRNA, according to findings [39].

III. **Regulation of protein stability:** Many studies have discovered that lncRNAs can influence protein stability through ubiquitination or phosphorylation. DINO, a damage-induced noncoding RNA (lncRNA) that is p53-dependent, affects p53 stability [40]. DINO participates in p53-mediated phenotypes such as Apoptosis and cell cycle arrest with respect to DNA damage. Eminently, DINO binds to and stabilises p53, allowing induced p53 to favourably regulate downstream targets like DINO. Because of its capacity to stabilise the p53 protein, DINO is an important component of the DNA damage-p53 regulation network. lncRNA GUARDIN is another paragon, which is likewise a p53-responsive lncRNA [41].

4.4 LncRNA-mediated regulation of protein activity

Several studies have discovered that lncRNAs can influence protein stability through ubiquitination or phosphorylation. DINO (lncRNA) has a function in phenotypes regulated by p53, such lncRNAs also regulate protein activity in mechanisms other than transcription. The *Caenorhabditis elegans* lncRNA rncs-1 found by Hellwig and Bass (2008) and functions in the processing of short RNAs by binding to and blocking the Dicer enzyme [42]. Marchese FP et al. established the involvement of lncRNA CONCR in sister chromatid cohesion control [43]. CONCR is a cell cycle-regulated lncRNA that is essential for DNA replication and cell cycle advancement and is activated by MYC. CONCR interacts with DDX11 (DNA-dependent transcription factor) and regulates its activity. ATPase and helicase have an impact on DNA replication and sister chromatid cohesion. Liu et al. showed how lncRNA regulates kinase signalling in the setting of metabolic stress response. The LKB1-AMPK pathway promotes the expression of lncRNA neighbour of BRCA1 gene 2 (NBR2), which has also been found to interact with AMPK in the context of energy stress [44]. The association

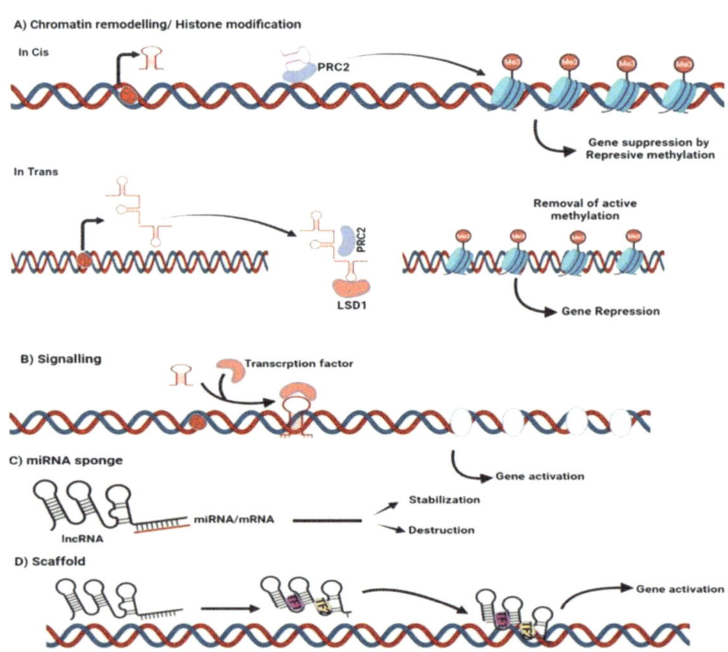

Figure 1.
Schematic representation of few mechanisms employed by lncRNAs in regulation gene expression. (A) Regulation by chromatin remodelling (B) Regulation through signalling (C) lncRNA sponging mRNA (D) By acting as scaffolds.

of lncRNA NBR2 with AMPK enhances its kinase activity under energy stress. AMPK activation is decreased in NBR2 loss, resulting in aberrant cell cycle, altered apoptosis/autophagy responses, and increase in tumour formation. The hypoxia-regulated lncRNA linc-p21 has been found to bind both HIF-1 and VHL, altering the VHL-HIF-1 interaction and increasing HIF-1 accumulation [45]. The importance of lincRNA-p21 in the control of the Warburg effect in tumour cells is highlighted by this positive feedback loop between HIF-1 and lincRNA-p21, which accelerates glycolysis under hypoxia. Certain lncRNAs control transcription factor activity in addition to impacting gene expression via mRNA interactions. As an alternatively spliced form of Evf-1 RNA, the lncRNA Evf2 is generated from the Dlx-5/6 ultra-conserved region. The lncRNA Evf2 forms a stable complex with the transcription factor Dlx2, boosting Dlx-5/6 enhancer transcriptional activation mediated by Dlx2 [46].

Despite the fact that lncRNAs are distinct from mRNAs exported to cytoplasm for protein synthesis [47, 48], few lncRNAs are confined in sub-nuclear compartments, suggesting possible activities in these compartments. The schematic figure that represents few mechanisms employed by lncRNAs in gene expression regulation (**Figure 1**).

5. Roles and functions of lncRNAs in different biological processes

An emerging view of lncRNAs is that they are key players in many biological processes. These lncRNAs have been discovered to be master regulators in different biological and pathological processes and their dysregulations leads to many life-threatening diseases including different cancers. Some of the pivotal roles and functions carried out by different lncRNAs are well documented.

5.1 Long non-coding RNAs in genomic imprinting: regulation of allelic expression

In layman's terms genomic imprinting represents a condition in which one of the alleles in an inherited paternal pair is active while the other one remains inactive. It is the parent of origin which will determines the differential expression of inherited parental alleles; in some cases, a genes allele is paternally imprinted, while in others, it is maternally imprinted.

Dna Methylation and Genomic imprinting: The process of adding a methyl (CH3) group to a cytosine known as DNA methylation is commonly located at CpG dinucleotides in mammals and is believed to regulate gene expression. CpG sites are very rare in the genome with the exceptions of CpG islands (which have high CpG amount/density). Generally found near or around promoter region these islands are usually unmethylated. Outside of CpG islands, CpG sites are often methylated, resulting in a bimodal methylation pattern across the genome. A family of DNA methyltransferases catalyses the acquisition of DNA methylation. DNMT1 is a DNA methyltransferase homologue that has an affinity for hemi-methylated DNA and is responsible for sustaining methylation following DNA replication. DNMT3A and DNMT3B catalyse de novo DNA methylation, while DNMT3L is a cofactor with no methyltransferase activity [49]. DNA methylation leads to epigenetic mechanisms and epigenetics leads to allow the transcriptional machinery of the cell to distinguish the two parental chromosomes at imprinted loci.

Imprinting is typically accomplished by altering the histone and/or DNA of a given locus, however lncRNAs have recently been identified to have a role in these phenomena [50]. Imprinted genes must be regulated by cis-regulatory mechanisms since expressed and repressed alleles share the same nucleus. The breakthrough in genomic imprinting was established with the discovery of gametic differentially methylated regions (these are actually control elements) that contain the "imprinting mark" acquired in oocytes and sperm. These markers are then transmitted down through the generations, guiding parental-specific allelic expression in children and embryos.

Control of imprinted lncRNAs is achieved by shared regulatory mechanisms such as parent-of-origin-dependent differentially methylated regions (DMRs) & lncRNAs within a single imprinted cluster [51]. Allele-specific DNA methylation occurs in a separate ICR in the germline in well-studied imprinted clusters, termed as principal DMRs or germline-derived DMRs and persists beyond fertilisation. Epigenetic changes (parent-of-origin-specific) such as DNA methylation, influence parentally inherited allele expression patterns in ICRs in imprinted clusters [52]. There are approximately 35 imprinted gDMRs in the human & 24 in Mouse genome (Monk et al., 2018). For embryonic development to govern imprinted gene expression, gDMRs must be established on paternal or maternal alleles [53]. In early primordial germ cells epigenetic markers including DNA methylation and histone modifications are substantially erased genome-wide. Depending on the parent-of-origin, DNA methylation of ICRs is reinstated in germline cells in gametes. After fertilisation, gDMRs are impervious to subsequent global epigenetic reprogramming. The data on DNA methylation at the ICRs of imprinted areas is retained. Imprinted loci gDMRs establish themselves strongly throughout germline development and are hence resistant to genomic reprogramming after fertilisation. Imprinting markings, on the other hand, are passed down from one generation to the next [54]. The allele-specific methylation statuses of gDMRs are generally identified by transcription regulators in maintaining parent-of-origin specific regulation of imprinted genes for example ZFP57 protein. The development of monoallelic gene expression requires differential methylation statuses of gDMRs on parental alleles. In early embryonic and adult lineages, imprinting control regions regulate DNA methylation and chromatin organisation, resulting in the survival of imprinting patterns through generations and their perpetuation in adult tissues [55].

To explain the control of gene regulation within an imprinted cluster, two fundamental methods have been proposed [56]. The lncRNA model is the earliest and arguably most frequent model. According to this concept, imprinted lncRNAs control imprinted gene expression. In this model, imprinted lncRNAs are closely linked to ICRs. Imprinted lncRNAs are defined by their ability to suppress imprinted genes in the same cluster [57]. As shown by the imprinted cluster Kcnq1/Kcnq1ot1. On paternal allele, the constantly expressed imprinted lncRNA Kcnq1ot1 can repress multiple imprinted genes bidirectionally throughout their gene area. The insulator paradigm, wherein parental allele-specific epigenetic changes at ICRs contribute to topological variations of imprinted gene areas, resulting in gene silence or activation of certain alleles, has been observed in additional imprinted regions. The insulin-like growth factor 2/H19 locus controls imprinted genes mechanistically, according to this concept. The following are some well-known lncRNAs and their roles in genomic imprinting:

I. **Airn lncRNA:** 108-kb nuclear-localised transcript that is synthesised in the opposite direction from 3.7-kb ICE of Igf type-2 receptor gene [58]. This lncRNA have been shown to influence the regulation of three parent of origin-specific genes viz. Igf2r, Slc22a2 & Slc22a3. Mice with an ICE deletion show biallelic expression of 3 genes (including Igf2r) and are smaller at birth [59].

II. **Kcnq1ot1:** Another lncRNA with a well-known involvement in imprinting is Kcnq1ot1. It is a 91-kilobyte RNA with many protein-coding genes that comes from the 1-megabyte Kcnq1/Cdkn1c locus on chromosome 7 [36, 60]. Because of CpG methylation, this lncRNA is suppressed on maternal chromosome and assumes paternal specific expression. The paternal chromosome specific expression is associated with inhibition of some 8–10 protein-coding genes that span many megabases. Kcnq1ot1, like Airn works in cis on the paternal chromosome to mute Phlda2, Kcnq1, Slc22a18, & Cdkn1c genes in all tissues (ubiquitously imprinted loci), Imprinting is a phenomenon that happens in a 600-kb region of mouse chromosome 7 called the imprinting cluster. H19 & Igf2, two genes in this cluster, are expressed maternally and paternally, respectively, and correlate to the human locus 11p15.5 [61, 62]. The H19 gene regulates expression of imprinted loci, forming the imprinted gene network, which is important for embryo development. H19 is a 2.3 kb lncRNA that has been demonstrated to generate an overgrowth phenotype and alleviate imprinting on Igf2 and other IGN genes when knocked out [63].

III. **DLK1-DIO3:** Human and mouse chromosome 14 & 12 respectvely both have a big imprinted cluster [imprinting status, in prototherians, metatherians and eutherians have also been determined] [64]. The paternally expressed genes DLK1 and DIO3 flank a 1 Mb area bordered by maternally expressed noncoding RNAs including the lncRNA MEG3 [65].

IV. **SNURF-SNRPN:** The SNURF-SNRPN area on chromosome 15q11-13, which spans over 2 Mb and has been related to the neurodevelopment diseases like Angel man Syndrome (AS) and Prader-Willi Syndrome (PWS) [66], is the biggest known imprinted cluster.

5.2 X-chromosome inactivation

Sex in most animals including humans is generally determined by X and Y chromosome system with men carrying XY and females XX chromosomes. In order to have the balance of products of sex-linked and autosomal genes, dosage compensation is required. X-chromosome inactivation (XCI) is a special kind of dosage compensation present in mammalian females involving random selection and transcriptional repression in one among the two X -chromosomes during the early stages of embryonic development [67, 68]. However, humans lack imprinted XCI and instead have XCD (X chromosome dampening) [69–71]. Most of the research with respect to this has been carried on mouse model and regulated by interactions of many lncRNAs [72]. At the heart of XCI/XCR (X-chromosome reactivation) regulation is a region of X chromosome namely Xic X-inactivation centre (containing many noncoding RNA genes whose expression is regulated by pluripotency factors) [73]. Developmental phase of mice includes two forms of XCI; one being imprinted and another random. Imprinted XCI, in which the paternally inherited X (Xp) is always inactivated, occurs during preimplantation development in the early embryo, when Xist becomes expressed on the Xp from the 2-cell stage onwards and is maintained in the placenta's extraembryonic tissues [74].

Xist lncRNA regulates all three stages (initiation, establishment, and maintenance) of XCI [75]. The X-linked minimum genetic region (XIC) contains many elements and genes like Tsix & Xist which are meant for XCI initiation [76]. Among the lncRNA loci reported in a 100–500 kb region of the mouse X chromosome and a 2.3 Mb syntenic region of the human X chromosome are RepA Jpx, Xist, Ftx, Tsix, & Xite [75, 76]. XIC contains the lncRNA Xist, and is located 15 kb downstream of Tsix antisense [77].

In first phase, complex factors Xite, OCT4, Tsix & CTCF among others bind Xi and Xa independently to promote X chromosome pairing and counting in the embryo following fertilisation [78]. After counting and pairing, Tsix, Xist, and other genes are elevated, which is regulated by a network of genetic interactions including OCT4, Jpx, Rnf12, and RepA Tsix, Sox2 & PRDM14 [79]. They use alternative transcription fates when full initiation of XCI occurs, with one becoming the Xa and the other Xi chromosome [72]. RNF12, Tsix, and RepA, as well as pluripotency factors (NANOG, OCT4, SOX2) impact lncRNA Xist activation and expression in Xi. Xist binds to Polycomb repressive complex 2 via Repeat A, producing the Xist-PRC2 complex, while YY1 tethers the PRC2-Xist complex to the Xi nucleation centre via Repeat C, where RNA polymerase II gets the lncRNA Xist-PRC2 complex [80]. Upon completion of initiation phase lncRNA Xist recruits different protein complex factors (including heterogeneous nuclear protein U, meant for lncRNA Xist localization, heterogeneous nuclear ribonucleoprotein K for Xist-mediated chromatin modifications) and gene-silencing factor Spen which binds to C, B, F, and A repeats at the 5′ end of the lncRNA Xist and causes the lncRNA Xist topologically associated domains meant for (epigenetic modification and chromatin compaction) to spread along the Xi chromosome at the established phase [76, 81]. ATRX directs PRC1 and PRC2 that cause epigenetic silencing by acetylation of histone H3 and H4 and methylation of CpG islands [56]. The protein complexes SHARP, HDAC3, LBR, Airn and Kcnq1ot1, U1 snRNP, Rsx, and CdK8 are all implicated in the lncRNA Xist spreading process. LncRNA Xist attracts restrictive complexes (like H3K27me3, H2AK119Ub, & the CpG island), which cause immediate histone modifications and DNA methylation, and coats the Xi to generate Xi [82]. Continuous synthesis of lncRNA Xist RNA in an inactive state has been used to establish and maintain the Xi.

6. Role of LncRNAs in cancer

The deadliest disease on the planet is linked to abnormal gene expression. Non-coding areas of the genome have been related to the majority of malignancies. Cancer genomic mutations are found in areas that do not code for proteins [83]. These areas, however, are frequently translated into long non-coding RNAs (lncRNAs). Anomalies in these lncRNAs is thought to have the tumour suppressor or carcinogenic effects and thus play a vital role in tumour establishment. Since lncRNAs have expression that are unique to a tissue, expressed in regulated manner and in association with other gene sets impact cell cycle regulations, immunological responses, survival etc. all of which affect cancer cell transformation [84]. The role of lncRNA is associated with their specific subcellular location. LncRNAs regulate gene expression by different interactions both in the nucleus as well as in the cytoplasm. In nucleus regulate expression at both epigenetic and transcriptional levels including histone modifications [24, 85], DNA methylation regulation [86], chromatin remodelling [87, 88], chromatin modification complexes [89, 90], transcription regulators [91] and proteins present in nucleus [92] while in the cytoplasm these lncRNAs regulate gene expression at both transcriptional and translational levels including interplay with proteins present in the cytoplasm [93], Control of mRNA metabolism [94], as endogenous competitive RNA (ceRNA) interacts with microRNA [95]. As a result, lncRNA play a significant role in cancer cell proliferation, transition, invasion, and treatment resistance [96, 97].

LncRNAs like LUCAT1, KCNQ1OT, HOTAIR, ANRIL, MALAT1(metastasis-associated lung adenocarcinoma transcript 1), Taurine-upregulated gene 1, LINC00152, RP11-385 J1.2 and TUBA4B bring different epigenetic modifiers at their respective loci and modify the chromatin shape and their dysregulation is strongly associated with establishment of different tumours including LUCAT1: digestive system tumours, ANRIL: prostate cancer, MALAT1: breast, liver, and colon cancer [98], HOTAIR: breast cancer KCNQ1OT1: colorectal cancer etc.

Some of known lncRNAs with links to cancer is represented below in a table:

Symbol/emblem	Cancer phenotype	Cancer association	Mechanism	Reference
HOTAIR	Promote metastasis	Upregulated in many cancers including those of liver, breast, lung and pancreas	By acting a platform for the PRC2 and LSD1 (chromatin repressors). By turning off *HOXD* and many other gene loci	[99]
MALAT1	Promotes both cell metastasis and proliferation	Overexpressed in non-small cell lung cancer, pancreatic, Colon, prostate, breast and hepatocellular carcinomas	Similar to alternative splicing and active transcription. Unique tRNA-like sequence at the 3′ end cleaved off and transformed to produce a short tRNA-like ncRNA (mascRNA)	[35, 98, 100]
PTENP1	Impede cell amplification, relocation and carcinoma establishment	Locus preferentially deleted in sporadic colon cancer, prostate and other different carcinomas	Inveigle for microRNAs that attack *PTEN*	[101]
PR-lncRNA-1	Impede cell amplification and stimulates Apoptosis	Suppressed in colorectal cancer	Upregulates the transcription of p53	[102]
LUCAT1(SCAL1)	Controls cellular events, programmed cell death and resistance to cisplatin in NSCLC cells by attacking IGF-2	Overexpressed in clear cell renal cell carcinoma ccRCC tissues	Engage in control of amplification, relocation, invasion and impedance to drugs in multiple tumours	[103]

One of the first lncRNAs to be discovered as having a functional role in cancer formation was the HOTAIR. HOTAIR lncRNAs enhance cancer spread by triggering epigenetic alterations in the chromatin status of tumour cells [104]. Interestingly, various lncRNAs have been reported to originate from the HOX locus, implying that it plays a global regulatory role [21]. In tumours, lncRNAs are also implicated in the control of the epithelial-mesenchymal transition (EMT) [99]. TGF-activated lncRNA (lncRNA-ATB) stimulated the EMT cascade by upregulating the levels of zinc finger

E-box-binding homeobox (ZEB1 and ZEB2) [105]. Recent research has discovered that the transcription factor PNUTS has a corresponding lncRNA-PNUTS, which plays a role in breast cancer metastasis by influencing the EMT process [106]. lncRNA human ortholog RNA of Dreh (hDREH), inhibitor of EMT is seen downregulated in many types of cancers. Some tumour suppressor lncRNAs, on the other hand, are expressed at low levels in tumours [107]. It is now possible to increase the expression of these lncRNAs in order to treat cancer. lncRNAs have been implicated in stemness-related signalling pathways in a number of studies. The tumour suppressor long noncoding RNA (TSLNC8), for example, inhibit the STAT3 signalling pathway and thus acted as a tumour suppressor [108]. lncRNA MST1/2-antagonising for YAP activation (MAYA) participate in the Hippo-YAP signalling pathway. These lncRNAs might be directly regulating cell stemness [109]. Thus, these lncRNAs act as potential targets for cancer treatment.

7. Role of LncRNAs in immunology

The study of lncRNA biology is still in its early stages, but it has already revealed key roles in the formation and functions of immune cells. However, because the functions of most lncRNAs are unknown, the field must fill a significant gap in order to comprehend the breadth of their roles in immunity. The function of non-long coding RNAs in the immunology of humans even though in its infancy stage has become hot topic in recent research. In immune system, lncRNAs have a role in immune cell formation, survival, cell fate determination, differentiation, amplification, and activation. Although the functions of most lncRNAs are unknown, novel protein-protein interactions or partnering with RNA or DNA have been discovered to influence innate and adaptive immune responses transcriptionally or post-transcriptionally. According to the recent research lncRNAs have been found in many immune cells including T cells and B cells. Regulation of these lncRNAs including expression levels is considered to be linked to immune cell development, differentiation, and activation [110].

To carry out their functions these IncRNAs can associate with transcription regulators and signalling molecules (NF-B, STAT3) [111, 112], RNA binding proteins including (hnRNP, HuR) [113, 114], and chromatin remodelling components (PRC2, WDR5).

7.1 Long non-coding RNA in T cells

LncRNAs, such as TMEVPG1 (also known as LincR-Ifng-3′AS), have been identified in both mouse and human CD8+ T cells and demonstrated to be positioned inside a cluster of cytokines genes, and have been shown to control Theiler's virus load in CNS infection [115]. T-bet/Stat, a transcription factor exclusive to Th1 cells that collaborates with TMEVPG1, promotes interferon gamma expression [116]. Interaction of lncRNA called NeST with WDR5, significant component of MLL H3K4 methyltransferases, leads to increase in methylation state of histones at Ifng gene in CD8+/Th1 cells [117]. Hundreds of lncRNAs were found in both CD8+ T cells of animal and human spleens after a genome-wide expression examination utilising a proprietary array, indicating that lncRNAs are important for lymphocyte differentiation and stimulation [118]. To get clearer picture of the role of lncRNAs in T cell growth and differentiation, Hu et al. used RNA-Seq to recognise 1524 genomic regions that produce lincRNAs in 42 subsets of mature peripheral T cells and thymocytes;

specific transcription regulators including T-bet, STAT4 for CD8+ descendants, & GATA-3 and STAT6 for CD4+ lineages seemed to be substantially responsible for lineage-specific expression of T cell lincRNAs (LincR-Ccr2-5′AS) [119].

7.2 Long non-coding RNA in B cells

B lymphocytes after being activated by antigen interaction, the major roles are to make antigen-specific antibodies, operate as APCs, and develop into memory cells. In compared to T cells, less is known regarding lncRNA roles in B cells. Bolland et al. [120] have documented how lncRNAs play their part in the chromatin remodelling that occurs during V/D/J gene recombination, which is required for the production of epitopes (Ig or TCR). Further study discovered that the synthesis of such antisense and sense lncRNAs is related to VH portions looping next to DJH areas during pro-B cell recombination, and as a result, it has been dubbed the Igh locus whole transcriptome of sense and antisense transcripts [121]. SAS-ZFAT gene expression which is restricted to CD19+ B cells of peripheral blood lymphocytes may be important for B cell function and AITD development [122].

7.3 Long non-coding RNA in macrophages

Macrophages are white blood cells that surround and destroy pathogens, destroy dead cells and stimulate other immune system cells. Macrophages as APCs also contribute to the optimal operation of both intrinsic and adaptive immune responses. LncRNA acknowledgement and purposes in monocytes/macrophages have received little attention. Macrophages have capital baseline level of ptprj/CD148 (a tyrosine phosphatase with tumour inhibitor-like role), as expected; its level is modulated by LPS, TLR, and CSF-1 treatments in various animals. Dave et al. investigated ptprj-as1, a 1006-nt lncRNA species that is produced antisense to ptprj. Transcripted ptprj-as1 is highly regulated in tissues augmented with macrophages that has been temporarily activated by TLR ligands, similar to ptprj [123]. Thus, the ptprj coding transcript may guide to inflammatory alteration that is promptly connected to macrophages. When myeloid and CD11c + dendritic cells are stimulated by lipopolysaccharide, a TLR4 signalling activator via NFkB, they express lncRNAs-COX2 (Ptgs2) [84]. Li et al. investigated how lincRNA expression changed when innate immune signalling was activated in THP1 macrophages and discovered that an unannotated LincRNA called THRIL was a critical factor in TNF- control and that its activity was clearly lower during the acute period of Kawasaki disease [114]. LncRNA has been observed to regulate healthy and pathological inflammatory immune responses through an RNA-protein complex with hnRNPL [124]. Many lncRNAs discovered as unique binding ally for lincRNA-cox2 in the nucleus and cytoplasm of macrophages, are key switch of immune genes [113].

7.4 Long non-coding RNA in natural-killer cells

Wright et al. uncovered an intron 2 promoter in many KIR genes that generate spliced antisense transcripts. KIR antisense lncRNA is found in progenitor cell lines, and its abundance in NK cells results in the under expression of KIR protein coding genes. KIR's antisense lncRNA corresponds to exons 1 and 2 of the KIR gene, and also the proximal promoter upstream of KIR. Myeloid zinc finger one (MZF-1) appears to impact KIR antisense lncRNA transcription, resulting in KIR silence via an unknown mechanism [125].

7.5 Functions of immune related lncRNAs

The following table represents the functions of some immune related lncRNAs:

S. no.	lncRNA	Functions	Reference
1	NEAT1	In response to viral infection, activates IL-8 transcription	[126]
2	Lnc-DC	Plays a role in transformation of monocytes of humans into dendritic cells	[112]
3	LincRNA-COX-2	increases the production of proinflammatory genes (IL-6) & suppresses the synthesis of anti-inflammation genes in non-stimulated cells	[113]
4	NeST	controls IFN-encoding chromatin epigenetic tagging, IFN-expression, and susceptibility to viral and bacterial pathogens	[117]
5	Hotair	Through epigenetic changes in the chromatin state, promotes cancer spread and progression	[127]
6	LincRCcr2–5′AS	In mouse CD4+ TH2 cells, it controls the synthesis of many chemokine receptor genes via STAT-6 pathway	[119]
7	LincRNA (THRIL)	Promotes TNF Transcription	[114]
8	IL1β	Modulation of chromatin	[128]
9	IL1β-RBT46	In monocytes regulates IL-1 homeostasis	[128]
10	IL1b-eRNA	Expression of CXCL8 and IL-1β (proinflammatory mediators)	[128]
11	Lethe	Activated during inflammation	[111]
12	NRAV	Transcriptional regulation of numerous interferon-stimulated genes (ISGs), including MxA and IFITM3	[129]
13	Morrbid	Control the longevity of myeloid cells with brief lives (neutrophils, eosinophils, and monocytes)	[130]
14	FAS AS1	Increase programmed cell death (Fas-driven) in B cell Carcinomas	[131]
15	lincRNA-EPS	Restriction of inflammation	[132]
16	TH2-LCR	Th2 cytokine gene transcription regulation	[133]
17	linc-MAF-4	Th1 cell differentiation	[134]
18	lnc-EGFR	Treg differentiation stimulation	[135]

8. LncRNAs in auto-immune diseases

Auto-immune diseases are conditions in which our immune system wrongly assaults our bodies, assumed to be the result of a complex interplay of genetic, immunological and environmental variables.

8.1 Systemic lupus erythematosus (SLE)

TLR4 signalling dysregulation has been connected to the progression of SLE. A lncRNA has been associated to SLE and is controlled by TLR4 signalling. Nuclear enriched abundant transcript 1 (NEAT1), a lncRNA, has been connected to the pathogenesis of SLE [136]. In a study NEAT1 levels were found to be elevated in PBMCs of SLE patients in comparison with healthy individual. In LPS-stimulated human monocytic cell lines, silencing NEAT1 with siRNA results in lower production of Interleukin-6, CCL2, and CXCL10, all of which have been related to SLE pathogenesis. NEAT1 regulates the stimulation of late mitogen-activated protein kinase signalling pathways, which play a role in the TLR4-driven inflammatory response. SLE patients have lower Gas5 expression in plasma, and in both CD4+ T cells and B cells than in healthy people [137].

8.2 Rheumatoid arthritis (RA)

Is an autoimmune illness characterised by inflammation and proliferation of synovial joint resulting in significant joint damage. Several recent investigations have found that dysregulated lncRNAs play a significant part in aetiology of RA. In 2015, Song et al. discovered that PBMCs and serum exosomes of RA patients have higher expression of HOTAIR than in the healthy controls. Furthermore, increasing HOTAIR increases active macrophage migration, whereas decreased HOTAIR suppresses the synthesis of matrix metalloproteinase (MMP)-2 and MMP-13 in developed osteoclasts and rheumatoid synoviocytes. These results suggest that abnormal HOTAIR expression could perform a part in the development of RA [138]. Low levels of lincRNA-p21 have been linked to increased NF-B activity in persons with Arthritis. Spurlock et al. observed that amount of phosphorylated p65, a hallmark of NF-B activation, was greater in the whole blood of patients suffering from RA however the expression of lincRNA-p21 was found to be downregulated. In comparison with MTX-treated RA patients, untreated counter parts had reduced levels of lincRNA-p21 activity and upregulated levels of p65 [139]. Lu et al. observed that T cells of patients suffering from RA have upregulated lncRNAs LOC100652951 and LOC100506036 in comparison with healthy individuals [140].

8.3 Sjogren's Syndrome (SS)

Chronic systemic auto-immune illness characterised by symptoms of driest mouth and eyes caused by gland inflammation (exocrine). The lncRNA Tmevpg1, which modulates Th1 responses, may have a role in the aetiology of SS, according to one research. The researchers discovered a connection between SS and the lncRNA Tmevpg1 [141].

8.4 Polymyositis and dermatomyositis (PM/DM)

Muscle inflammatory illness that is persistent. PM/DM has been connected to the expression of the RNA component of signal recognition particles, lncRNA 7SL [142]. Using microarray research, Peng et al. discovered 1198 differently transcribed lncRNAs in diabetes patients muscles compared to normal ones. uc011ihb.2, ENST00000583156.1, ENST00000551761.1, ENST00000541196.1 & linc-DGCR6-1, were among the five lncRNAs confirmed. As per their computational predictions, the linc-DGCR6-1 gene controls USP18, a kind of type 1 interferon-inducible gene found predominantly in the perifascicular portions of muscle fibres of diabetes patients [143].

9. Conclusion

Although there has been immense research going on to understand the role of lncRNAs, still there are many questions that need to be addressed. Efforts are being carried out to elucidate the role of lncRNAs as potential regulators in different biological and pathological processes. The advancement in technologies will further help to pave way in clarifying the mechanisms underlying of lncRNA influence in different diseases. Studying lncRNA role in regulation of host-pathogen interactions can be helpful in identifying different lncRNAs that can serve as potential drug targets and can also serve as novel biomarkers.

Author details

Ishteyaq Majeed Shah[1], Mashooq Ahmad Dar[2,3], Kaiser Ahmad Bhat[4], Tashook Ahmad Dar[4], Fayaz Ahmad[1] and Syed Mudasir Ahmad[3]*

1 Department of Zoology, University of Kashmir, Kashmir, India

2 Department of Biochemistry/Clinical Biochemistry, University of Kashmir, Kashmir, India

3 Division of Animal Biotechnology, Faculty of Veterinary Sciences and Animal Husbandry, Sher-e-Kashmir University of Agricultural Sciences and Technology, Kashmir, India

4 School of Biosciences and Biotechnology, Baba Ghulam Shah Badshah University, Rajouri, India

*Address all correspondence to: mudasirbio@gmail.com

References

[1] Hon CC, Ramilowski JA, Harshbarger J, Bertin N, Rackham OJ, Gough J, et al. An atlas of human long non-coding RNAs with accurate 5′ ends. Nature. 2017;**543**(7644):199-204

[2] Kapusta A, Feschotte C. Volatile evolution of long noncoding RNA repertoires: Mechanisms and biological implications. Trends in Genetics. 2014;**30**(10):439-452

[3] Uszczynska-Ratajczak B, Lagarde J, Frankish A, Guigó R, Johnson R. Towards a complete map of the human long non-coding RNA transcriptome. Nature Reviews Genetics. 2018;**19**(9):535-548

[4] Fang S, Zhang L, Guo J, Niu Y, Wu Y, Li H, et al. NONCODEV5: A comprehensive annotation database for long non-coding RNAs. Nucleic Acids Research. 2018;**46**(D1):D308-D314

[5] Quinn JJ, Chang HY. Unique features of long non-coding RNA biogenesis and function. Nature Reviews Genetics. 2016;**17**(1):47-62

[6] Jarroux J, Morillon A, Pinskaya M. History, discovery, and classification of lncRNAs. Long Non Coding RNA Biology. 2017;**1008**:1-46

[7] Huarte M. The emerging role of lncRNAs in cancer. Nature Medicine. 2015;**21**(11):1253-1261

[8] Kornienko AE, Guenzl PM, Barlow DP, Pauler FM. Gene regulation by the act of long non-coding RNA transcription. BMC Biology. 2013;**11**(1):1-14

[9] Akerman I, Tu Z, Beucher A, Rolando DM, Sauty-Colace C, Benazra M, et al. Human pancreatic β cell lncRNAs control cell-specific regulatory networks. Cell Metabolism. 2017;**25**(2):400-411

[10] Wu H, Yang L, Chen LL. The diversity of long noncoding RNAs and their generation. Trends in Genetics. 2017;**33**(8):540-552

[11] Vicens Q, Westhof E. Biogenesis of circular RNAs. Cell. 2014;**159**(1):13-14

[12] Chen LL. The biogenesis and emerging roles of circular RNAs. Nature Reviews Molecular Cell Biology. 2016;**17**(4):205-211

[13] Naganuma T, Hirose T. Paraspeckle formation during the biogenesis of long non-coding RNAs. RNA Biology. 2013;**10**(3):456-461

[14] Krol J. Paraspeckles: Nuclear nests helping to raise mature miRNAs. Nature Structural & Molecular Biology. 2017;**24**(10):783-784

[15] Kutter C, Watt S, Stefflova K, Wilson MD, Goncalves A, Ponting CP, et al. Rapid turnover of long noncoding RNAs and the evolution of gene expression. PLoS Genetics. 2012;**8**(7):e1002841

[16] Kaessmann H. Origins, evolution, and phenotypic impact of new genes. Genome Research. 2010;**20**(10):1313-1326

[17] Kapusta A, Kronenberg Z, Lynch VJ, Zhuo X, Ramsay L, Bourque G, et al. Transposable elements are major contributors to the origin, diversification, and regulation of vertebrate long noncoding RNAs. PLoS Genetics. 2013;**9**(4):e1003470

[18] Ponting CP, Oliver PL, Reik W. Evolution and functions of long

noncoding RNAs. Cell. 2009;**136**(4):629-641

[19] Gribnau J, Grootegoed JA. Origin and evolution of X chromosome inactivation. Current Opinion in Cell Biology. 2012;**24**(3):397-404

[20] Elisaphenko EA, Kolesnikov NN, Shevchenko AI, Rogozin IB, Nesterova TB, Brockdorff N, et al. A dual origin of the Xist gene from a protein-coding gene and a set of transposable elements. PLoS One. 2008;**3**(6):e2521

[21] Rinn JL, Chang HY. Genome regulation by long noncoding RNAs. Annual Review of Biochemistry. 2012;**81**:145-166

[22] Mao YS, Sunwoo H, Zhang B, Spector DL. Direct visualization of the co-transcriptional assembly of a nuclear body by noncoding RNAs. Nature Cell Biology. 2011;**13**(1):95-101

[23] Plath K, Fang J, Mlynarczyk-Evans SK, Cao R, Worringer KA, Wang H, et al. Role of histone H3 lysine 27 methylation in X inactivation. Science. 2003;**300**(5616):131-135

[24] da Rocha ST, Boeva V, Escamilla-Del-Arenal M, Ancelin K, Granier C, Matias NR, et al. Jarid2 is implicated in the initial Xist-induced targeting of PRC2 to the inactive X chromosome. Molecular Cell. 2014;**53**(2):301-316

[25] Rinn JL, Kertesz M, Wang JK, Squazzo SL, Xu X, Brugmann SA, et al. Functional demarcation of active and silent chromatin domains in human HOX loci by noncoding RNAs. Cell. 2007;**129**(7):1311-1323

[26] Lee JT. Gracefully ageing at 50, X-chromosome inactivation becomes a paradigm for RNA and chromatin control. Nature Reviews Molecular Cell Biology. 2011;**12**(12):815-826

[27] Wongtrakoongate P, Riddick G, Fucharoen S, Felsenfeld G. Association of the long non-coding RNA steroid receptor RNA activator (SRA) with TrxG and PRC2 complexes. PLoS Genetics. 2015;**11**(10):e1005615

[28] Hu X, Feng Y, Zhang D, Zhao SD, Hu Z, Greshock J, et al. A functional genomic approach identifies FAL1 as an oncogenic long noncoding RNA that associates with BMI1 and represses p21 expression in cancer. Cancer Cell. 2014;**26**(3):344-357

[29] Li W, Notani D, Rosenfeld MG. Enhancers as non-coding RNA transcription units: Recent insights and future perspectives. Nature Reviews Genetics. 2016;**17**(4):207-223

[30] Kim TK, Hemberg M, Gray JM, Costa AM, Bear DM, Wu J, et al. Widespread transcription at neuronal activity-regulated enhancers. Nature. 2010;**465**(7295):182-187

[31] Andersson R, Gebhard C, Miguel-Escalada I, Hoof I, Bornholdt J, Boyd M, et al. An atlas of active enhancers across human cell types and tissues. Nature. 2014;**507**(7493):455-461

[32] Tsai MC, Manor O, Wan Y, Mosammaparast N, Wang JK, Lan F, et al. Long noncoding RNA as modular scaffold of histone modification complexes. Science. 2010;**329**(5992):689-693

[33] Luco RF, Pan Q, Tominaga K, Blencowe BJ, Pereira-Smith OM, Misteli T. Regulationofalternativesplicingbyhistone modifications.Science.2010;**327**(5968):996-1000

[34] Dykes IM, Emanueli C. Transcriptional and post-transcriptional gene regulation by long non-coding RNA. Genomics, Proteomics & Bioinformatics. 2017;**15**(3):177-186

[35] Tripathi V, Ellis JD, Shen Z, Song DY, Pan Q, Watt AT, et al. The nuclear-retained noncoding RNA MALAT1 regulates alternative splicing by modulating SR splicing factor phosphorylation. Molecular Cell. 2010;**39**(6):925-938

[36] Pandey RR, Mondal T, Mohammad F, Enroth S, Redrup L, Komorowski J, et al. Kcnq1ot1 antisense noncoding RNA mediates lineage-specific transcriptional silencing through chromatin-level regulation. Molecular Cell. 2008;**32**(2):232-246

[37] Gonzalez I, Munita R, Agirre E, Dittmer TA, Gysling K, Misteli T, et al. A lncRNA regulates alternative splicing via establishment of a splicing-specific chromatin signature. Nature Structural & Molecular Biology. 2015;**22**(5):370-376

[38] Lan Y, Xiao X, He Z, Luo Y, Wu C, Li L, et al. Long noncoding RNA OCC-1 suppresses cell growth through destabilizing HuR protein in colorectal cancer. Nucleic Acids Research. 2018;**46**(11):5809-5821

[39] Huang J, Zhang A, Ho TT, Zhang Z, Zhou N, Ding X, et al. Linc-RoR promotes c-Myc expression through hnRNP I and AUF1. Nucleic Acids Research. 2016;**44**(7):3059-3069

[40] Schmitt AM, Garcia JT, Hung T, Flynn RA, Shen Y, Qu K, et al. An inducible long noncoding RNA amplifies DNA damage signaling. Nature Genetics. 2016;**48**(11):1370-1376

[41] Hu WL, Jin L, Xu AN, Wang YF, Thorne RF, Zhang XD, et al. GUARDIN is a p53-responsive long non-coding RNA that is essential for genomic stability. Nature Cell Biology. 2018;**20**(4):492-502

[42] Hellwig S, Bass BL. A starvation-induced noncoding RNA modulates expression of dicer-regulated genes. Proceedings of the National Academy of Sciences. 2008;**105**(35):12897-12902

[43] Marchese FP, Grossi E, Marín-Béjar O, Bharti SK, Raimondi I, González J, et al. A long noncoding RNA regulates sister chromatid cohesion. Molecular Cell. 2016;**63**(3):397-407

[44] Liu X, Xiao ZD, Han L, Zhang J, Lee SW, Wang W, et al. LncRNA NBR2 engages a metabolic checkpoint by regulating AMPK under energy stress. Nature Cell Biology. 2016;**18**(4):431-442

[45] Yang F, Zhang H, Mei Y, Wu M. Reciprocal regulation of HIF-1α and lincRNA-p21 modulates the Warburg effect. Molecular Cell. 2014;**53**(1):88-100

[46] Feng J, Bi C, Clark BS, Mady R, Shah P, Kohtz JD. The Evf-2 noncoding RNA is transcribed from the Dlx-5/6 ultraconserved region and functions as a Dlx-2 transcriptional coactivator. Genes & Development. 2006;**20**(11):1470-1484

[47] Kanduri C. Kcnq1ot1: a chromatin regulatory RNA. Seminars in Cell & Developmental Biology. 2011;**22**(4): 343-350

[48] Clark MB, Johnston RL, Inostroza-Ponta M, Fox AH, Fortini E, Moscato P, et al. Genome-wide analysis of long noncoding RNA stability. Genome Research. 2012;**22**(5):885-898

[49] Adalsteinsson BT, Ferguson-Smith AC. Epigenetic control of the genome—Lessons from genomic imprinting. Genes. 2014;**5**(3):635-655

[50] Kanduri C. Long noncoding RNAs: Lessons from genomic imprinting. Biochimica et Biophysica Acta (BBA)-Gene Regulatory Mechanisms. 2016;**1859**(1):102-111

[51] Peters J. The role of genomic imprinting in biology and disease:

An expanding view. Nature Reviews Genetics. 2014;**15**(8):517-530

[52] da Rocha ST, Gendrel AV. The influence of DNA methylation on monoallelic expression. Essays in Biochemistry. 2019;**63**(6):663-676

[53] Elbracht M, Mackay D, Begemann M, Kagan KO, Eggermann T. Disturbed genomic imprinting and its relevance for human reproduction: Causes and clinical consequences. Human Reproduction Update. 2020;**26**(2):197-213

[54] Henckel A, Chebli K, Kota SK, Arnaud P, Feil R. Transcription and histone methylation changes correlate with imprint acquisition in male germ cells. The EMBO Journal. 2012;**31**(3):606-615

[55] Monk D, Mackay DJ, Eggermann T, Maher ER, Riccio A. Genomic imprinting disorders: Lessons on how genome, epigenome and environment interact. Nature Reviews Genetics. 2019;**20**(4):235-248

[56] Chen Z, Zhang Y. Maternal H3K27me3- dependent autosomal and X chromosome imprinting. Nature Reviews Genetics. 2020;**21**(9):555-571

[57] Tucci V, Isles AR, Kelsey G, Ferguson-Smith AC, Bartolomei MS, Benvenisty N, et al. Genomic imprinting and physiological processes in mammals. Cell. 2019;**176**(5):952-965

[58] Wutz A, Barlow DP. Imprinting of the mouse Igf2r gene depends on an intronic CpG island. Molecular and Cellular Endocrinology. 1998;**140**(1-2):9-14

[59] Sleutels F, Zwart R, Barlow DP. The non-coding air RNA is required for silencing autosomal imprinted genes. Nature. 2002;**415**(6873):810-813

[60] Mohammad F, Mondal T, Guseva N, Pandey GK, Kanduri C. Kcnq1ot1 noncoding RNA mediates transcriptional gene silencing by interacting with Dnmt1. Development. 2010;**137**(15):2493-2499

[61] Ripoche MA, Kress C, Poirier F, Dandolo L. Deletion of the H19 transcription unit reveals the existence of a putative imprinting control element. Genes & Development. 1997;**11**(12):1596-1604

[62] Monnier P, Martinet C, Pontis J, Stancheva I, Ait-Si-Ali S, Dandolo L. H19 lncRNA controls gene expression of the imprinted gene network by recruiting MBD1. Proceedings of the National Academy of Sciences. 2013;**110**(51):20693-20698

[63] Brannan CI, Dees EC, Ingram RS, Tilghman SM. The product of the H19 gene may function as an RNA. Molecular and Cellular Biology. 1990;**10**(1):28-36

[64] Edwards CA, Mungall AJ, Matthews L, Ryder E, Gray DJ, Pask AJ, et al. The evolution of the DLK1-DIO3 imprinted domain in mammals. PLoS Biology. 2008;**6**(6):e135

[65] McMurray EN, Schmidt JV. Identification of imprinting regulators at the Meg3 differentially methylated region. Genomics. 2012;**100**(3):184-194

[66] Royo H, Cavaillé J. Non-coding RNAs in imprinted gene clusters. Biology of the Cell. 2008;**100**(3):149-166

[67] Bar S, Seaton LR, Weissbein U, Eldar-Geva T, Benvenisty N. Global characterization of X chromosome inactivation in human pluripotent stem cells. Cell Reports. 2019;**27**(1):20-29

[68] Strehle M, Guttman M. Xist drives spatial compartmentalization of DNA

and protein to orchestrate initiation and maintenance of X inactivation. Current Opinion in Cell Biology. 2020;**64**:139-147

[69] Wang F, Shin J, Shea JM, Yu J, Bošković A, Byron M, et al. Regulation of X-linked gene expression during early mouse development by Rlim. eLife. 2016;**5**:e19127

[70] Wu H, Luo J, Yu H, Rattner A, Mo A, Wang Y, et al. Cellular resolution maps of X chromosome inactivation: Implications for neural development, function, and disease. Neuron. 2014;**81**(1):103-119

[71] Gendrel AV, Heard E. Noncoding RNAs and epigenetic mechanisms during X-chromosome inactivation. Annual Review of Cell and Developmental Biology. 2014;**30**:561-580

[72] Vallot C, Rougeulle C. Long non-coding RNAs and human X-chromosome regulation: A coat for the active X chromosome. RNA Biology. 2013;**10**(8):1262-1265

[73] Payer B, Lee JT. Coupling of X-chromosome reactivation with the pluripotent stem cell state. RNA Biology. 2014;**11**(7):798-807

[74] Huynh KD, Lee JT. Inheritance of a pre-inactivated paternal X chromosome in early mouse embryos. Nature. 2003;**426**(6968):857-862

[75] Sidorenko J, Kassam I, Kemper KE, Zeng J, Lloyd-Jones LR, Montgomery GW, et al. The effect of X-linked dosage compensation on complex trait variation. Nature Communications. 2019;**10**(1):1-11

[76] Loda A, Heard E. Xist RNA in action: Past, present, and future. PLoS Genetics. 2019;**15**(9):e1008333

[77] Monfort A, Wutz A. The B-side of Xist. 2020;**F1000Research**:9

[78] Kung JT, Kesner B, An JY, Ahn JY, Cifuentes-Rojas C, Colognori D, et al. Locus-specific targeting to the X chromosome revealed by the RNA interactome of CTCF. Molecular Cell. 2015;**57**(2):361-375

[79] Khamlichi AA, Feil R. Parallels between mammalian mechanisms of monoallelic gene expression. Trends in Genetics. 2018;**34**(12):954-971

[80] Chigi Y, Sasaki H, Sado T. The 5′ region of Xist RNA has the potential to associate with chromatin through the A-repeat. RNA. 2017;**23**(12):1894-1901

[81] Dossin F, Pinheiro I, Żylicz JJ, Roensch J, Collombet S, Le Saux A, et al. SPEN integrates transcriptional and epigenetic control of X-inactivation. Nature. 2020;**578**(7795):455-460

[82] Mira-Bontenbal H, Gribnau J. New Xist-interacting proteins in X-chromosome inactivation. Current Biology. 2016;**26**(8):R338-R342

[83] Maurano MT, Humbert R, Rynes E, Thurman RE, Haugen E, Wang H, et al. Systematic localization of common disease-associated variation in regulatory DNA. Science. 2012;**337**(6099):1190-1195

[84] Guttman M, Amit I, Garber M, French C, Lin MF, Feldser D, et al. Chromatin signature reveals over a thousand highly conserved large non-coding RNAs in mammals. Nature. 2009;**458**(7235):223-227

[85] Li L, Liu B, Wapinski OL, Tsai MC, Qu K, Zhang J, et al. Targeted disruption of Hotair leads to homeotic transformation and gene derepression. Cell Reports. 2013;**5**(1):3-12

[86] Venkatraman A, He XC, Thorvaldsen JL, Sugimura R, Perry JM, Tao F, et al. Maternal imprinting at

the H19–Igf2 locus maintains adult haematopoietic stem cell quiescence. Nature. 2013;**500**(7462):345-349

[87] Zhang J, Zhang P, Wang L, Piao HL, Ma L. Long non-coding RNA HOTAIR in carcinogenesis and metastasis. Acta Biochimica et Biophysica Sinica. 2014;**46**(1):1-5

[88] Chen D, Zhang Z, Mao C, Zhou Y, Yu L, Yin Y, et al. ANRIL inhibits p15INK4b through the TGFβ1 signaling pathway in human esophageal squamous cell carcinoma. Cellular Immunology. 2014;**289**(1-2):91-96

[89] Hasegawa Y, Brockdorff N, Kawano S, Tsutui K, Tsutui K, Nakagawa S. The matrix protein hnRNP U is required for chromosomal localization of Xist RNA. Developmental Cell. 2010;**19**(3):469-476

[90] Hacisuleyman E, Goff LA, Trapnell C, Williams A, Henao-Mejia J, Sun L, et al. Topological organization of multichromosomal regions by the long intergenic noncoding RNA firre. Nature Structural & Molecular Biology. 2014;**21**(2):198-206

[91] Jiang W, Liu Y, Liu R, Zhang K, Zhang Y. The lncRNA DEANR1 facilitates human endoderm differentiation by activating FOXA2 expression. Cell Reports. 2015;**11**(1):137-148

[92] Li M, Gou H, Tripathi BK, Huang J, Jiang S, Dubois W, et al. An Apela RNA-containing negative feedback loop regulates p53-mediated apoptosis in embryonic stem cells. Cell Stem Cell. 2015;**16**(6):669-683

[93] Chu C, Zhang QC, Da Rocha ST, Flynn RA, Bharadwaj M, Calabrese JM, et al. Systematic discovery of Xist RNA binding proteins. Cell. 2015;**161**(2):404-416

[94] Giovarelli M, Bucci G, Ramos A, Bordo D, Wilusz CJ, Chen CY, et al. H19 long noncoding RNA controls the mRNA decay promoting function of KSRP. Proceedings of the National Academy of Sciences. 2014;**111**(47):E5023-E5028

[95] Kallen AN, Zhou XB, Xu J, Qiao C, Ma J, Yan L, et al. The imprinted H19 lncRNA antagonizes let-7 microRNAs. Molecular Cell. 2013;**52**(1):101-112

[96] Zhang J, Liu SC, Luo XH, Tao GX, Guan M, Yuan H, et al. Exosomal long noncoding RNA s are differentially expressed in the Cervicovaginal lavage samples of cervical cancer patients. Journal of Clinical Laboratory Analysis. 2016;**30**(6):1116-1121

[97] Xia T, Chen S, Jiang Z, Shao Y, Jiang X, Li P, et al. Long noncoding RNA FER1L4 suppresses cancer cell growth by acting as a competing endogenous RNA and regulating PTEN expression. Scientific Reports. 2015;**5**(1):1-9

[98] Gutschner T, Hämmerle M, Diederichs S. MALAT1—A paradigm for long noncoding RNA function in cancer. Journal of Molecular Medicine. 2013;**91**(7):791-801

[99] Gupta RA, Shah N, Wang KC, Kim J, Horlings HM, Wong DJ, et al. Long non-coding RNA HOTAIR reprograms chromatin state to promote cancer metastasis. Nature. 2010;**464**(7291):1071-1076

[100] Wilusz JE, Freier SM, Spector DL. 3′ end processing of a long nuclear-retained noncoding RNA yields a tRNA-like cytoplasmic RNA. Cell. 2008;**135**(5):919-932

[101] Poliseno L, Haimovic A, Christos PJ. Deletion of PTENP1 pseudogene in human melanoma. The Journal of Investigative Dermatology. 2011;**131**(12):2497

[102] Sánchez Y, Segura V, Marín-Béjar O, Athie A, Marchese FP, González J, et al. Genome-wide analysis of the human p53 transcriptional network unveils a lncRNA tumour suppressor signature. Nature Communications. 2014;**5**(1):1-13

[103] Zheng Z, Zhao F, Zhu D, Han J, Chen H, Cai Y, et al. Long non-coding RNA LUCAT1 promotes proliferation and invasion in clear cell renal cell carcinoma through AKT/GSK-3β signaling pathway. Cellular Physiology and Biochemistry. 2018;**48**(3):891-904

[104] Guffanti A, Iacono M, Pelucchi P, Kim N, Soldà G, Croft LJ, et al. A transcriptional sketch of a primary human breast cancer by 454 deep sequencing. BMC Genomics. 2009;**10**(1):1-17

[105] Yuan JH, Yang F, Wang F, Ma JZ, Guo YJ, Tao QF, et al. A long noncoding RNA activated by TGF-β promotes the invasion-metastasis cascade in hepatocellular carcinoma. Cancer Cell. 2014;**25**(5):666-681

[106] Grelet S, Link LA, Howley B, Obellianne C, Palanisamy V, Gangaraju VK, et al. A regulated PNUTS mRNA to lncRNA splice switch mediates EMT and tumour progression. Nature Cell Biology. 2017;**19**(9):1105-1115

[107] Huang JF, Guo YJ, Zhao CX, Yuan SX, Wang Y, Tang GN, et al. Hepatitis B virus X protein (HBx)-related long noncoding RNA (lncRNA) down-regulated expression by HBx (Dreh) inhibits hepatocellular carcinoma metastasis by targeting the intermediate filament protein vimentin. Hepatology. 2013;**57**(5):1882-1892

[108] Zhang J, Li Z, Liu L, Wang Q, Li S, Chen D, et al. Long noncoding RNA TSLNC8 is a tumor suppressor that inactivates the interleukin-6/STAT3 signaling pathway. Hepatology. 2018;**67**(1):171-187

[109] Li C, Wang S, Xing Z, Lin A, Liang K, Song J, et al. A ROR1–HER3–lncRNA signalling axis modulates the hippo–YAP pathway to regulate bone metastasis. Nature Cell Biology. 2017;**19**(2):106-119

[110] Atianand MK, Fitzgerald KA. Long non-coding RNAs and control of gene expression in the immune system. Trends in Molecular Medicine. 2014;**20**(11):623-631

[111] Rapicavoli NA, Qu K, Zhang J, Mikhail M, Laberge RM, Chang HY. A mammalian pseudogene lncRNA at the interface of inflammation and anti-inflammatory therapeutics. elife. 2013;**2**:e00762

[112] Wang P, Xue Y, Han Y, Lin L, Wu C, Xu S, et al. The STAT3-binding long noncoding RNA lnc-DC controls human dendritic cell differentiation. Science. 2014;**344**(6181):310-313

[113] Carpenter S, Aiello D, Atianand MK, Ricci EP, Gandhi P, Hall LL, et al. A long noncoding RNA mediates both activation and repression of immune response genes. Science. 2013;**341**(6147):789-792

[114] Li Z, Chao TC, Chang KY, Lin N, Patil VS, Shimizu C, et al. The long noncoding RNA THRIL regulates TNFα expression through its interaction with hnRNPL. Proceedings of the National Academy of Sciences. 2014;**111**(3):1002-1007

[115] Vigneau S, Rohrlich PS, Brahic M, Bureau JF. Tmevpg1, a candidate gene for the control of Theiler's virus persistence, could be implicated in the regulation of gamma interferon. Journal of Virology. 2003;**77**(10):5632-5638

[116] Collier SP, Collins PL, Williams CL, Boothby MR, Aune TM. Cutting edge: Influence of Tmevpg1, a long intergenic noncoding RNA, on the expression of Ifng by Th1 cells. The Journal of Immunology. 2012;**189**(5):2084-2088

[117] Gomez JA, Wapinski OL, Yang YW, Bureau JF, Gopinath S, Monack DM, et al. The NeST long ncRNA controls microbial susceptibility and epigenetic activation of the interferon-γ locus. Cell. 2013;**152**(4):743-754

[118] Pang KC, Dinger ME, Mercer TR, Malquori L, Grimmond SM, Chen W, et al. Genome-wide identification of long noncoding RNAs in CD8+ T cells. The Journal of Immunology. 2009;**182**(12):7738-7748

[119] Hu G, Tang Q, Sharma S, Yu F, Escobar TM, Muljo SA, et al. Expression and regulation of intergenic long noncoding RNAs during T cell development and differentiation. Nature Immunology. 2013;**14**(11):1190-1198

[120] Bolland DJ, Wood AL, Johnston CM, Bunting SF, Morgan G, Chakalova L, et al. Antisense intergenic transcription in V (D) J recombination. Nature Immunology. 2004;**5**(6):630-637

[121] Verma-Gaur J, Torkamani A, Schaffer L, Head SR, Schork NJ, Feeney AJ. Noncoding transcription within the Igh distal VH region at PAIR elements affects the 3D structure of the Igh locus in pro-B cells. Proceedings of the National Academy of Sciences. 2012;**109**(42):17004-17009

[122] Shirasawa S, Harada H, Furugaki K, Akamizu T, Ishikawa N, Ito K, et al. SNPs in the promoter of a B cell-specific antisense transcript, SAS-ZFAT, determine susceptibility to autoimmune thyroid disease. Human Molecular Genetics. 2004;**13**(19):2221-2231

[123] Dave RK, Dinger ME, Andrew M, Askarian-Amiri M, Hume DA, Kellie S. Regulated expression of PTPRJ/CD148 and an antisense long noncoding RNA in macrophages by proinflammatory stimuli. PLoS One. 2013;**8**(6):e68306

[124] Huarte M, Guttman M, Feldser D, Garber M, Koziol MJ, Kenzelmann-Broz D, et al. A large intergenic noncoding RNA induced by p53 mediates global gene repression in the p53 response. Cell. 2010;**142**(3):409-419

[125] Wright PW, Huehn A, Cichocki F, Li H, Sharma N, Dang H, et al. Identification of a KIR antisense lncRNA expressed by progenitor cells. Genes & immunity. 2013;**14**(7):427-433

[126] Imamura K, Akimitsu N. Long non-coding RNAs involved in immune responses. Frontiers in Immunology. 2014;**5**:573

[127] Bei L, Lu Y, Bellis SL, Zhou W, Horvath E, Eklund EA. Identification of a HoxA10 activation domain necessary for transcription of the gene encoding β3 integrin during myeloid differentiation. Journal of Biological Chemistry. 2007;**282**(23):16846-16859

[128] Ilott NE, Heward JA, Roux B, Tsitsiou E, Fenwick PS, Lenzi L, et al. Long non-coding RNAs and enhancer RNAs regulate the lipopolysaccharide-induced inflammatory response in human monocytes. Nature Communications. 2014;**5**(1):1-14

[129] Campbell M, Kim KY, Chang PC, Huerta S, Shevchenko B, Wang DH, et al. A lytic viral long noncoding RNA modulates the function of a latent protein. Journal of Virology. 2014;**88**(3):1843-1848

[130] Kotzin JJ, Spencer SP, McCright SJ, Kumar DBU, Collet MA, Mowel WK, et al.

The long non-coding RNA Morrbid regulates Bim and short-lived myeloid cell lifespan. Nature. 2016;**537**(7619):239-243

[131] Sehgal L, Mathur R, Braun FK, Wise JF, Berkova Z, Neelapu S, et al. FAS-antisense 1 lncRNA and production of soluble versus membrane FAS in B-cell lymphoma. Leukemia. 2014;**28**(12):2376-2387

[132] Atianand MK, Hu W, Satpathy AT, Shen Y, Ricci EP, Alvarez-Dominguez JR, et al. A long noncoding RNA lincRNA-EPS acts as a transcriptional brake to restrain inflammation. Cell. 2016;**165**(7):1672-1685

[133] Spurlock CF, Tossberg JT, Guo Y, Collier SP, Crooke PS, Aune TM. Expression and functions of long noncoding RNAs during human T helper cell differentiation. Nature Communications. 2015;**6**(1):1-12

[134] Ranzani V, Rossetti G, Panzeri I, Arrigoni A, Bonnal RJ, Curti S, et al. The long intergenic noncoding RNA landscape of human lymphocytes highlights the regulation of T cell differentiation by linc-MAF-4. Nature Immunology. 2015;**16**(3):318-325

[135] Jiang R, Tang J, Chen Y, Deng L, Ji J, Xie Y, et al. The long noncoding RNA lnc-EGFR stimulates T-regulatory cells differentiation thus promoting hepatocellular carcinoma immune evasion. Nature Communications. 2017;**8**(1):1-15

[136] Zhang F, Wu L, Qian J, Qu B, Xia S, La T, et al. Identification of the long noncoding RNA NEAT1 as a novel inflammatory regulator acting through MAPK pathway in human lupus. Journal of Autoimmunity. 2016;**75**:96-104

[137] Wu GC, Li J, Leng RX, Li XP, Li XM, Wang DG, et al. Identification of long non-coding RNAs GAS5, linc0597 and lnc-DC in plasma as novel biomarkers for systemic lupus erythematosus. Oncotarget. 2017;**8**(14):23650

[138] Song J, Kim D, Han J, Kim Y, Lee M, Jin EJ. PBMC and exosome-derived Hotair is a critical regulator and potent marker for rheumatoid arthritis. Clinical and Experimental Medicine. 2015;**15**(1):121-126

[139] Spurlock CF III, Tossberg JT, Matlock BK, Olsen NJ, Aune TM. Methotrexate inhibits NF-κB activity via long intergenic (noncoding) RNA–p21 induction. Arthritis & Rheumatology. 2014;**66**(11):2947-2957

[140] Lu MC, Yu HC, Yu CL, Huang HB, Koo M, Tung CH, et al. Increased expression of long noncoding RNAs LOC100652951 and LOC100506036 in T cells from patients with rheumatoid arthritis facilitates the inflammatory responses. Immunologic Research. 2016;**64**(2):576-583

[141] Wang J, Peng H, Tian J, Ma J, Tang X, Rui K, et al. Upregulation of long noncoding RNA TMEVPG1 enhances T helper type 1 cell response in patients with Sjögren syndrome. Immunologic Research. 2016;**64**(2):489-496

[142] Satoh T, Okano T, Matsui T, Watabe H, Ogasawara T, Kubo K, et al. Novel autoantibodies against 7SL RNA in patients with polymyositis/dermatomyositis. The Journal of Rheumatology. 2005;**32**(9):1727-1733

[143] Peng QL, Zhang YM, Yang HB, Shu XM, Lu X, Wang GC. Transcriptomic profiling of long non-coding RNAs in dermatomyositis by microarray analysis. Scientific Reports. 2016;**6**(1):1-11

Chapter 3

Advantages of Noncoding RNAs in Molecular Diagnosis

Tomomi Fujii, Tomoko Uchiyama and Maiko Takeda

Abstract

Noncoding RNAs contribute to physiological processes by regulating many intracellular molecules participating in the life-supporting mechanisms of development, differentiation, and regeneration as well as by disrupting various signaling mechanisms such as disease development and progression and tumor growth. Because microRNAs (miRNAs) target and regulate the functions of key proteins, it is very useful to identify specific miRNAs that contribute to cellular functions and to clarify the roles of their target molecules as diagnostic and therapeutic strategies for cancer prognosis and treatment. In this section, the roles of miRNAs in various cancers and the processes leading to the identification of their target molecules are described, and the latest diagnostic strategies using miRNAs are discussed with specific examples.

Keywords: microRNA, cancer, molecular diagnosis

1. Introduction

Noncoding RNAs (ncRNAs) comprise the majority of gene transcripts in eukaryotes. ncRNAs play little biological role, but microRNAs (miRNAs), first reported in 1993, have important roles in gene expression [1, 2]. One of the most well-known miRNAs, let-7, a heterochronic gene in C. elegans, is considered important for developmental differentiation and regulates the larva-to-adult transition during larval development [3]. As a summary of the biosynthetic process of miRNAs, double-stranded RNA, the source of RNA interference, is sequentially processed into single-stranded RNA fragments of 21–23 nucleotides (nt) by the action of various enzymes [4, 5]. Let-7 encodes a small 21-nt ncRNA that binds to the 3′-untranslated region (UTR) of lin genes, resulting in RNA–RNA interactions and negative regulation of mRNA [6]. More than 30,000 miRNAs have been identified from more than 250 species, ranging from prokaryotes to eukaryotes, invertebrates to vertebrates, and even viruses [7, 8]. More than 5000 of these miRNAs have been identified in humans [miRBase: The microRNA database; cited 2018 Aug; Available from: http://www.mirbase.org].

miRNAs function as posttranscriptional regulators (negative regulators) of various gene expressions by binding to complementary sequences, primarily in the 3′-UTR of their target genes. miRNAs can target a large number of genes, and the mRNAs targeted by miRNAs mRNAs targeted by miRNAs account for more than 60% of all genes. Most miRNAs are encoded within the introns of coding mRNAs, but some can also be found within the 3′-UTR sequences of noncoding or coding mRNAs but can also be found in the 3′-UTR sequence of noncoding or coding mRNAs [9]. When miRNAs bind to target mRNAs, these are destabilized by deadenylation factors becoming more susceptible to degradation. As a result, mRNA is degraded; however, sometimes the mRNA is not degraded and translation is regulated, a mechanism that is not yet unclear. Alterations in the genetic structure of miRNA-associated regions are known to occur in many pathologies, especially cancer. Such chromosomal aberrations include amplifications (e.g. miR-26a in gliomas), deletions (e.g. miR-15a/16–1 in chronic lymphocytic leukemia), mutations (e.g. miR-125a in breast cancer), translocations [e.g. miR-125b in acute myeloid leukemia with t(2;11)(p21;q23)], single-nucleotide polymorphisms (e.g. miR-608 in colorectal adenocarcinoma), and heterozygous deletions (such as the 14q32 cluster in acute lymphoblastic leukemia) [10–15]. These changes can occur not only in the sequence of the mature miRNA itself but also in the promoter region/primary transcript (pri-miRNA) sequence or in the miRNA binding site of the target gene, and as somatic or germline mutations [16–18]. A number of transcription factors, as well as vital protein-coding genes, influence the expression levels of miRNAs, and this regulatory action is assumed to be particularly important for tissue specificity and developmental stage control. Conversely, loss of Dicer, DGCR8, Drosha, and Argonaute2(Ago2), components of pathways involved in the miRNA biosynthesis mechanism, is known to result in the inability to sustain life and early pregnancy death due to severe developmental defects. [19–22]. Loss of reproductive function due to the deletion of components involved in miRNA biosynthesis, and developmental defects in the heart, lungs, and neuromuscular tissue have been reported [23–30]. Dicer mutations have also been reported to cause tumor development and progression [31, 32]. Dysfunction of the miRNA biogenesis pathway causes the disruption of important life-support mechanisms associated with various diseases, among which cancer development and progression are strongly influenced. In particular, abnormal expression of Dicer and Drosha is known to lead to poor prognosis in various cancers [33–39]. Although there is a vast amount of evidence that miRNAs play fundamental roles in the mechanisms of many diseases, including cancer, unfortunately, they have not yet been fully exploited in diagnostic and therapeutic settings. It is therefore necessary to determine how miRNAs can potentially be utilized in clinical practice in the future. miRNAs likely have the greatest and most direct potential as novel biomarkers of diagnosis and prognosis, as well as predictors of therapeutic efficacy. It is also clear that miRNAs regulate or disrupt the expression of numerous target mRNAs, resulting in maintenance of vital activity or disease, which cannot be resolved by a single miRNA. Therefore, gene expression analysis by miRNA expression profiling in disease must accurately discriminate between disease diagnosis and tumor stage of development [40].

A more accurate diagnosis of tumors can be obtained by morphological histopathology using formalin-fixed paraffin-embedded (FFPE) tissues and profiling of expressed proteins via immunohistochemical staining. Genetic analysis using FFPE is also emerging as being important for therapeutic selection. However, the degradation of nucleic acids is a problem for FFPE, and nucleic acids extracted from aged tissues are degraded [41]. A particularly attractive property of miRNAs is their stability against chemical and enzymatic degradation. This implies that they can be purified from routinely prepared FFPE biopsy materials and measured robustly [42]. As a result, retrospective miRNA expression studies are underway, using FFPE as a conserved and valuable resource. The stability and clinical utility of miRNAs are due to their presence in extracellular biological fluids, including blood, as well as in tissues and cells. Tumor-associated miRNAs are found at higher levels in the serum and plasma of cancer patients than in healthy controls. Therefore, the use of miRNAs as potential noninvasive biomarkers of disease has attracted much attention, and miRNAs have been detected in many biological fluids, including plasma, serum, tears, urine, cerebrospinal fluid, breast milk, and saliva [43, 44]. The widespread use of biomarker testing, which is noninvasive and more reliable than the conventional histopathological diagnosis of cancer that invasive to the patient, could pave the way for screening programs, improve the early detection rate of disease, and enhance cancer prevention. Despite the growing functional importance of miRNAs as diagnostic and therapeutic strategies for cancer, there are still many knowledge gaps despite the potential to develop miRNA markers in the future.

2. Role of miRNAs as oncogenes and tumor suppressor genes

The role of miRNAs in regulating the genes involved in cancer growth and progression may be to suppress cancer progression primarily through suppressing target gene expression or to inhibit the function of genes that suppress cancer progression, therefore positively affecting cancer progression. The results obtained by detailed profiling of miRNA expression in cancer according to organ or cancer differentiation level revealed that the expression pattern of miRNAs varies depending on the organ, histological type, and differentiation level of cancer, indicating that the role of miRNAs is highly segmented [40]. Many miRNAs function in a suppressive manner in cancer. The expression of the aforementioned let-7 miRNA is downregulated in lung cancer, targeting and suppressing the expression of Ras, an important oncogene. This indicates that let-7 may function as a cancer suppressor gene [45]. The expression of miR-15 and miR-16 is absent or decreased in chronic lymphocytic leukemia, suggesting they act in a tumor-suppressive manner by targeting B cell lymphoma-2, an antiapoptotic factor [46]. Human miR-373 binds to the E-cadherin (CDH1) promoter and induces gene expression [47]. In addition to gene silencing through base pairing with DNA and mRNA target sequences, miRNAs are known to inhibit the function of regulatory proteins (decoy activity). miR-328 binds to poly C-binding protein 2 (PCBP2), also known as heterogeneous ribonucleoprotein E2. This binding does not involve the seed region of the miRNA, but it inhibits its interaction with the target mRNA. In chronic myeloid leukemia, downregulation of miR-328 inhibits myeloid differentiation via PCBP2, leading to tumor progression [48]. It is also important to understand the molecular mechanisms of miRNAs to define the mechanism of their suppressive properties against cancer. miRNAs primarily target the 3′-UTR of mRNAs and downregulate the cytoplasmic expression of protein-coding genes. As evidence for this, miRNAs are usually localized in the nucleus [49]. In addition to the 3′-UTR, other genetic regions at the DNA and RNA levels, that is, the 5′-UTR, promoter, and coding regions, as well as proteins can be targeted (**Figure 1**) [50–52]. By binding to various functional regions of genes, miRNAs can upregulate or downregulate gene expression, interact with other ncRNAs and RNA transcripts, and modulate biological networks [53, 54]. It has become clear that the actions of these miRNAs on their target molecules lead to the regulation of gene expression [55]. It has been shown that miRNAs not only bind to key sites in other RNAs but also to promoter regions at the DNA level, thereby affecting transcriptional activity. As a specific example, in terms of localization sites, miRNAs have been shown to function both in the cytoplasm and nucleus [56]. Investigation of the subcellular localization of miR-29b revealed

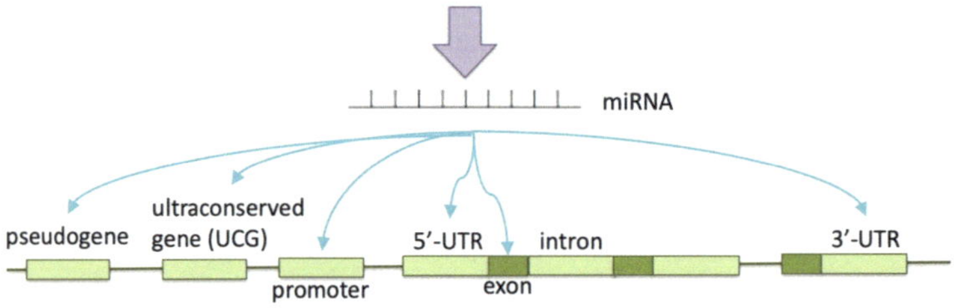

Figure 1.
Predicted binding sites for miRNAs in genes. miRNAs have binding sites not only in the 3′UTR but also in every site of the gene.

it was mostly localized to the nucleus. The characteristic hexanucleotide terminal motif of miR-29b functions as a metastable nuclear localization element that induces the nuclear localization of the miRNA or small-interference RNA to which it binds [49]. It has been shown that miRNAs bind to adenylate-uridylate-rich elements and upregulate translation in cells that have undergone cell cycle arrest. This suggests that miRNAs can affect not only cell differentiation and proliferation stages in a broad sense but also the cell cycle [57].

3. Expression dynamics of miRNAs in cancer and expectations for clinical application

Cancer is a malignant disease in which a population of cells with genetically abnormal protein expression proliferate autonomously, destroying host tissues as they grow, metastasize, and settle in other organs via vascular flow. As a result, cancer causes the dysfunction of normal tissues and ultimately leads to organ failure. There is evidence that carcinogenesis is a multistep process in which malignant cells accumulate epigenetic and genetic changes that gradually transform normal cells into malignant cells. Triggers for carcinogenesis include tobacco, chemical exogenous stimuli such as chemicals and dust from air pollution, and accumulation of genetic damage due to the aging of individual cells [58]. The proliferation of cancer cells progresses by causing structural changes in genes that promote cancer cell proliferation (oncogenes), genes that prevent their proliferation (tumor suppressor genes), and abnormal gene expression [59–62]. Malignant cells lose cell discipline in morphology and differentiation and acquire autonomous proliferation, antiapoptosis, and invasiveness properties. miRNAs have been analyzed in various human malignant tumors and can be involved in the pathophysiology of benign and malignant tumors in various ways. Although there are differences in miRNA expression profiles between normal and tumor tissues, many of these miRNAs are only indirectly altered by genetic changes that occur during carcinogenesis, epigenomic dynamics, and physiological changes in cell biology and do not directly trigger tumor development. Differentially expressed miRNAs between tumor and normal tissues have been identified in lymphomas, breast cancer, lung cancer, papillary thyroid cancer, glioblastoma, hepatocellular carcinoma, pancreatic tumor, pituitary adenoma, cervical cancer, brain tumors, prostate cancer (PCa), kidney and bladder cancer, and colon cancer [63–76]. The involvement of miRNAs in the carcinogenic process may involve changes in the components of miRNA biosynthesis pathway, and overall suppression of miRNA maturation by mutations in DROSHA, DGCR8, or DICER has been shown to affect the transcription and translation of multiple mRNAs, ultimately promoting cell transformation and tumorigenesis [77–79]. The fact that conditional loss of DICER or DGCR8 inhibits bone and cartilage growth and differentiation in mice and in vitro has been demonstrated, suggesting that components involved in the miRNA biosynthesis mechanism are also key molecules in carcinogenesis and cancer progression [80, 81]. The expression of Dicer, Exportin-5, TRKRA, TARBP2, DGCR8, and Argonaut-2 changes dynamically with changes in miRNA expression during the oncogenic phase in pancreatic cancer, suggesting that these miRNA biosynthesis-related molecules can cause cellular changes, including carcinogenesis [82]. Decreased expression of some components that play an important role in miRNA biogenesis, such as DICER, is associated with cancer prognosis and sensitivity to molecularly targeted drugs and has been shown to correlate with short survival in non-small cell lung cancer while increasing sensitivity to gefitinib [36, 83]. The methylation of DICER and DROSHA is also a potential biomarker for lung cancer [84]. Some miRNA precursors, known as mirtrons, have the unique feature of entering the miRNA biosynthesis pathway without undergoing Drosha-mediated cleavage while mimicking the structural features of pre-miRNAs. They are susceptible to epigenetic regulation and have been shown to exert epigenetic effects through interactions between various miRNAs and host genes in urothelial cell carcinoma [85–87]. Breast cancer susceptibility gene 1 (BRCA1) promotes the processing of primary miRNA transcripts and increases the expression of both precursors and mature forms of let-7a-1, miR-16-1, miR-145, and miR-34a [88]. BRCA1 interacts with Smad3, p53, and DHX9 RNA helicases by directly binding to DROSHA and DDX5 in the DROSHA microprocessor complex that regulates miRNA maturation and recognizes RNA secondary structures through its DNA-binding domain, which interacts with pri-miRNA via the DNA-binding domain.

Thus, from their discovery to the present, miRNAs have brought great promise and success in cancer diagnosis, prognosis, and treatment both in clinical practice and experimental medicine. Powerful technologies, such as miRNA arrays, short RNA deep sequencing, specific quantitative polymerase chain reaction (PCR) of miRNAs, and antisense technologies, have revealed the functions of numerous miRNAs. It is expected that they will continue to have a major impact on clinical oncology in terms of cancer diagnosis and prognostic treatment. Because miRNAs are important factors that define cellular characteristics, direct detection of miRNAs and miRNA target molecules from algorithms based on the vast amount of data obtained by profiling analysis could be used as a valuable tool for cancer diagnosis. miRNA expression profiling has been considered more efficient and informative than conventional mRNA profiling in classifying tumors with respect to their tissue of origin and differentiation [89–93]. These findings indicate that in clinical practice, miRNAs are useful biomarkers for tracking the tissue of origin of tumors [94–97]. miRNA expression profiles can be an important source of information for cancer progression prediction and prognosis. It has been shown that high expression of miR-21 and miR-155 in lung cancer and colorectal cancer (CRC) predicts efficient recurrence, poor prognosis, and reduced survival [98–101]. Functional analysis of miRNAs through experimental processes has been found to be valuable for therapeutic strategies based on the regulation of miRNA activity. As a therapeutic strategy against miRNAs acting as oncogenes (oncomirs), anti-miRNAs are expected to exert therapeutic effects by blocking oncomirs through the action of oligonucleotides that are complementary to miRNAs. For them to function stably, they must be chemically modified to enhance their stability and deliverability to the target organs. As is the case with many drugs used in cancer therapy, issues related to the delivery of miRNA-containing compounds, their stability in vivo, and biological defense measures against toxicity are important issues that must be resolved as miRNAs progress from experimental to clinical trials. However, because miRNAs have multiple targets, inhibition of target molecules by miRNAs may cause serious side effects. These issues are expected to be resolved and applied clinically in the future.

4. Functions of miRNAs in various organs

Given their properties, miRNAs have many target molecules and each performs different functions during cell differentiation and proliferation. Therefore, miRNAs are expected to perform characteristic functions in various organs. Here, the functions of miRNAs in typical cancers are introduced.

4.1 Breast cancer

miRNA profiling studies in breast cancer have been conducted from various perspectives. The first miRNA shown to be highly expressed in metastatic breast cancer was miR-10b (using mouse and human cells), with clinical correlation in primary breast cancer [102]. Subsequent studies confirmed the elevated levels of miR-10b, miR-34a, and miR-155 in patients with metastatic breast cancer [103]. Furthermore, miR-10b and miR-373 were recently shown to be upregulated in lymph node-positive breast cancer [104]. In addition, miRNAs from previous miRNA profiling studies have been shown to play potential roles as tumor suppressor genes or oncogenes in breast cancer [65, 105, 106]. The decreased expression of many genes involved in cancer development and progression has become evident, and miRNAs and their target molecules that are downregulated in breast cancer tissues and cell lines have become the focus of research. Breast cancer is a cancerous tissue with high histopathological heterogeneity. Identifying miRNAs and their target molecules that are specifically expressed and function in this context and have diagnostic value is therefore difficult. miRNA profiling should facilitate the accurate classification of tumor subtypes and provide useful additional information to complement current classification methods and guide therapeutic decisions. Studies have nested to predict miRNAs in accordance with previous subtype classifications. Recent analyses of miRNAs have identified predicted miRNAs corresponding to hormone receptor and HER2 subtypes, including ER (miR-342, miR-299, miR-217, miR-190, miR-135b, and miR-218), PR (miR-520g, miR-377, miR- 527-518a, miR-520f-520c), and HER2 (miR-520d, miR-181c, miR-302c, miR-376b, and miR-30e). These expression kinetics classified cases with 100% accuracy compared to immunohistochemistry results [107]. Further classification is expected to increase miRNA profiling accuracy and the development of new diagnostic markers and therapeutic strategies based on miRNA target molecules.

4.2 Prostate cancer

Prostate cancer (PCa) is one of the most common causes of cancer-related death in men. Although most PCa progress very slowly and remain within the primary tumor, some have an aggressive behavior that can spread to other organs via the vascular system. Prostate-specific antigen (PSA) and prostate acid phosphatase (PAP) are useful tumor markers for prostate cancer. However, PAP has low specificity and PSA, despite its superior specificity, is inadequate for predicting the tumor types in which it is not elevated and histological differentiation and progression. Many studies have indicated that miRNAs are involved in the development of PCa [108–112]. Aberrant expression of miRNAs has been detected in PCa cell lines, in experimental carcinogenesis using cancer xenografts, and in clinical samples obtained from patients [113–118]. These changes suggest that miRNAs play an important role in the pathogenesis of PCa.

Many miRNAs are expressed as oncogenes. For example, miR-375, miR-106a, and miR-194 have been reported to play important roles in tumor formation, proliferation, and progression [119–121]. When the expression of tumor suppressor miRNAs decreases, the expression of oncogenes increases, promoting cancer growth and progression. Experimental introduction of precursors of these miRNAs into cells and overexpression of these miRNAs to reproduce normal expression patterns suppressed the growth, invasion, clonogenesis, and metastatic potential of PCa cells. The most well-known miRNAs are miR-149-5p, miR-7-5p, miR-122, miR-124-3p, miR-188, and miR-129 [122–127]. Downregulation of these miRNAs is associated with increased cell proliferation, migration, and chemotherapy resistance, primarily through the regulation of cell growth and proliferation via the mitogen-activated protein kinase pathway.

Clinically practical markers in PCa include serum PSA measurement and digital rectal examination; however, their diagnostic value is limited and does not extend to prognostic prediction based on cancer progression or assessment of differentiation related to tumor growth potential. Human glandular kallikrein 2, urokinase plasminogen activator and its receptor, transforming growth factor-β1, and interleukin 6 and its receptor are biomarkers with high sensitivity and specificity for the early diagnosis of PCa. miRNAs are also clinically promising diagnostic markers for this cancer. miRNAs can be used as diagnostic and disease-monitoring markers for the presence of minimal residual disease and early detection of recurrence. Furthermore, the establishment of a diagnostic algorithm combining multiple oncomir and tumor suppressor miRNAs is expected to enable a more stepwise diagnosis of PCa. In this cancer, histopathological diagnosis by biopsy is highly invasive and often fails to detect microscopic cancers owing to the extremely small amount of visible tissue. To compensate for the shortcomings of local biopsy pathology diagnosis, the availability of profiling tests with circulating miRNAs has the potential to predict the onset of cancer and the degree of differentiation through its combination algorithm. From the time of diagnosis and initiation of treatment, the detection of circulating miRNAs could contribute to the early detection of hormone refractory PCa. The role of cancer stem cells in PCa has been elucidated in previous studies. The CD44-positive PCa stem cell population has tumorigenic and metastatic potential, which has been mentioned in conjunction with other useful markers for cancer stem cells [128]. Functional analysis of miRNAs has shown that miR-9-5p, miR-34a, miR-373, miR-708, and miR-520c directly target CD44 suppressing its expression [129–133]. The fact that the expression levels of these miRNAs are decreased in PCa suggests an increased potential for tumor invasion and metastasis. Profiling of miRNAs in PCa holds promise as a more precise diagnostic tool before performing prostate biopsy.

4.3 CRC

CRC is a common cancer worldwide and is the second most common cause of cancer-related deaths in the Western world. Although the 5-year survival rate for early-stage cancer exceeds 90%, it decreases to approximately 70% for advanced cancer and to approximately 10% when distant metastases are present. Although it is certainly a carcinoma for which early diagnosis is very useful, in reality early detection is less than 40% due to insufficient noninvasive screening. Although direct diagnosis by endoscopy is most effective in CRC, it often relies on a fecal occult blood test because of its invasive nature. However, the fecal occult blood reaction can be positive even for inflammatory or nonneoplastic polyps and lacks specificity in terms of cancer diagnosis. If CRC can be found to have miRNA expression characteristics, analysis of miRNAs using stool and the detection of circulating miRNAs may be useful in detecting marginally present tumor cells. Therefore, we searched for miRNAs that were significantly elevated in CRC using stool and plasma and found a number of miRNAs, including miR-17, miR-18a, miR-19a, miR-21, miR-92a, miR-200c, miR-221, and miR-106a as diagnostic markers [134–138]. miR-141 is a miRNA that functions in an inhibitory manner against colon cancer cells in terms of cell proliferation, invasiveness, and migration [139–142]. As a circulating miRNA, miR-141, together with miR-200 and miR-143, could be an independent prognostic marker for advanced CRC [143, 144].

CRC progresses from adenoma to colorectal adenocarcinoma as precancerous lesions. Investigation of miRNA expression in staged histological types has revealed that the expression of several miRNAs is altered in precancerous lesions, adenomas, and CRC tissues compared to that in normal colorectal tissue. This suggests that some miRNAs are involved in the process of CRC and may be important biomarkers in the transition of tumor tissue from benign to malignant. In addition, miRNAs are now being extracted from stored FFPE tissue specimens and retrospectively profiled for miRNA expression using next-generation sequencing (NGS) to understand the origin of CRC development and metastatic disease in cases with multiple lesions. The most studied miRNAs with respect to clinical prognosis are miR-21, miR-143, and miR-145. Although miR-21 suppresses the expression of various tumor suppressor genes, it also affects cell proliferation, apoptosis, invasion, and tumor progression. Increased miR-21 expression in CRC tumor tissue correlates with increased metastatic potential of the primary tumor and is associated with shorter disease-free and overall survival. Owing to the antiapoptotic effect of miR-21, its overexpression was also found to affect therapeutic efficacy by reducing the efficacy of 5-fluorouracil (5-FU) chemotherapy [145–150]. Decreased expression of miR-143 and miR-145 in CRC tumor tissue has been observed in several studies, suggesting that they behave as tumor suppressors [132, 151–154]. Their decreased expression has been associated with increased tumor growth and angiogenesis, and it is clinically associated with shorter disease-free survival. The expression of miR-143 directly correlates with the sensitivity of the colon cancer cell line HCT116 to 5-FU treatment. miR-215 is involved in the cell proliferative capacity of CRC and is sensitive to chemotherapy and molecular-targeted therapy. miR-215 is also involved in the prognostic prediction of CRC [155–160].

Although biomarker analysis using stool as a method to directly capture tumor cells in CRC is open for consideration, the establishment of a methodology for good-quality nucleic acid extraction that enables good analysis and sample quality maintenance is required to obtain reliable data due to the heterogeneity of sample processing.

In contrast, for the prediction of treatment potential and prognosis for advanced cancer, miRNA profiling can be performed by nucleic acid extraction from FFPE of excised tumor tissue, and sufficient technology is being established for accuracy and reliability.

5. Analysis of circulating miRNAs for their usefulness as biomarkers

In addition to serum and plasma, various body fluids, such as saliva, cerebrospinal fluid, and body cavity fluid, are candidates as analyzable materials for the detection of circulating miRNAs. However, in samples of these fluids from cancer patients, not only tumor cells but also blood cells, macrophages, exosomes, and microparticles are present; where the miRNAs are present, there is also the issue of how many of the targeted tumor-derived miRNAs are included or how reliable the analysis is based on which miRNAs are included. Nevertheless, regardless of the members, each of whom may possess miRNAs, if the changes caused by the coexistence of cancer can be captured for cancer patients, the usefulness of profiling will be well maintained. It is well known that analysis of exosome-derived miRNAs can detect more cancer-relevant miRNAs than analysis using untreated serum. An interesting aspect of the quantitative analysis of miRNAs in exosomes and microparticles is that they may be involved in cell–cell interactions, stimulate intracellular signaling, and modulate metabolic functions and homeostasis in a small number of stem cells. Quantitative analysis of circulating miRNAs is most useful for miRNAs quantitative real-time PCR (qRT-PCR), because it detects miRNAs from a very small amount of nucleic acids. Although NGS is superior for expression profiling, it requires a sufficient amount of nucleic acids and is likely to lack reliability due to detection errors or low sensitivity. Therefore, a single-miRNA assay using the TaqMan method should be performed on miRNAs with presumed abnormal expression at the transcriptional level, as detected from microarray analysis or NGS analysis based on FFPE, followed by qRT-PCR validation. Capturing abnormal miRNA expression in cancer is a highly useful diagnostic strategy but, because capturing circulating miRNAs involves sampling a physiological diverse environment, we may be quantifying miRNAs derived not only from cancer but also from blood or other organs. In addition, miRNAs derived not only from cancer but also from coexisting diseases may be captured; therefore, it is not always the case that miRNAs of cancer cells are captured. In other words, the possibility of observing the dynamics of miRNAs in a broad sense, including in the cancer microenvironment, must be fully understood. Nevertheless, the analysis of circulating miRNAs is highly useful as a potential candidate for blood-based biomarkers that can be tested repeatedly. Circulating miRNAs are promising diagnostic biomarkers owing to their high information content and disease-specific regulation. miRNAs inhibit the translation of various proteins involved in disease-related signaling pathways, including malignant and benign diseases, and alterations in physiological states, thereby inhibiting specific signaling pathways. Therefore, the analysis of the complex profiling of multiple miRNAs involved in complex pathways is expected to provide more specific diagnostic algorithms.

Biomarker development involves several important issues. The use of various analytical technology platforms, serum or plasma samples, extraction of miRNAs from whole serum/plasma or exosomes/microvesicles separated by specific disease-related markers, and sample collection, storage, and processing, all need to be addressed. Depending on the time point of blood sample collection (presurgery, during surgery, and posttreatment) and patient treatment (surgery, chemotherapy, immunotherapy, and/or drug therapy), the expression profile of circulating miRNAs may change. It is also important to establish endogenous miRNA control and assess its consistency with the patient's clinicopathological data to assess prognosis.

6. Conclusions

miRNA expression profiling for cancer diagnosis can be subdivided into miRNA expression patterns based on signaling common to cancer, such as cell proliferation, invasion, migration, and antiapoptotic effects, and miRNA expression patterns according to various organ or tumor differentiation levels and tissue types. In addition, the expression patterns of miRNAs in cancers of various organs are different according to cancer differentiation levels and tissue types. In addition, the degree of differentiation and tissue classification are often heterogeneous among cancers of various organs, and the estimation of miRNAs based on the differentiation of each organ or developmental stage and the miRNAs that may be targeted may be important determinants for organ identification in so-called primary unknown cancers. A vast number of miRNA expression analyses in various cancers are expected to be reported in the near future. As more cancer-specific miRNAs become known, they will be systematically classified and miRNA expression profiling consistent with conventional immunohistochemical staining of cancer tissues is expected to have practical application.

Acknowledgements

We thank Aya Sugimoto for her excellent research skills and support of our work.

Conflict of interest

The authors declare no conflict of interest.

Author details

Tomomi Fujii*, Tomoko Uchiyama and Maiko Takeda
Department of Diagnostic Pathology, Nara Medical University School of Medicine, Nara, Japan

*Address all correspondence to: fujiit@naramed-u.ac.jp

References

[1] Lee RC, Feinbaum RL, Ambros V, The C. Elegans heterochronic gene lin-4 encodes small RNAs with antisense complementarity to lin-14. Cell. 1993;**75**(5):843-854

[2] Wightman B, Ha I, Ruvkun G. Posttranscriptional regulation of the heterochronic gene lin-14 by lin-4 mediates temporal pattern formation in C. elegans. Cell. 1993;**75**(5):855-862

[3] Reinhart BJ, Slack FJ, Basson M, Pasquinelli AE, Bettinger JC, Rougvie AE, et al. The 21-nucleotide let-7 RNA regulates developmental timing in Caenorhabditis elegans. Nature. 2000;**403**(6772):901-906

[4] Fire A, Xu S, Montgomery MK, Kostas SA, Driver SE, Mello CC. Potent and specific genetic interference by double-stranded RNA in Caenorhabditis elegans. Nature. 1998;**391**(6669):806-811

[5] Zamore PD, Tuschl T, Sharp PA, Bartel DP. RNAi: Double-stranded RNA directs the ATP-dependent cleavage of mRNA at 21 to 23 nucleotide intervals. Cell. 2000;**101**(1):25-33

[6] Pasquinelli AE, Reinhart BJ, Slack F, Martindale MQ, Kuroda MI, Maller B, et al. Conservation of the sequence and temporal expression of let-7 heterochronic regulatory RNA. Nature. 2000;**408**(6808):86-89

[7] Fan R, Xiao C, Wan X, Cha W, Miao Y, Zhou Y, et al. Small molecules with big roles in microRNA chemical biology and microRNA-targeted therapeutics. RNA Biology. 2019;**16**(6):707-718

[8] Griffiths-Jones S, Grocock RJ, van Dongen S, Bateman A, Enright AJ. miRBase: microRNA sequences, targets and gene nomenclature. Nucleic Acids Research. 2006;**34**, (Database issue):D140-D144

[9] Rodriguez A, Griffiths-Jones S, Ashurst JL, Bradley A. Identification of mammalian microRNA host genes and transcription units. Genome Research. 2004;**14**(10A):1902-1910

[10] Agueli C, Cammarata G, Salemi D, Dagnino L, Nicoletti R, La Rosa M, et al. 14q32/miRNA clusters loss of heterozygosity in acute lymphoblastic leukemia is associated with up-regulation of BCL11a. American Journal of Hematology. 2010;**85**(8):575-578

[11] Bousquet M, Quelen C, Rosati R, Mansat-De Mas V, La Starza R, Bastard C, et al. Myeloid cell differentiation arrest by miR-125b-1 in myelodysplastic syndrome and acute myeloid leukemia with the t(2;11)(p21;q23) translocation. The Journal of Experimental Medicine. 2008;**205**(11):2499-2506

[12] Calin GA, Dumitru CD, Shimizu M, Bichi R, Zupo S, Noch E, et al. Frequent deletions and down-regulation of micro- RNA genes miR15 and miR16 at 13q14 in chronic lymphocytic leukemia. Proceedings of the National Academy of Sciences of the United States of America. 2002;**99**(24):15524-15529

[13] Huse JT, Brennan C, Hambardzumyan D, Wee B, Pena J, Rouhanifard SH, et al. The PTEN-regulating microRNA miR-26a is amplified in high-grade glioma and facilitates gliomagenesis in vivo. Genes & Development. 2009;**23**(11):1327-1337

[14] Li W, Duan R, Kooy F, Sherman SL, Zhou W, Jin P. Germline mutation of microRNA-125a is associated with breast

cancer. Journal of Medical Genetics. 2009;**46**(5):358-360

[15] Lin M, Gu J, Eng C, Ellis LM, Hildebrandt MA, Lin J, et al. Genetic polymorphisms in MicroRNA-related genes as predictors of clinical outcomes in colorectal adenocarcinoma patients. Clinical Cancer Research. 2012;**18**(14):3982-3991

[16] Abelson JF, Kwan KY, O'Roak BJ, Baek DY, Stillman AA, Morgan TM, et al. Sequence variants in SLITRK1 are associated with Tourette's syndrome. Science. 2005;**310**(5746):317-320

[17] Calin GA, Ferracin M, Cimmino A, Di Leva G, Shimizu M, Wojcik SE, et al. A MicroRNA signature associated with prognosis and progression in chronic lymphocytic leukemia. The New England Journal of Medicine. 2005;**353**(17):1793-1801

[18] Calin GA, Sevignani C, Dumitru CD, Hyslop T, Noch E, Yendamuri S, et al. Human microRNA genes are frequently located at fragile sites and genomic regions involved in cancers. Proceedings of the National Academy of Sciences of the United States of America. 2004;**101**(9):2999-3004

[19] Bernstein E, Kim SY, Carmell MA, Murchison EP, Alcorn H, Li MZ, et al. Dicer is essential for mouse development. Nature Genetics. 2003;**35**(3):215-217

[20] Kao SH, Cheng WC, Wang YT, Wu HT, Yeh HY, Chen YJ, et al. Regulation of miRNA biogenesis and histone modification by K63-Polyubiquitinated DDX17 controls Cancer stem-like features. Cancer Research. 2019;**79**(10):2549-2563

[21] Morita S, Horii T, Kimura M, Goto Y, Ochiya T, Hatada I. One Argonaute family member, Eif2c2 (Ago2), is essential for development and appears not to be involved in DNA methylation. Genomics. 2007;**89**(6):687-696

[22] Wang Y, Medvid R, Melton C, Jaenisch R, Blelloch R. DGCR8 is essential for microRNA biogenesis and silencing of embryonic stem cell self-renewal. Nature Genetics. 2007;**39**(3):380-385

[23] Chapnik E, Sasson V, Blelloch R, Hornstein E. Dgcr8 controls neural crest cells survival in cardiovascular development. Developmental Biology. 2012;**362**(1):50-56

[24] Chen Z, Wu J, Yang C, Fan P, Balazs L, Jiao Y, et al. DiGeorge syndrome critical region 8 (DGCR8) protein-mediated microRNA biogenesis is essential for vascular smooth muscle cell development in mice. The Journal of Biological Chemistry. 2012;**287**(23):19018-19028

[25] da Costa Martins PA, Bourajjaj M, Gladka M, Kortland M, van Oort RJ, Pinto YM, et al. Conditional dicer gene deletion in the postnatal myocardium provokes spontaneous cardiac remodeling. Circulation. 2008;**118**(15):1567-1576

[26] Gonzalez G, Behringer RR. Dicer is required for female reproductive tract development and fertility in the mouse. Molecular Reproduction and Development. 2009;**76**(7):678-688

[27] Harris KS, Zhang Z, McManus MT, Harfe BD, Sun X. Dicer function is essential for lung epithelium morphogenesis. Proceedings of the National Academy of Sciences of the United States of America. 2006;**103**(7):2208-2213

[28] O'Donnell KA, Wentzel EA, Zeller KI, Dang CV, Mendell JT.

c-Myc-regulated microRNAs modulate E2F1 expression. Nature. 2005; **435**(7043):839-843

[29] Shin D, Shin JY, McManus MT, Ptacek LJ, Fu YH. Dicer ablation in oligodendrocytes provokes neuronal impairment in mice. Annals of Neurology. 2009;**66**(6):843-857

[30] Tao J, Wu H, Lin Q, Wei W, Lu XH, Cantle JP, et al. Deletion of astroglial dicer causes non-cell-autonomous neuronal dysfunction and degeneration. The Journal of Neuroscience. 2011;**31**(22):8306-8319

[31] Kumar MS, Lu J, Mercer KL, Golub TR, Jacks T. Impaired microRNA processing enhances cellular transformation and tumorigenesis. Nature Genetics. 2007;**39**(5):673-677

[32] Yang Z, Jin P, Xu S, Zhang T, Yang X, Li X, et al. Dicer reprograms stromal fibroblasts to a pro-inflammatory and tumor-promoting phenotype in ovarian cancer. Cancer Letters. 2018;**415**:20-29

[33] Chiosea S, Jelezcova E, Chandran U, Acquafondata M, McHale T, Sobol RW, et al. Up-regulation of dicer, a component of the MicroRNA machinery, in prostate adenocarcinoma. The American Journal of Pathology. 2006;**169**(5):1812-1820

[34] Faber C, Horst D, Hlubek F, Kirchner T. Overexpression of dicer predicts poor survival in colorectal cancer. European Journal of Cancer. 2011;**47**(9):1414-1419

[35] Guo X, Liao Q, Chen P, Li X, Xiong W, Ma J, et al. The microRNA-processing enzymes: Drosha and dicer can predict prognosis of nasopharyngeal carcinoma. Journal of Cancer Research and Clinical Oncology. 2012;**138**(1):49-56

[36] Karube Y, Tanaka H, Osada H, Tomida S, Tatematsu Y, Yanagisawa K, et al. Reduced expression of dicer associated with poor prognosis in lung cancer patients. Cancer Science. 2005;**96**(2):111-115

[37] Khoshnaw SM, Rakha EA, Abdel-Fatah TM, Nolan CC, Hodi Z, Macmillan DR, et al. Loss of dicer expression is associated with breast cancer progression and recurrence. Breast Cancer Research and Treatment. 2012;**135**(2):403-413

[38] Lin RJ, Lin YC, Chen J, Kuo HH, Chen YY, Diccianni MB, et al. microRNA signature and expression of dicer and Drosha can predict prognosis and delineate risk groups in neuroblastoma. Cancer Research. 2010;**70**(20):7841-7850

[39] Merritt WM, Lin YG, Han LY, Kamat AA, Spannuth WA, Schmandt R, et al. Dicer, Drosha, and outcomes in patients with ovarian cancer. The New England Journal of Medicine. 2008;**359**(25):2641-2650

[40] Lu J, Getz G, Miska EA, Alvarez-Saavedra E, Lamb J, Peck D, et al. MicroRNA expression profiles classify human cancers. Nature. 2005;**435**(7043):834-838

[41] Fujii T, Uchiyama T, Matsuoka M, Myojin T, Sugimoto S, Nitta Y, et al. Evaluation of DNA and RNA quality from archival formalin-fixed paraffin-embedded tissue for next-generation sequencing - retrospective study in Japanese single institution. Pathology International. 2020;**70**(9):602-611

[42] Lawrie CH, Soneji S, Marafioti T, Cooper CD, Palazzo S, Paterson JC, et al. MicroRNA expression distinguishes between germinal center B cell-like and activated B cell-like subtypes of diffuse

large B cell lymphoma. International Journal of Cancer. 2007;**121**(5):1156-1161

[43] Lawrie CH, Gal S, Dunlop HM, Pushkaran B, Liggins AP, Pulford K, et al. Detection of elevated levels of tumour-associated microRNAs in serum of patients with diffuse large B-cell lymphoma. British Journal of Haematology. 2008;**141**(5):672-675

[44] Weber JA, Baxter DH, Zhang S, Huang DY, Huang KH, Lee MJ, et al. The microRNA spectrum in 12 body fluids. Clinical Chemistry. 2010;**56**(11): 1733-1741

[45] Johnson SM, Grosshans H, Shingara J, Byrom M, Jarvis R, Cheng A, et al. RAS is regulated by the let-7 microRNA family. Cell. 2005;**120**(5):635-647

[46] Calin GA, Cimmino A, Fabbri M, Ferracin M, Wojcik SE, Shimizu M, et al. MiR-15a and miR-16-1 cluster functions in human leukemia. Proceedings of the National Academy of Sciences of the United States of America. 2008;**105**(13):5166-5171

[47] Place RF, Li LC, Pookot D, Noonan EJ, Dahiya R. MicroRNA-373 induces expression of genes with complementary promoter sequences. Proceedings of the National Academy of Sciences of the United States of America. 2008;**105**(5):1608-1613

[48] Eiring AM, Harb JG, Neviani P, Garton C, Oaks JJ, Spizzo R, et al. miR-328 functions as an RNA decoy to modulate hnRNP E2 regulation of mRNA translation in leukemic blasts. Cell. 2010;**140**(5):652-665

[49] Hwang HW, Wentzel EA, Mendell JT. A hexanucleotide element directs microRNA nuclear import. Science. 2007;**315**(5808):97-100

[50] Forman JJ, Legesse-Miller A, Coller HA. A search for conserved sequences in coding regions reveals that the let-7 microRNA targets dicer within its coding sequence. Proceedings of the National Academy of Sciences of the United States of America. 2008;**105**(39):14879-14884

[51] Lytle JR, Yario TA, Steitz JA. Target mRNAs are repressed as efficiently by microRNA-binding sites in the 5' UTR as in the 3' UTR. Proceedings of the National Academy of Sciences of the United States of America. 2007;**104**(23):9667-9672

[52] Tay Y, Zhang J, Thomson AM, Lim B, Rigoutsos I. MicroRNAs to Nanog, Oct4 and Sox2 coding regions modulate embryonic stem cell differentiation. Nature. 2008;**455**(7216):1124-1128

[53] Salmena L, Poliseno L, Tay Y, Kats L, Pandolfi PP. A ceRNA hypothesis: The Rosetta stone of a hidden RNA language? Cell. 2011;**146**(3):353-358

[54] Vasudevan S, Tong Y, Steitz JA. Switching from repression to activation: microRNAs can up-regulate translation. Science. 2007;**318**(5858):1931-1934

[55] Fukao A, Aoyama T, Fujiwara T. The molecular mechanism of translational control via the communication between the microRNA pathway and RNA-binding proteins. RNA Biology. 2015;**12**(9):922-926

[56] Stavast CJ, Erkeland SJ. The non-canonical aspects of MicroRNAs: Many roads to gene regulation. Cell. 2019;**8**:11

[57] Vasudevan S, Tong Y, Steitz JA. Cell-cycle control of microRNA-mediated translation regulation. Cell Cycle. 2008;**7**(11):1545-1549

[58] Fujii T, Shimada K, Nakai T, Ohbayashi C. MicroRNAs in

smoking-related carcinogenesis: Biomarkers, functions, and therapy. Journal of Clinical Medicine. 2018;**7**:5

[59] Saikia M, Paul S, Chakraborty S. Role of microRNA in forming breast carcinoma. Life Sciences. 2020;**259**:118256

[60] Shenouda SK, Alahari SK. MicroRNA function in cancer: Oncogene or a tumor suppressor? Cancer Metastasis Reviews. 2009;**28**(3-4):369-378

[61] Svoronos AA, Engelman DM, Slack FJ. OncomiR or tumor suppressor? The duplicity of MicroRNAs in Cancer. Cancer Research. 2016;**76**(13):3666-3670

[62] Volinia S, Calin GA, Liu CG, Ambs S, Cimmino A, Petrocca F, et al. A microRNA expression signature of human solid tumors defines cancer gene targets. Proceedings of the National Academy of Sciences of the United States of America. 2006;**103**(7):2257-2261

[63] Bedewy AML, Elmaghraby SM, Shehata AA, Kandil NS. Prognostic value of miRNA-155 expression in B-cell non-Hodgkin lymphoma. Turkish Journal of Haematology. 2017;**34**(3):207-212

[64] Gierlikowski W, Broniarek K, Cheda L, Rogulski Z, Kotlarek-Lysakowska M. MiR-181a-5p regulates NIS expression in papillary thyroid carcinoma. International Journal of Molecular Sciences. 2021;**22**(11):6067

[65] Iorio MV, Ferracin M, Liu CG, Veronese A, Spizzo R, Sabbioni S, et al. MicroRNA gene expression deregulation in human breast cancer. Cancer Research. 2005;**65**(16):7065-7070

[66] Komoll RM, Hu Q, Olarewaju O, von Dohlen L, Yuan Q, Xie Y, et al. MicroRNA-342-3p is a potent tumour suppressor in hepatocellular carcinoma. Journal of Hepatology. 2021;**74**(1):122-134

[67] Kong X, Xu R, Wang W, Zeng M, Li Y, Lin M, et al. CircularLRRC7 is a potential tumor suppressor associated with miR-1281 and PDXP expression in glioblastoma. Frontiers in Molecular Biosciences. 2021;**8**:743417

[68] Liang G, Meng W, Huang X, Zhu W, Yin C, Wang C, et al. miR-196b-5p-mediated downregulation of TSPAN12 and GATA6 promotes tumor progression in non-small cell lung cancer. Proceedings of the National Academy of Sciences of the United States of America. 2020;**117**(8):4347-4357

[69] Pellatt DF, Stevens JR, Wolff RK, Mullany LE, Herrick JS, Samowitz W, et al. Expression profiles of miRNA subsets distinguish human colorectal carcinoma and Normal colonic mucosa. Clinical and Translational Gastroenterology. 2016;**7**:e152

[70] Shen P, Yang T, Chen Q, Yuan H, Wu P, Cai B, et al. CircNEIL3 regulatory loop promotes pancreatic ductal adenocarcinoma progression via miRNA sponging and A-to-I RNA-editing. Molecular Cancer. 2021;**20**(1):51

[71] Sommerova L, Frankova H, Anton M, Jandakova E, Vojtesek B, Hrstka R. Expression and functional characterization of miR-34c in cervical Cancer. Klinická Onkologie. 2018;**31**(Suppl. 2):82-87

[72] Wang ZY, Zhang W, Yang JJ, Song DK, Wei JX. Expression of miRNA-630 in bladder urothelial carcinoma and its clinical significance. Journal of Huazhong University of Science and Technology. Medical Sciences. 2016;**36**(5):705-709

[73] Yang J, Lai CC, Xian ZM, Wang WQ, Xu BL. Preliminary results indicate

increased expression of miR-184 in patients with renal carcinoma. European Review for Medical and Pharmacological Sciences. 2019;**23**(16):6878-6887

[74] Yi D, Wang R, Shi X, Xu L, Yilihamu Y, Sang J. METTL14 promotes the migration and invasion of breast cancer cells by modulating N6methyladenosine and hsamiR146a5p expression. Oncology Reports. 2020;**43**(5):1375-1386

[75] Zhang Q, Wang Y, Zhou Y, Zhang Q, Xu C. Potential biomarkers of miRNA in non-functional pituitary adenomas. World Journal of Surgical Oncology. 2021;**19**(1):270

[76] Zhang R, Li F, Wang Y, Yao M, Chi C. Prognostic value of microRNA-20b expression level in patients with prostate cancer. Histology and Histopathology. 2020;**35**(8):827-831

[77] Gurtner A, Falcone E, Garibaldi F, Piaggio G. Dysregulation of microRNA biogenesis in cancer: The impact of mutant p53 on Drosha complex activity. Journal of Experimental & Clinical Cancer Research. 2016;**35**:45

[78] Babu KR, Tay Y. The Yin-Yang regulation of reactive oxygen species and MicroRNAs in Cancer. International Journal of Molecular Sciences. 2019;**20**(21):5335

[79] Krell J, Stebbing J, Carissimi C, Dabrowska AF, de Giorgio A, Frampton AE, et al. TP53 regulates miRNA association with AGO2 to remodel the miRNA-mRNA interaction network. Genome Research. 2016;**26**(3):331-341

[80] Kobayashi T, Papaioannou G, Mirzamohammadi F, Kozhemyakina E, Zhang M, Blelloch R, et al. Early postnatal ablation of the microRNA-processing enzyme, Drosha, causes chondrocyte death and impairs the structural integrity of the articular cartilage. Osteoarthritis and Cartilage. 2015;**23**(7):1214-1220

[81] Sugatani T, Hruska KA. Impaired micro-RNA pathways diminish osteoclast differentiation and function. The Journal of Biological Chemistry. 2009;**284**(7):4667-4678

[82] Rachagani S, Macha MA, Menning MS, Dey P, Pai P, Smith LM, et al. Changes in microRNA (miRNA) expression during pancreatic cancer development and progression in a genetically engineered KrasG12D;Pdx1-Cre mouse (KC) model. Oncotarget. 2015;**6**(37):40295-40309

[83] Chen JC, Su YH, Chiu CF, Chang YW, Yu YH, Tseng CF, et al. Suppression of dicer increases sensitivity to gefitinib in human lung cancer cells. Annals of Surgical Oncology. 2014;**21**(Suppl. 4):S555-S563

[84] Szczyrek M, Grenda A, Kuznar-Kaminska B, Krawczyk P, Sawicki M, Batura-Gabryel H, et al. Methylation of DROSHA and DICER as a biomarker for the detection of lung Cancer. Cancers (Basel). 2021;**13**(23):6139

[85] Butkyte S, Ciupas L, Jakubauskiene E, Vilys L, Mocevicius P, Kanopka A, et al. Splicing-dependent expression of microRNAs of mirtron origin in human digestive and excretory system cancer cells. Clinical Epigenetics. 2016;**8**:33

[86] Dudziec E, Miah S, Choudhry HM, Owen HC, Blizard S, Glover M, et al. Hypermethylation of CpG islands and shores around specific microRNAs and mirtrons is associated with the phenotype and presence of bladder

cancer. Clinical Cancer Research. 2011;**17**(6):1287-1296

[87] Sibley CR, Seow Y, Saayman S, Dijkstra KK, El Andaloussi S, Weinberg MS, et al. The biogenesis and characterization of mammalian microRNAs of mirtron origin. Nucleic Acids Research. 2012;**40**(1):438-448

[88] Kawai S, Amano A. BRCA1 regulates microRNA biogenesis via the DROSHA microprocessor complex. The Journal of Cell Biology. 2012;**197**(2):201-208

[89] Hayes J, Peruzzi PP, Lawler S. MicroRNAs in cancer: Biomarkers, functions and therapy. Trends in Molecular Medicine. 2014;**20**(8):460-469

[90] Hussen BM, Hidayat HJ, Salihi A, Sabir DK, Taheri M, Ghafouri-Fard S. MicroRNA: A signature for cancer progression. Biomedicine & Pharmacotherapy. 2021;**138**:111528

[91] Iorio MV, Croce CM. MicroRNA dysregulation in cancer: Diagnostics, monitoring and therapeutics. A comprehensive review. EMBO Mol Med. 2012;**4**(3):143-159

[92] Lee YS, Dutta A. MicroRNAs in cancer. Annual Review of Pathology. 2009;**4**:199-227

[93] Munker R, Calin GA. MicroRNA profiling in cancer. Clinical Science (London, England). 2011;**121**(4):141-158

[94] Barker EV, Cervigne NK, Reis PP, Goswami RS, Xu W, Weinreb I, et al. microRNA evaluation of unknown primary lesions in the head and neck. Molecular Cancer. 2009;**8**:127

[95] Ferracin M, Pedriali M, Veronese A, Zagatti B, Gafa R, Magri E, et al. MicroRNA profiling for the identification of cancers with unknown primary tissue-of-origin. The Journal of Pathology. 2011;**225**(1):43-53

[96] Laprovitera N, Riefolo M, Porcellini E, Durante G, Garajova I, Vasuri F, et al. MicroRNA expression profiling with a droplet digital PCR assay enables molecular diagnosis and prognosis of cancers of unknown primary. Molecular Oncology. 2021;**15**(10):2732-2751

[97] Varadhachary GR, Spector Y, Abbruzzese JL, Rosenwald S, Wang H, Aharonov R, et al. Prospective gene signature study using microRNA to identify the tissue of origin in patients with carcinoma of unknown primary. Clinical Cancer Research. 2011;**17**(12):4063-4070

[98] Lan J, Sun L, Xu F, Liu L, Hu F, Song D, et al. M2 macrophage-derived exosomes promote cell migration and invasion in Colon Cancer. Cancer Research. 2019;**79**(1):146-158

[99] Wang Y, Li J, Tong L, Zhang J, Zhai A, Xu K, et al. The prognostic value of miR-21 and miR-155 in non-small-cell lung cancer: A meta-analysis. Japanese Journal of Clinical Oncology. 2013;**43**(8):813-820

[100] Xue X, Liu Y, Wang Y, Meng M, Wang K, Zang X, et al. MiR-21 and MiR-155 promote non-small cell lung cancer progression by downregulating SOCS1, SOCS6, and PTEN. Oncotarget. 2016;7(51):84508-84519

[101] Yang M, Shen H, Qiu C, Ni Y, Wang L, Dong W, et al. High expression of miR-21 and miR-155 predicts recurrence and unfavourable survival in non-small cell lung cancer. European Journal of Cancer. 2013;**49**(3):604-615

[102] Ma L, Teruya-Feldstein J, Weinberg RA. Tumour invasion and

metastasis initiated by microRNA-10b in breast cancer. Nature. 2007;**449**(7163):682-688

[103] Roth C, Rack B, Muller V, Janni W, Pantel K, Schwarzenbach H. Circulating microRNAs as blood-based markers for patients with primary and metastatic breast cancer. Breast Cancer Research. 2010;**12**(6):R90

[104] Chen W, Cai F, Zhang B, Barekati Z, Zhong XY. The level of circulating miRNA-10b and miRNA-373 in detecting lymph node metastasis of breast cancer: Potential biomarkers. Tumour Biology. 2013;**34**(1):455-462

[105] Bertoli G, Cava C, Castiglioni I. MicroRNAs: New biomarkers for diagnosis, prognosis, therapy prediction and therapeutic tools for breast Cancer. Theranostics. 2015;**5**(10):1122-1143

[106] Rahman MM, Brane AC, Tollefsbol TO. MicroRNAs and epigenetics strategies to reverse breast Cancer. Cell. 2019;**8**:10

[107] Lowery AJ, Miller N, Devaney A, McNeill RE, Davoren PA, Lemetre C, et al. MicroRNA signatures predict oestrogen receptor, progesterone receptor and HER2/neu receptor status in breast cancer. Breast Cancer Research. 2009;**11**(3):R27

[108] Chen QY, Des Marais T, Costa M. Deregulation of SATB2 in carcinogenesis with emphasis on miRNA-mediated control. Carcinogenesis. 2019;**40**(3):393-402

[109] Culig Z. miRNA as regulators of prostate carcinogenesis and endocrine and Chemoresistance. Current Cancer Drug Targets. 2021;**21**(4):283-288

[110] Deng JH, Deng Q, Kuo CH, Delaney SW, Ying SY. MiRNA targets of prostate cancer. Methods in Molecular Biology. 2013;**936**:357-369

[111] Liu Y, Ao X, Ding W, Ponnusamy M, Wu W, Hao X, et al. Critical role of FOXO3a in carcinogenesis. Molecular Cancer. 2018;**17**(1):104

[112] Vlaeminck-Guillem V. Extracellular vesicles in prostate Cancer carcinogenesis, diagnosis, and management. Frontiers in Oncology. 2018;**8**:222

[113] Che Y, Shi X, Shi Y, Jiang X, Ai Q, Shi Y, et al. Exosomes derived from miR-143-overexpressing MSCs inhibit cell migration and invasion in human prostate Cancer by downregulating TFF3. Mol Ther Nucleic Acids. 2019;**18**:232-244

[114] Du C, Lv C, Feng Y, Yu S. Activation of the KDM5A/miRNA-495/YTHDF2/m6A-MOB3B axis facilitates prostate cancer progression. Journal of Experimental & Clinical Cancer Research. 2020;**39**(1):223

[115] Fujii T, Shimada K, Tatsumi Y, Fujimoto K, Konishi N. Syndecan-1 responsive microRNA-126 and 149 regulate cell proliferation in prostate cancer. Biochemical and Biophysical Research Communications. 2015;**456**(1):183-189

[116] Fujii T, Shimada K, Tatsumi Y, Tanaka N, Fujimoto K, Konishi N. Syndecan-1 up-regulates microRNA-331-3p and mediates epithelial-to-mesenchymal transition in prostate cancer. Molecular Carcinogenesis. 2016;**55**(9):1378-1386

[117] Meng XF, Liu AD, Li SL. SNHG1 promotes proliferation, invasion and EMT of prostate cancer cells through miR-195-5p. European Review for Medical and Pharmacological Sciences. 2020;**24**(19):9880-9888

[118] Wu M, Huang Y, Chen T, Wang W, Yang S, Ye Z, et al. LncRNA MEG3 inhibits the progression of prostate cancer by modulating miR-9-5p/QKI-5 axis. Journal of Cellular and Molecular Medicine. 2019;**23**(1):29-38

[119] Fernandes RC, Toubia J, Townley S, Hanson AR, Dredge BK, Pillman KA, et al. Post-transcriptional gene regulation by MicroRNA-194 promotes neuroendocrine Transdifferentiation in prostate Cancer. Cell Reports. 2021;**34**(1):108585

[120] Lu J, Mu X, Yin Q, Hu K. miR-106a contributes to prostate carcinoma progression through PTEN. Oncology Letters. 2019;**17**(1):1327-1332

[121] Szczyrba J, Nolte E, Wach S, Kremmer E, Stohr R, Hartmann A, et al. Downregulation of Sec23A protein by miRNA-375 in prostate carcinoma. Molecular Cancer Research. 2011;**9**(6):791-800

[122] Liu H, Hou T, Ju W, Xing Y, Zhang X, Yang J. MicroRNA122 downregulates Rhoassociated protein kinase 2 expression and inhibits the proliferation of prostate carcinoma cells. Molecular Medicine Reports. 2019;**19**(5):3882-3888

[123] Ma J, Wei H, Li X, Qu X. Hsa-miR-149-5p suppresses prostate carcinoma malignancy by suppressing RGS17. Cancer Management and Research. 2021;**13**:2773-2783

[124] Xiao H. MiR-7-5p suppresses tumor metastasis of non-small cell lung cancer by targeting NOVA2. Cellular & Molecular Biology Letters. 2019;**24**:60

[125] Xu S, Yi XM, Zhang ZY, Ge JP, Zhou WQ. miR-129 predicts prognosis and inhibits cell growth in human prostate carcinoma. Molecular Medicine Reports. 2016;**14**(6):5025-5032

[126] Zhang Y, Zhang W, Xu A, Tian Y, Liang C, Wang Z. MicroRNA-188 inhibits proliferation migration and invasion of prostate carcinoma by targeting at MARCKS. American Journal of Translational Research. 2019;**11**(8):5019-5028

[127] Zhang Z. MiR-124-3p suppresses prostatic carcinoma by targeting PTGS2 through the AKT/NF-kappaB pathway. Molecular Biotechnology. 2021;**63**(7):621-630

[128] Shimada K, Anai S, Fujii T, Tanaka N, Fujimoto K, Konishi N. Syndecan-1 (CD138) contributes to prostate cancer progression by stabilizing tumour-initiating cells. The Journal of Pathology. 2013;**231**(4):495-504

[129] Iczkowski KA. Cell adhesion molecule CD44: Its functional roles in prostate cancer. American Journal of Translational Research. 2010;**3**(1):1-7

[130] Liu C, Kelnar K, Liu B, Chen X, Calhoun-Davis T, Li H, et al. The microRNA miR-34a inhibits prostate cancer stem cells and metastasis by directly repressing CD44. Nature Medicine. 2011;**17**(2):211-215

[131] Saini S, Majid S, Shahryari V, Arora S, Yamamura S, Chang I, et al. miRNA-708 control of CD44(+) prostate cancer-initiating cells. Cancer Research. 2012;**72**(14):3618-3630

[132] Wang X, Cai J, Zhao L, Zhang D, Xu G, Hu J, et al. NUMB suppression by miR-9-5P enhances CD44(+) prostate cancer stem cell growth and metastasis. Scientific Reports. 2021;**11**(1):11210

[133] Yan X, Tang B, Chen B, Shan Y, Yang H, Reproducibility Project: Cancer,

B. Replication study: The microRNA miR-34a inhibits prostate cancer stem cells and metastasis by directly repressing CD44. eLife. 2019;**8**:e43511

[134] Koga Y, Yamazaki N, Yamamoto Y, Yamamoto S, Saito N, Kakugawa Y, et al. Fecal miR-106a is a useful marker for colorectal cancer patients with false-negative results in immunochemical fecal occult blood test. Cancer Epidemiology, Biomarkers & Prevention. 2013;**22**(10):1844-1852

[135] Koga Y, Yasunaga M, Takahashi A, Kuroda J, Moriya Y, Akasu T, et al. MicroRNA expression profiling of exfoliated colonocytes isolated from feces for colorectal cancer screening. Cancer Prevention Research (Philadelphia, Pa.). 2010;**3**(11):1435-1442

[136] Link A, Balaguer F, Shen Y, Nagasaka T, Lozano JJ, Boland CR, et al. Fecal MicroRNAs as novel biomarkers for colon cancer screening. Cancer Epidemiology, Biomarkers & Prevention. 2010;**19**(7):1766-1774

[137] Ng EK, Chong WW, Jin H, Lam EK, Shin VY, Yu J, et al. Differential expression of microRNAs in plasma of patients with colorectal cancer: A potential marker for colorectal cancer screening. Gut. 2009;**58**(10):1375-1381

[138] Wu CW, Ng SS, Dong YJ, Ng SC, Leung WW, Lee CW, et al. Detection of miR-92a and miR-21 in stool samples as potential screening biomarkers for colorectal cancer and polyps. Gut. 2012;**61**(5):739-745

[139] Liang Z, Li X, Liu S, Li C, Wang X, Xing J. MiR-141-3p inhibits cell proliferation, migration and invasion by targeting TRAF5 in colorectal cancer. Biochemical and Biophysical Research Communications. 2019;**514**(3):699-705

[140] Long ZH, Bai ZG, Song JN, Zheng Z, Li J, Zhang J, et al. miR-141 inhibits proliferation and migration of colorectal Cancer SW480 cells. Anticancer Research. 2017;**37**(8):4345-4352

[141] Tong SJ, Zhang XY, Guo HF, Yang J, Qi YP, Lu S. Study on effects of miR-141-3p in proliferation, migration, invasion and apoptosis of colon cancer cells by inhibiting Bcl2. Clinical & Translational Oncology. 2021;**23**(12):2526-2535

[142] Xing Y, Jing H, Zhang Y, Suo J, Qian M. MicroRNA-141-3p affected proliferation, chemosensitivity, migration and invasion of colorectal cancer cells by targeting EGFR. The International Journal of Biochemistry & Cell Biology. 2020;**118**:105643

[143] Ardila HJ, Sanabria-Salas MC, Meneses X, Rios R, Huertas-Salgado A, Serrano ML. Circulating miR-141-3p, miR-143-3p and miR-200c-3p are differentially expressed in colorectal cancer and advanced adenomas. Mol Clin Oncol. 2019;**11**(2):201-207

[144] Ding M, Zhang T, Li S, Zhang Y, Qiu Y, Zhang B. Correlation analysis between liver metastasis and serum levels of miR200 and miR141 in patients with colorectal cancer. Molecular Medicine Reports. 2017;**16**(5):7791-7795

[145] Ding T, Cui P, Zhou Y, Chen C, Zhao J, Wang H, et al. Antisense oligonucleotides against miR-21 inhibit the growth and metastasis of colorectal carcinoma via the DUSP8 pathway. Mol Ther Nucleic Acids. 2018;**13**:244-255

[146] Igder S, Mohammadiasl J, Mokarram P. Altered miR-21, miRNA-148a expression in relation to KRAS mutation status as Indicator of adenoma-carcinoma transitional pattern in colorectal adenoma and

carcinoma lesions. Biochemical Genetics. 2019;**57**(6):767-780

[147] Li G, Wang Q, Li Z, Shen Y. Serum miR-21 and miR-210 as promising non-invasive biomarkers for the diagnosis and prognosis of colorectal cancer. Revista Española de Enfermedades Digestivas. 2020;**112**(11):832-837

[148] Liang G, Zhu Y, Ali DJ, Tian T, Xu H, Si K, et al. Engineered exosomes for targeted co-delivery of miR-21 inhibitor and chemotherapeutics to reverse drug resistance in colon cancer. J Nanobiotechnology. 2020;**18**(1):10

[149] Liu Q, Yang W, Luo Y, Hu S, Zhu L. Correlation between miR-21 and miR-145 and the incidence and prognosis of colorectal cancer. Journal of BUON. 2018;**23**(1):29-35

[150] Shan L, Ji Q, Cheng G, Xia J, Liu D, Wu C, et al. Diagnostic value of circulating miR-21 for colorectal cancer: A meta-analysis. Cancer Biomarkers. 2015;**15**(1):47-56

[151] Gomes SE, Simoes AE, Pereira DM, Castro RE, Rodrigues CM, Borralho PM. miR-143 or miR-145 overexpression increases cetuximab-mediated antibody-dependent cellular cytotoxicity in human colon cancer cells. Oncotarget. 2016;**7**(8):9368-9387

[152] Kent OA, Fox-Talbot K, Halushka MK. RREB1 repressed miR-143/145 modulates KRAS signaling through downregulation of multiple targets. Oncogene. 2013;**32**(20):2576-2585

[153] Li C, Yan G, Yin L, Liu T, Li C, Wang L. Prognostic roles of microRNA 143 and microRNA 145 in colorectal cancer: A meta-analysis. The International Journal of Biological Markers. 2019;**34**(1):6-14

[154] Li JM, Zhao RH, Li ST, Xie CX, Jiang HH, Ding WJ, et al. Down-regulation of fecal miR-143 and miR-145 as potential markers for colorectal cancer. Saudi Medical Journal. 2012;**33**(1):24-29

[155] Caritg O, Navarro A, Moreno I, Martinez-Rodenas F, Cordeiro A, Munoz C, et al. Identifying high-risk stage II Colon Cancer patients: A three-MicroRNA-based score as a prognostic biomarker. Clinical Colorectal Cancer. 2016;**15**(4):e175-e182

[156] Karaayvaz M, Pal T, Song B, Zhang C, Georgakopoulos P, Mehmood S, et al. Prognostic significance of miR-215 in colon cancer. Clinical Colorectal Cancer. 2011;**10**(4):340-347

[157] Milanesi E, Dobre M, Bucuroiu AI, Herlea V, Manuc TE, Salvi A, et al. miRNAs-based molecular signature for KRAS mutated and wild type colorectal Cancer: An explorative study. Journal of Immunology Research. 2020;**2020**:4927120

[158] Slattery ML, Herrick JS, Mullany LE, Valeri N, Stevens J, Caan BJ, et al. An evaluation and replication of miRNAs with disease stage and colorectal cancer-specific mortality. International Journal of Cancer. 2015;**137**(2):428-438

[159] Svoboda M, Sana J, Fabian P, Kocakova I, Gombosova J, Nekvindova J, et al. MicroRNA expression profile associated with response to neoadjuvant chemoradiotherapy in locally advanced rectal cancer patients. Radiation Oncology. 2012;**7**:195

[160] Zhang JX, Song W, Chen ZH, Wei JH, Liao YJ, Lei J, et al. Prognostic and predictive value of a microRNA signature in stage II colon cancer: A microRNA expression analysis. The Lancet Oncology. 2013;**14**(13):1295-1306

Chapter 4

Role of Non-Coding RNAs in Lung Cancer

Maksat Babayev and Patricia Silveyra

Abstract

Lung cancer is the most common cancer worldwide, and the leading cancer killer in both men and women. Globally, it accounts for 11.6% of all cancer cases and is responsible for 18.4% of cancer-related deaths. The mechanisms underlying lung cancer development and progression have been widely studied, and roles for non-coding RNAs (ncRNAs) have been identified. Non-coding RNAs are a type of RNA molecules that are not translated into proteins. The main types of ncRNAs include transfer RNAs (tRNAs), microRNAs (miRNAs), small interfering RNAs (siRNAs), piwi-interacting RNAs (piRNAs), small nucleolar/nuclear RNAs (snoRNAs, snRNAs), extracellular RNAs (exRNAs), tRNA fragments, and long non-coding RNAs (lncRNAs). In the past few years, there has been an increased interest in the role of ncRNAs in oncology, and lung cancer tumorigenesis specifically. Multiple ncRNAs were identified as tumor suppressors: tRNA fragments, snoRNAs, and piRNAs while others were reported to have tumor-promoting functions: circular RNAs (circRNAs), snoRNAs, piRNAs, YRNAs, natural antisense transcripts (NATs) and pseudogene transcripts. In this chapter, we discuss the latest body of knowledge regarding the role of ncRNAs in lung cancer pathogenesis as well as their potential use as biomarkers or therapies against lung cancer.

Keywords: lung cancer, miRNAs, adenocarcinoma, squamous cell carcinoma, NSCLC, SCLC, small RNAs, non-coding RNAs

1. Introduction

Lung cancer is responsible for 19% of cancer-related deaths, making it the number one cause of cancer-related mortality worldwide. A recent global cancer statistics report has estimated that approximately 2.2 million new cases and 1.8 million deaths were reported in 2020 [1, 2]. Similarly, in the United States, 230,000 new cases of lung cancer and 132,000 deaths were reported in the same year [1].

While smoking is a well-investigated major risk factor, responsible for approximately 80% of total lung cancer fatalities, not all lung cancers are associated with smoking, particularly in women [3]. Other environmental and occupational factors have been linked to lung cancer development, including second hand smoke exposure, ionizing radiation, arsenic in drinking water, and radon, silica, asbestos, heavy metals, and air pollution exposures. Moreover, genetic factors and other comorbidities such as

IntechOpen

chronic obstructive pulmonary disease (COPD) have been identified as risk factors for lung cancer [4].

Lung cancer is defined as a cancer that starts in lung tissue. The condition is divided into two main types, small cell lung cancer (SCLC) and non-small cell lung cancer (NSCLC). The NSCLC type represents around 85% of all lung cancer cases, whereas the SCLC represents the remaining 15% [5, 6]. The NSCLC is further divided into several subtypes which include lung adenocarcinoma (LAC), squamous cell carcinoma (SCC), and large cell carcinoma (LCC). The World Health Organization (WHO) has classified lung tumors into multiple subtypes. This classification relies on the use of immunohistochemical characterization and microscopy and provides standardized criteria and terminology for diagnosis on small biopsies and cytology [7]. It also provides guidance for molecular testing, recognizing the therapeutic importance of targetable genetic alterations.

The molecular basis of lung cancer development is complex and involves a combination of genetic and epigenetic alterations that regulate tumor development. Multiple pro-oncogenic and tumor suppressor genes, as well as growth factors, transcription factors and other regulatory molecules are involved. Recent studies describing the pathways involved in lung cancer tumorigenesis have identified non-coding RNAs (ncRNAs) as important players in its pathogenesis regulation. Non-coding RNAs are a subtype of RNA molecules that regulate gene expression at the transcriptional and post-transcriptional level but are not translated into proteins. These ncRNAs are divided into two categories, short non-coding RNAs (less than 200 bp) an long non-coding RNAs (lncRNAs, more than 200 bp) [8]. The category of short ncRNAs consists of microRNA (miRNA), piwi-interacting RNA (piRNA), small interfering RNA (siRNA), small nucleolar RNA (snoRNA), tRNA-derived stress-induced RNA (tiRNA), YRNA and transfer RNA-derived RNA fragment (tRF). Further, the lncRNA makes up a heterogeneous category, which includes long intergenic non-coding RNAs (lincRNAs), bidirectional lncRNAs, intronic lncRNAs, overlapping sense lncRNAs, circular intronic RNAs (ciRNAs), T-UCR lncRNAs (transcribed from ultra-conserved regions), antisense transcripts, and enhancer RNAs [9, 10]. The lncRNAs display additional subtypes, and can also act as precursors to smaller ncRNAs such as snoRNAs, miRNAs, piRNAs, or siRNAs [10]. A summary of known non-coding RNA subtypes is provided in **Table 1**.

2. Role of ncRNAs in non-small cell lung cancer

2.1 Role of ncRNAs in NSCLC development

Lung adenocarcinoma is the most common lung cancer subtype, representing 40% of all lung NSCLC cases [11]. It is also the most common subtype diagnosed in never smokers. This subtype of lung cancer usually occurs in the lung periphery, evolving from mucosal glands, but can also be found in scars or areas of chronic inflammation [12].

In early 2000, Hanahan and Weinberg proposed a set of molecular and biochemical principles, that the most of human cancers share based on the knowledge accumulated at the time. The initial list of six traits included apoptosis evasion, self-sufficiency in growth signaling, insensitivity to anti-growth signals, sustained angiogenesis, limitless replicative potential with tissue invasion and metastasis [13]. Two decades later, new traits and principles were introduced in the list of hallmarks with

ncRNA	Full name
miRNA	microRNA
piRNA	PIWI interacting RNA
snoRNA	small nucleolar RNA
snRNA	small nuclear RNA
lncNRA	long non-coding RNA
circRNA	circular RNA
siRNA	small interfering RNA
tRNA	transfer RNA
tRF	tRNA fragments
tiRNA	tRNA-derived stress-induced RNA
TERC	Telomerase RNA Component
NAT	Natural Antisense Transcript
T-UCR	Transcribed ultra-conserved noncoding RNA

Table 1.
Common ncRNAs and standard nomenclature.

the latest set containing emerging hallmarks and cancer enabling characteristics (**Figure 1**). The enabling characteristics involve unlocking phenotypic plasticity, non-mutational epigenetic reprogramming, senescent cells, and polymorphic microbiomes.

The last few decades have seen a steep increase in interest and consequent number of studies related to ncRNAs role in lung cancer development. Significant attention is given to main ncRNA groups such as miRNAs, lncRNAs, snoRNAs, piRNAs and as well as tRNAs with its derivatives. In the next few sections, we will be discussing the roles that some groups within ncRNAs families play in lung cancer tumorigenesis, diagnosis, prognosis, and therapy.

2.1.1 MicroRNAs

MiRNAs are the most studied group of ncRNAs involved in lung cancer. MiRNAs make up a family of small noncoding RNAs with length of 21–25 nucleotides that can promote mRNA degradation by inhibiting their translation [15].

Several miRNAs can act on the same target mRNA, but a single miRNA can also regulate several different target mRNAs. Studies estimate that 30% of genes are regulated by miRNAs, and they participate various processes, such as gene regulation, apoptosis, cell differentiation and hematopoietic development [15, 16]. One of the hallmarks of cancer is sustained cell proliferation and unsuppressed cell growth [14]. Proteins such as kinases and kinase receptors play an important role in cell proliferation processes. For example, epidermal growth factor (EGF) and transforming growth factor-α (TGF-α) can attach to EGF receptor (EGFR), activating it, and causing further signaling pathway activation downstream. This leads to activation of the Ras/Raf/MEK/ERK and PI3K/Akt/mTOR pathways, two major signaling pathways, that play role in cell cycle progression and proliferation [17]. The EGFR is a direct target of numerous miRNAs, thus they play an important role in cell proliferation processes.

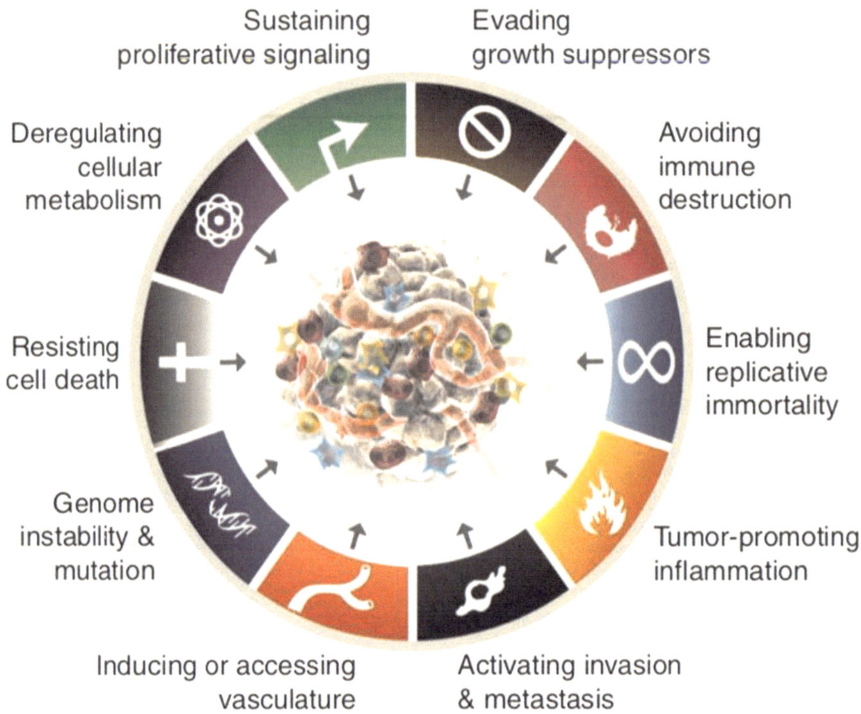

Figure 1.
The schematic representation of hallmarks of cancer (from Hanahan and Weinberg) [14].

These include, miR-146, miR-149, miR-7, miR-133, miR-27a-3p, miR-30, miR-34, miR-134, miR-145, miR-218, and miR-542-5p [15, 18–21].

The fusion proteins EML4 and ALK are also able to induce PI3K/Akt/mTOR and Ras/Raf/MEK/ERK pathways. The EML4 and ALK getting more interest as potential targets in NSCLC therapy, and miR-96 was shown to suppress ALK post-transcriptionally in a cell model [22]. The miR-760 had negative impact on cell proliferation in NSCLC cell lines by downregulating ROS1 expression, another potential therapeutic target. Same as previous kinase proteins, ROS1 promotes cell proliferation and survival via SHP-1/SHP-2, JAK/STAT, PI3K/Akt/mTOR, and MEK/ERK pathways [23, 24].

The Kirsten rat sarcoma 2 virus (KRAS) gene, encodes for K-Ras, which also acts through EGFR, ALK and ROS to activate Ras/Raf/MEK/ERK pathway [25, 26]. In a recent study, miR-193a-3p was reported to inhibit KRAS-mutated lung tumor growth by targeting KRAS directly [27]. Similarly, miR-181a-5p was reported to suppress A549 lung epithelial cells proliferation and migration by downregulating KRAS [28]. In addition, miR-148a-3p was found to suppress cell proliferation in NSCLC by downregulating SOS1, a protein involved in the Ras signaling pathway [29]. The miR-1258 was reported to suppress tumor progression by targeting GRB2/Ras/Erk pathway, while miR-520-3p was found to be involved in PI3K/Akt/mTOR pathway in vitro [30, 31].

The highly expressed miR-15a and miR-16 suppress cyclin D1, an important regulator of cell cycle progression. Cyclin D1 acts upstream of retinoblastoma (RB) pathway, and its suppression leads to RB upregulation and cell cycle arrest, which is a necessary step leading to cell senescence or apoptosis [32]. The E2F3 gene, which encodes for transcription factor E2F3, is a target of miR-449a and has low expression levels in tumor tissues. The miR-449a upregulation suppresses E2F3 with consequent cell cycle blockage and cell senescence [33]. Finally, miR-641 and miR-660 were reported to promote lung cancer cells apoptosis through suppressing the p53 pathway by targeting MDM2 [34, 35]. **Figure 2** summarizes the list of miRNAs involved in pathways associated with cancer hallmarks.

In addition to regulating genes involved in cancer-related pathways, miRNAs are also involved in enabling cancer cells with unlimited replicative immortality. The miRNAs from the miR-29 family demonstrated tumor-suppressing effect in lung cancer cells in vitro by targeting DNMT3A and DNMT3B [36]. These DNA methyltransferases (DNMT) play a role in controlling telomere length similar to telomerase, being involved in cell replicative potential.

Another critical cancer feature that involves miRNAs is metastasis. An important factor in cancer metastasis is epithelial-to-mesenchymal transition (EMT), that normally takes place in the embryonic development stage. The EMT involves the loss of

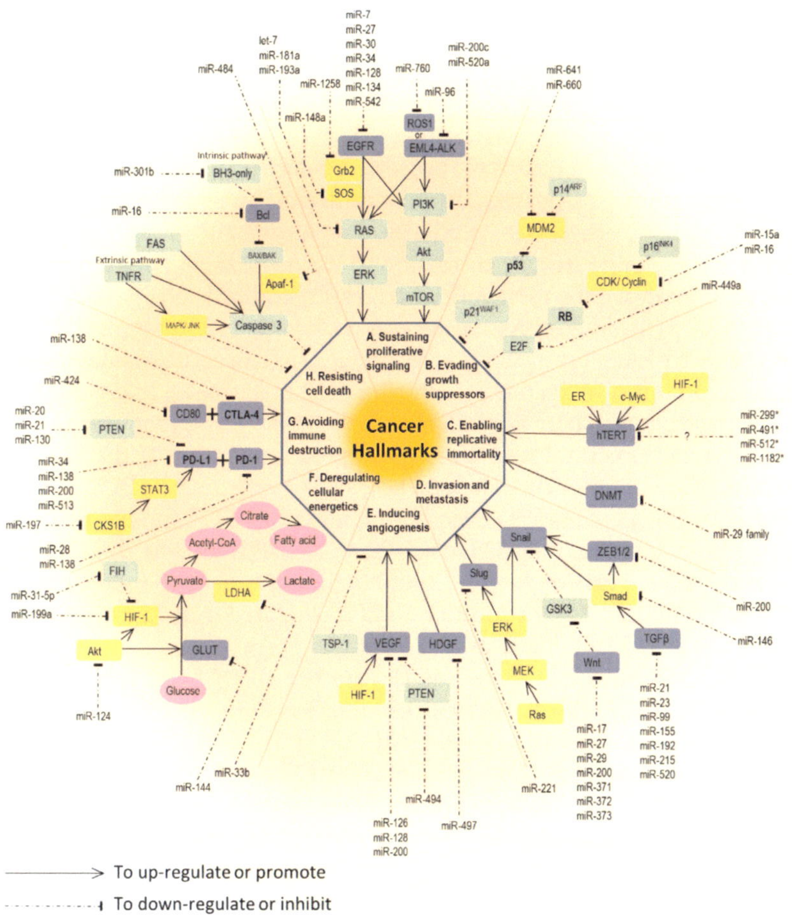

Figure 2.
A schematic diagram of miRNAs and their involvement in cancer hallmarks pathways (from Wu [15]).

E-cadherin-mediated cell adhesion and increased cell motility, which in turn promotes tumor invasion and metastasis. The miRNA 15a was reported to inhibit metastasis in NSCLC by targeting BCL2L2, and its overexpression significantly inhibited cell viability, invasion and migration [37]. There are several main transcription factors (TFs) related to epithelial-to-mesenchymal (EMT) transition that are directly targeted by miRNAs. These TFs are Snail, Slug, ZEB1, ZEB2 and Twist [38]. For example, miR-126 was reported to regulate NSCLC cell invasion and migration suppressing EMT by directly targeting PI3K/AKT/Snail pathway [39]. MiR-346 is upregulated in NSCLC and it promotes cell proliferation, metastasis and hinders apoptosis by targeting XPC/ERK/SNAIL/E-cadherin pathway [40]. Interestingly, miR-22 and miR-30a are downregulated in NSCLC, and they regulate EMT by directly targeting Snail [41–43].

In order to grow and spread, tumor cells require nutrients and oxygen, and that requires angiogenesis. Vascular endothelial growth factors (VEGFs) are the most studied group involved in angiogenesis process. MiRNAs from the miR-200 family were reported to suppress neovascularization in lung cancer cell lines by targeting the VEGF [44, 45]. Additionally, miR-126 and miR-128 were observed to target VEGF-A and VEGF-C, respectively, and inhibit angiogenesis in vitro when upregulated [46, 47]. When overexpressed, miR-497 was found to suppress angiogenesis in lung cancer by targeting an HDGF, and inducing a independent pathway [48]. However, there are miRNAs that promote angiogenesis as well. The miR-494 enhances angiogenesis by targeting a VEGF suppressor PTEN [49, 50]. Besides that, miR-23a activates VEGF pathway by targeting PHD1 and PHD2, inducing HIF-1α, and consequently promoting neovascularization [50].

Apoptosis, a programmed cell death process, is another cancer hallmark that miRNAs are involved in. The dysregulation of miRNAs can lead to downregulation of genes involved in apoptosis, as well as other tumor suppressor genes. Apoptosis can take place via two major pathways, extrinsic and intrinsic; the intrinsic pathway is triggered by genotoxic agents, metabolic aberrations, and transcriptional signals, while the extrinsic pathway is triggered by extracellular apoptotic signals [15]. These mentioned cues are picked up by BH3-only proteins, which results in deactivation of BCL-2 regulator proteins, with consequent activation of caspases, and eventual cell death [51]. In this context, there are miRNAs that can have antiapoptotic or proapoptotic effects. As central regulators of apoptosis, members of the BCL-2 family can be targets of several miRNAs in lung cancer cells. For example, BCL-2 is a direct target of miR-7 in NSCLC cells [52]. Another member of BCL-2 family, BCL-W was identified as a direct target of miR-335 in A549 and NCI-H1299 cells [53]. The miRNA-15a, that was mentioned earlier, besides inhibiting metastasis, also induces cell apoptosis by targeting BC2L2 [37]. In addition to BCL-2 related miRNAs, miR-608 has been identified as BCL-XL-induced miRNA and was found to be involved in regulating apoptosis in A549 and SK-LU-1 cells [54]. Another miRNA that induces apoptosis in lung cancer cells (A549, H460, and 95D cell lines) is miR-192. This miRNA acts by targeting the retinoblastoma 1 (RB1) gene [55].

When it comes to miRNAs with antiapoptotic effect, the activation of PPAR-γ/VEGF pathway by miR-130b leads to indirect Bcl-2 targeting and consequent suppression of NSCLC cell apoptosis [56]. A study showed that miR-214 modulates NSCLC cells radiotherapy response through regulation of p38 MAPK, apoptosis, and senescence [57]. Similarly, miR-197 is upregulated in cancer tissue, and miR-197 knockdown in NIH-H460 and A549 cells promotes apoptosis induction. It was also shown that miR-197 can act on the p53 pathway on various levels to hinder apoptosis, and to promote cell proliferation [58]. Other miRNAs known to have antiapoptotic properties in lung cancer are miR-21, miR-212, miR-17-5p and miR-20a. The miR-21 targets negative regulators of the RAS pathway and targets proapoptotic genes in NSCLC [59].

MiRNAs also participate in cellular energetics deregulation processes in cancer cells. For example, a decreased expression of miR-144 in vitro can increase glucose uptake by upregulating the glucose transporter (GLUT1) expression [60]. Besides, miR-33b was found to suppress cell growth in NSCLC by downregulating an enzyme participating in glucose metabolism lactate dehydrogenase A (LDHA) [61]. MiR-199a impacts glycolytic pathways by suppressing HIF-1α and consequently inhibits cancer growth [62]. MiR-31-5p also supports glycolysis through downregulation of the inhibitor of HIF-1α (FIH) gene, thus promoting cancer development [63].

2.1.2 Long noncoding RNAs

Long noncoding RNAs include transcripts with sizes that exceed 200 nt and they make up the majority of ncRNAs [64]. There are several subgroups of lncRNAs which are involved in lung cancer. Among the lncRNAs that have gained more attention among investigators, natural antisense transcripts (NATs), transcribed ultra-conserved region RNAs (T-UCR), telomerase RNA components (TERC), circular RNAs (circRNAs), and pseudogenes transcripts are the ones that stand out.

LncRNAs cover a wide range of functions such as cell and tissue differentiation, gene imprinting, interaction with transcription mechanisms, regulation of mRNA splicing and degradation, protein translation modulation and sponging of miRNAs to name a few [65]. Given a wide range of biological functions, lncRNAs are also involved in lung cancer mechanisms as well, with members having tumorigenic or tumor suppressor properties.

One of the most studied lncRNAs in lung cancer is MALAT1 and it is known to have carcinogenic properties through modulation of miR-124/STAT3. It is reported to be overexpressed in lung cancer and to promote carcinogenesis via miR-124 sponging which is a STAT3 suppressor [66]. The MALAT1 was also reported to promote epithelial-mesenchymal transition and metastasis through miR-204/SLUG axis [67]. Another closely studied lncRNA is XIST, which was reported to inhibit NSCLC development when downregulated by activating miR-335/SOD2/ROS signal pathway [68]. The XIST was also reported to control NSCLC proliferation and invasion by modulating miR-186-5p [69]. Its silencing suppressed cell proliferation, migration, and invasion, and promoted apoptosis through regulation of miR449a and Bcl-2 [70]. Another reported lncRNA with pro-tumor effect is HOTAIR, which is overexpressed in a various cancer types, including NSCLC [71].

Natural antisense transcripts (NATs), are a group of lncRNAs that have transcript complementarity with other RNA transcripts [72]. The NATs NKX2–1-AS1, WRAP53, FAM83A and AFAP1-AS1 were found to be upregulated in lung cancer, with first two increasing lung malignant cell proliferation rates [73, 74], FAM83A promoting lung cancer cell progression [75], and AFAP1-AS1 promoting cell migration in NSCLC [76]. On top of that, pseudogene transcripts such as DUXAP8 and DUXAP10 were reported to be upregulated while SFTA1P was found to be downregulated in NSCLC [77–79]. Other lncRNAs that have been reported as involved in lung cancer are T-UCRs. For example, Uc.338 and Uc.339 increase malignant cell cycle progression and migration in cells, and they are upregulated in NSCLC, while Uc.454, having the same biological role is downregulated [80–82].

CircRNAs make up a large group of ncRNAs and are produced through an unconventional splicing event called back-splicing. CircRNAs are part of the lncRNAs with coding potential, they possess important biological functions such as acting as miRNA and protein inhibitors and regulating protein function [83]. Circular RNAs can have several action mechanisms: interact with chromatin histones, act as miRNA sponges, entrap transcription factors to prevent gene transcription, attach themselves to RNA polymerase, and encircle protein-coding exons [84].

The role of the interaction between circRNA, miRNA and mRNA in lung cancer development is gaining more attention. A study reported that circRAD23B is overexpressed in lung tumors compared to healthy adjacent tissue. In these tumors, the circRAD23B sponged miR-593-3p and miR-653-5p, and normalized the expression levels mRNAs CCND2 and TIAM1, respectively [85]. Similarly, the circRNA100146 sponged miR-361-3p and miR-615-5p as a result of its overexpression. The sponging of miRNAs leads to upregulation of their respective targets, miR-361-3p targeting COL1A1, NFAT5, and TRAF3, and miR-615-5p targeting MEF2C in H460 NSCLC cells [86]. Another finding shows how an apoptotic resistance takes place in NSCLC due to sponging of miR-497, a BCL-2 (anti-apoptotic gene) suppressor by circPVT1 [87]. On the other hand, some circular RNAs such as circHIPK3 can have tumor-promoting effect by binding miR-193, miR-124, miR-654, and miR-379. The non-coding RNA hsa_circ_0007385 behaves as a competing endogenous RNA to miR-181 and is an oncogenic circRNA. One of the contributors to the cancer proliferation and improved invasion capacity in lung adenocarcinoma is the upregulation of hsa_circ_001358 [88]. Another circRNA that acts as an oncogene is circ_0000735. It is upregulated in lung cancer tissue compared to normal tissue, and it sponges tumor suppressor miRNAs miR-11,179 and miR-1182. The association of circ_0000735 with the lung cancer cells capacity to self-renew was also reported [89].

Table 2 provides a list of studies that investigated the role of circRNA-miRNA-mRNA axis in the context of lung cancer. There are circular RNAs that can convey tumor-suppressing capabilities utilizing their ability to sponge pro-carcinogenic microRNAs. One example is circ-ITCH, a circRNA with tumor suppressing ability that stems from its interaction with miR-7 and miR-214 [97].

2.1.3 Transfer RNAs

Transfer RNAs are a type of small ncRNA that plays a major role in protein synthesis by serving as a link between mRNA and the growing chain of amino acids [98]. Besides its known conventional function, tRNA dysregulated expression has been found in some malignancies. Transfer RNAs can be cleaved by ANG (angiogenin) and form tRNA-derived stress-induced RNAs (tiRNAs), which in turn can be further changed into tRNA-derived fragments (tRFs) [99]. As an example of tRNA dysregulation, the tiRNAs ts-3676 and ts-4521 were found to be downregulated in a lung tumor tissue when compared with healthy tissue [100]. Also, ts-46 and ts-47, tiRNAs with tumor suppressing properties were found to be downregulated in lung cancer. The introduction of mentioned tiRNAs in two lung cancer cell lines demonstrated their ability to negatively impact cell proliferation rate and self-renewal capacity in tumor cells.

An association between the tiRNAs ts-101 and ts-53 and PiwiL2, a protein that plays an important role in silencing transposons, was also found in lung cancer [101]. The tRNAs-Leu and tRNAs-Val were found to be overexpressed in lung tumor tissue,

circRNA	Targeted miRNA(s)	Indirect target(s)	Biological effect(s)	Reference
circ-RAD23B	miR-593-3p	CCND2	↑ Cell invasion	[85]
	miR-653-5p	TIAM1		
circRNA 100,146	miR-361-3p	NFAT5, COL1A1, TRAF3	↑ Cell invasion ↑ proliferation	[86]
	miR-615-5p	MEF2C		
circPVT1	miR-497	BCL-2	↑ apoptosis ↓ cell proliferation	[87]
	miR-125b	E2F1	↑ tumorigenesis	[90]
circFGFR3	miR-22-3p	Gal-1, p-AKT, and p-ERK1/2	↑ cell invasion	[91]
circ_0004015	miR-1183	PDPK1	↓ survival ↑ cell viability ↑ proliferation ↑ cell invasion ↓ drug (gefitinib) resistance	[92]
circPUM1	miR-326	CCND1 and BCL-2	↑ cell proliferation ↑ cell invasion ↑ cell migration	[93]
circFLI1	miR-584-3p	ROCK1	↑ Metastasis	[94]
circABCB10	miR-1252	FOXR2	↑ cell proliferation ↑ cell migration	[95]
circHIPK3	miR-124	SphK1, STAT3 and CDK4	↑ Cell proliferation ↓ apoptosis	[96]

Table 2.
Oncogenic circRNAs acting as miRNA sponges in NSCLC, and their biological effects (adapted from Braicu et al. [84]).

in 37% and 26% of samples, respectively. On the other hand, tRF-Leu-CAG was found to be overexpressed in not only lung tumor tissue, but also in serum and cell lines. The involvement of tRF-Leu-CAG in cell cycle progression and cell proliferation was reported, and its overexpression was shown to be associated with NSCLC progression. This tRF seems to interact with protein AURKA and its role in lung cancer needs further investigation [102].

2.1.4 Small nucleolar RNAs

Small nucleolar RNAs (snoRNAs) are a class of noncoding RNAs that guide the chemical modifications of ribosomal RNAs, transfer RNAs and small nuclear RNAs. SnoRNAs are located in the region of introns of genes that code for proteins or lncRNAs [84]. The snoRNAs also known to be a source of piRNAs (piR30840) [103]. The analysis of The Cancer Genome Atlas (TCGA) data has revealed that snoRNAs U60, U51, U28, U63, U104, HBI-100, U59B, HBII-419, HBII-142, and U30 are overexpressed, and HBII-420 is under-expressed, in lung cancer. Interestingly, SNORD15A was found to be significantly downregulated in non-smoker lung tissue with an overall difference pattern better distinguished in non-smokers compared to smokers [104]. The fact that SNORD78 is overexpressed in vitro, leads to cell proliferation, promotes EMT and consequently leads to enhanced invasion capacity, adds to the critical role snoRNAs play in NSCLC development [105]. Additionally, SNORD116–26 was found to be downregulated in tumor-initiating cells, while SNRA42 and SNORA3 were upregulated in the same cell type. Silencing of SNORA42 in cancer stem cells (CSCs) results in lower levels of tumorigenesis in lung cancer cells, while decreased expression of SNORA3 and SNORA42 in patients with lung tumors is associated with improved overall survival rate [106].

2.1.5 PIWI-interacting RNAs

The P-Element induced wimpy testis (PIWI) are a type of proteins highly conserved in plants and animals which are responsible for stem cell and germ cell differentiation [107]. The PIWI-interacting RNAs (piRNAs) make up the largest group of noncoding RNAs in animal cells and they originate from transposable elements (TE), mRNA and lncRNA (**Table 3**) [84, 113–115].

Type of ncRNA	Transcript	Expression in tumor vs. control	Biological function	Reference
piRNA	piR-34,871, piR-52,200	↑	↑ apoptosis ↑ cell proliferation	[108]
	piR-35,127, piR-46,545	↓	None	[108]
	piR-L-163	↓	↓ cell migration ↓ cell cycle progression	[109]
tRNA fragments	ts-46, ts-47, ts-101 and ts-53	↓	↓ cell proliferation	[101]
	tRF-Leu-CAG1	↑	↑ cell cycle progression ↑ cell proliferation	[102]
	tRF-Leu-CAG2			
YRNA	hY4 RNA	↑	↑ cell proliferation	[110]
SNORD	SNORA42	↑	Preserve tumor initiating make-up of cancer cells.	[106]
	U60, U63, U28, U51, U104, HBII-419, U59B, HBII-142, HBI-100, U30	↑	None	[104]
	HBII-420	↓		
	SNORD78	↑	↑ in vivo tumorigenesis ↑ lung tumor cell proliferation	[105]
	SNORA47, SNORA68, SNORA78, SNORA21, SNORD28 SNORD66	↑	None	[111]
	SNORD33, SNORD66 SNORD76	↑	None	[112]

Type of ncRNA	Transcript	Expression in tumor vs. control	Biological function	Reference
NAT	NKX2–1-AS1	↑	↑ lung malignant cell proliferation.	[73]
	WRAP53		↑ lung malignant cell proliferation	[74]
	FAM83A		↑ tumor progression	[75]
	AFAP1-AS1		↑ cell invasion and metastasis	[76]
Pseudogene transcripts	SFTA1P	↓	↓ cell migration and invasion	[79]
	DUXAP8	↑	↑ malignant cell survival, proliferation, tumorigenesis	[77]
	DUXAP10		↑ malignant cell survival, proliferation, migration, tumorigenesis	[78]
T-UCR	Uc.338	↑	↑ malignant cell cycle progression, invasion, and migration.	[80]
	Uc.339	↑	↑ malignant cell cycle progression, and migration.	[81]
	Uc.454	↓	↓ malignant cell cycle progression, invasion, and migration	[82]

Table 3.
Examples of ncRNA involved in lung cancer and their biological effects (adapted from Braicu et al. [84]).

2.2 Role of ncRNAs in NSCLC diagnosis and prognosis

2.2.1 MicroRNAs

When diagnosing a lung cancer, several miRNAs can be used to determine the cancer subtype. As an example, miR-205 can be utilized to distinguish SCC from other lung cancer NSCLC subtypes, whereas miR-124a is known for its specificity to LAC [116, 117]. In addition, four upregulated miRNAs (miR-93, miR-221 miR-30e, and miR-205,) show specificity to SCC, while another five upregulated miRNAs (miR-100, let-7e, miR-125a-5p, miR-29b and miR-29c) are specific to LAC [118]. Being able to distinguish primary lung tumor from metastatic tumor plays an important role for diagnosis and prognosis. The high levels of miR-182 were reported to be associated with primary lung tumors, while overexpression of miR-126 points to tumors of metastatic nature [119]. In a similar fashion, overexpression of miR-552 and miR-592 helps to distinguish primary LAC from metastatic colorectal adenocarcinoma [120].

The possibility of performing diagnosis based on miRNA expression in bodily fluids (blood, plasma, sputum) remains a topic of high interest for researchers due to feasibility and high potential as a diagnostic tool. One of the suggestions is utilizing a set of miRNAs, a miR-test kit comprising of 13 miRNAs which include miR-140-5p miR30b-5p, miR148a-3p, let-7d-5p, miR-191-5p, miR-30c-5p, miR-328-3p, miR-331-3p, miR-374a-5p, miR-29a-3p, miR-484, miR-223-3p, and miR-92a-3p [121]. A commercially available kit named microRNA signature classifier (MSC) uses the expression ratio among 24 miRNAs in lung cancer as a diagnostic tool [122].

MiRNAs play an important role as prognosis tools as well. For example, under-expression [123] of let-7 miRNA is associated with shortened postoperative survival. Another study reported that miR-21 and miR-155 were associated with poor recurrence-free survival for NSCLC patients [124].

2.2.2 Long noncoding RNAs

Regarding lncRNAs in the context of lung cancer diagnosis and prognosis, a number of lncRNAs were found to be of use. For example, the overexpression of HOTAIR promotes metastasis and indicates a poor prognosis for NSLC patients [71]. Similarly, MALAT1 in conjunction with protein thymosin beta 4 can be used to predict metastasis and survival in early-stage NSCLC determined using early stage and metastasized tumor tissue removed with surgery [125]. The lncRNA CDKN2B-AS1 with a more common name as antisense noncoding RNA in the INK4 locus (ANRIL) is associated with advanced lymph node metastasis and poor overall survival. A high expression of large intergenic RNA (lincRNA) PVT1 was shown to be associated with tumor advanced stage and advanced stage of tumor-node-metastasis (TNM) in NSCLC tissues, with consequent poor prognosis [126]. Other lncRNAs associated with poor NSCLC prognosis are listed in the **Table 4**.

LncRNA	**Expression in NSCLC (vs. normal tissue)**	**Clinical association**	**Reference**
MALAT1	↑	Poor prognosis	[125]
HOTAIR	↑	Poor survival and prognosis	[71]
SPRY4-IT1	↓	Poor prognosis	[128]
CDKN2B-AS1	↑	Poor survival	[129]
CCAT2	↑	Poor prognosis	[130]
PVT1	↑	Poor prognosis	[131]
IRAIN	↓	Poor prognosis	[132]
LCAL1	↑	Poor prognosis	[133]
SOX2OT	↑	Poor survival and prognosis	[134]
AFAP1-AS1	↑	Poor prognosis	[135]
TATDN1	↑	Poor prognosis	[136]
FOXD2-AS1	↑	Poor prognosis	[137]
SNHG1	↑	Poor survival and prognosis	[138]
ARHGAP27P1	↑	Aggressive tumorigenesis and poor prognosis	[139]
UCA1	↑	Poor prognosis	[140, 141]
HOXA11-AS	↑	Poor prognosis	[142]
LINC00473	↑	Poor prognosis	[143]

LncRNA	Expression in NSCLC (vs. normal tissue)	Clinical association	Reference
LINC00673	↑	Poor prognosis	[144]
BC087858	↓	Poor prognosis	[145]

Table 4.
LncRNAs associated with poor NSCLC prognosis (adapted from Osielska et al. [127]).

2.2.3 YRNAs

YRNAs and YRNA-derived small RNAs (YsRNAs) are also found in NSCLC patients, and they are gaining traction as potential lung cancer biomarkers. When assessed in A549 NSCLC cell lines, Ys4RNA was significantly downregulated. On the other hand, a deep sequencing expression analysis of small RNAs in plasma extracellular vesicles from LAC patients, SCC patients and healthy individuals showed upregulation of Ys4RNA [110]. The finding shows it may be used as a potential circulating biomarker for NSCLC diagnosis.

2.3 Role of ncRNAs in NSCLC therapy

The last two decades have seen a significant change in lung cancer management and treatment. Achievements in tumor genotyping and other molecular approaches helped to develop tools for personalized medicine adding targeted therapy and immunotherapy to traditional chemotherapy and radiation therapy. Investigation of PD-L1 status and genetic mutations within tumor helps to predict the most appropriate targeted therapy or immune checkpoint blockers (ICBs). The combination of platinum-based doublet therapy has served as a standard for advanced stage NSCLC patients [146]. Surgical resection remains as the most effective therapy for NSCLC in stages I and II, however, there is a high percentage of tumor recurrence, with varying 5-year overall survival rate depending on the NSCLC stage [147, 148]. In this section, we will discuss the roles of noncoding RNAs in NSCLC therapy.

2.3.1 MicroRNAs

Owing to their role that they play in gene regulation, miRNAs do also impact the response to cancer radiotherapy, chemotherapy, and targeted therapy [149]. MiRNAs have been shown to modify the sensitivity and resistance to the most common platinum-based therapy. For example, cisplatin sensitivity in NSCLC in vitro was reported to increase as a result of miR-106b overexpression, its further suppression of polycystin 2 (PKD2) levels, and consequent downregulation of P-glycoprotein [150]. Another study reported how miR-503 blocked drug efflux mechanism and suppressed a number of proteins associated with drug resistance (MRP1, MDR1, survivin, Bcl-2 and ERCC1), consequently improving cisplatin sensitivity [151]. Interestingly, the upregulation of miR-196 had an opposite effect on the same proteins, thus promoting drug efflux and cisplatin resistance [152]. When it comes to radiation therapy, miR-200c was shown to have a positive impact on radiotherapy by suppressing oxidative response genes and inhibiting DNA repair [153]. The upregulation of miRNA-138 was reported to induce radio-sensitization in NSCLC cells [154]. Similarly, miR-25 modulated the radio-sensitivity in lung cancer cells by directly inhibiting BTG2 expression [155].

In the context of molecular targeted therapy, miR-21 were reported to induce resistance to gefitinib through activation of ALK and ERK and inhibiting PTEN in lung cancer [156, 157]. The ALK resistance is another aspect where miRNAs play a role, and it was reported that histone H3 lysine 27 acetylation (H3K27ac) loss and inhibition of miR-34a is one the ways how ALK-positive lung cancer acquire ALK inhibitor resistance [158]. Another study observed a fingerprint of 7 circulating miRNAs (miR-493-5p, miR-411-3p, miR-494-3p, miR-215-5p, miR-495-3p, miR-93-3p and miR-548j-5p) to have a strong association with improved survival in lung cancer patients following the nivolumab treatment.

Currently, the most studied therapeutic miRNAs are let-7, miR-150, miR-29b, miR-200c, miR-34, and miR-145. The miR-34a alters the p53/mir-34/PD-L1 pathway by targeting PD-L1 and liposomal mimic MRX34 is a first miRNA that was used in phase I clinical trials initially showing promising antitumor activity [159]. However, the trials had to be terminated due to adverse effects [18]. **Table 5** summarizes the list of miRNAs associated with drug therapy and radiation sensitivity and resistance.

miRNA	Target/Pathway	Reference	miRNA	Target/Pathway	Reference
Chemo-sensitive			**Chemo-resistant**		
let-7	LIN28	[160]	miR-15b	PEBP4	[161]
miR-7	EGFR	[162]	miR-21	PTEN, SMAD7	[163, 164]
miR-17, 20a, 20b	TGFβR2	[165]			
miR-17 and miR-92 family	CDKN1A, RAD21	[166]	miR-27a	RKIP	[167]
miR-34a	PEBP4	[168]	miR-92a	PTEN	[169]
miR-101	ROCK2	[170]	miR-106a	Unknown	[171]
miR-106b	PKD2	[150]			
miR-135b	FZD1	[172]	miR-181c	WIF1, Wnt/β-catenin pathway	[173]
miR-137	NUCKS1	[174]			
miR-138	ZEB2	[175]	miR-196	MDR1, MRP1, ERCC1,	[152]
miR-146a	CCNJ	[176]		Survivin and Bcl-2	
miR-181b	TGFβR1/Smad signaling pathway	[177]	miR-205	PTEN, Mcl-1 and Survivin	[178, 179]
miR-184	Bcl-2	[180]	miR-488	eIF3a-mediated NER signaling pathway	[181]
miR-218	RUNX2	[182]			
mir-296	CX3CR1	[183]			
miR-379	EIF4G2	[184]			
miR-451	c-Myc-survivin/rad-51 signaling	[185]			
miR-503	Down-regulation of MDR1, MRP1, ERCC1,	[151]			
	Survivin and Bcl-2				

miRNA	Target/Pathway	Reference	miRNA	Target/Pathway	Reference
miR-9600	STAT3	[186]			
Radio-sensitive			**Radio-resistant**		
miR-29c	Bcl-2, Mcl-1	[187]	miR-21	PTEN, HIF1α, PDCD4	[163, 188]
miR-138	SENP1	[154]	miR-25	BTG2	[155]
miR-200c	PRDX2, GAPB/ Nrf2, and SESN1	[153]	miR-210	HIF1	[189]
miR-328	γ-H2AX	[190]	miR-1323	PRKDC	[191]
miR-449a	Unknown	[192]			
miR-451	c-Myc-survivin/ rad-51 signaling	[185]			
EGFR TKI-sensitive			**EGFR TKI-resistant**		
miR-126	Akt and ERK pathways	[193]	miR-21	PTEN, PDCD4	[194]
miR-134/miR-487b/miR-655 cluster	MAGI2	[195]	miR-23a	PTEN/PI3K/Akt pathway	[196]
miR-200c	PI3K/Akt pathway	[197]	miR-30 family	PI3K-SIAH2	[198]
miR-223	IGF1R/PI3K/Akt pathway	[199]	miR-214	PTEN/AKT pathway	[200]
miR-483-3p	integrin β3/ FAK/Erk pathway	[201]			
ALK TKI-sensitive					
miR-200c	ZEB1	[202]			

Table 5.
miRNAs associated with lung cancer therapy and radiation sensitivity or resistance (adapted from Wu et al.) [15].

2.3.2 Long noncoding RNAs

The MALAT1 is the first lncRNA used in targeted therapy studies with lncRNAs molecules. The targeted therapy decreased the amount of MALAT1 using antisense oligonucleotides (ASOs), consequently reducing lung cancer metastasis in a murine model [203]. The protein STAT3 can impact the MRP1 transcription by binding upstream, thus STAT3 activation is associated with MRP1 and MDR1 upregulation, which in turn enhances lung tumor cells resistance to cisplatin [204, 205]. In similar manner, the lncRNA KCNQ1OT1 expression was shown to be positively correlated with MDR1 expression, and KCNQ1OT1 knockdown can improve paclitaxel sensitivity in LAC cells [206]. A different study has demonstrated the ability of the lncRNA XIST to act as a competing endogenous RNA by sponging miR-144-3p, and thus regulating the expression of MRP1 [207]. In another study, the lncRNA SNHG14 was found to regulate the DDP-resistance of NSCLC cell through miR-133a/HOXB12 pathway [208].

The EGFR-tyrosine kinase inhibitors (EGFR-TKIs) prevent the lung cancer cells growth by inhibiting EGFR activity. The lncRNA LINC00460 eliminates miR-769-5p, which in turn promotes EGFR expression and therefore enhances NSCLC cells resistance to Gefitinib. The association between expression of LINC00460 and expression of proteins with multidrug-resistance, such as BCRP, P-gp, and MRP1 was reported [209]. The lncRNA colon cancer-associated transcript-1 (CCAT1), targets the miR-130a-3p/SOX4 axis and promotes cisplatin resistance in NSCLC in vitro [210]. Another lncRNA that induces cisplatin resistance in NSCLC is SNHG7, and it does it by upregulating MRD1 and BCRP via PI3K/AKT pathway [211]. A larger list of lncRNAs involved in drug resistance in NSCLC can be found in **Table 6**.

Drug	lncRNA	Effect on NSCLC	miRNA Target	Expression in tumor vs. control	Reference
Gefitinib	LINC00460	Promote	miR-769-5p	↑	[205]
	LINC00665		EZH2		[213]
	RHN1-AS1	Inhibit	miR-299-3p	↓	[214]
Cisplatin	MALAT1	Promote	STAT3	↑	[215]
	CCAT1		miR-130a-3p		[207]
	SNHG7		PI3K/AKT		[211]
	ROR		Akt/mTOR		[216]
	LINC00485		miR-195		[217]
	BLACAT		miR-17		[218]
	XIST		miR-17		[219]
	HOXA-AS3		HOXA3		[220]
	PAX6		PI3K/AKT		[221]
	PVT1		miR-216b		[222]
	NBAT1	Inhibit	PSMD10	↓	[223]
	TUG1		miR-221		[224]
	MEG3		p53, Bcl-xl		[225]
Vincristine	MEG3	Inhibit	miR-650	↓	[226]
Paclitaxel	KCNQ1OT1	Promote	Not known	↑	[227]
	NEAT1		Akt/mTOR		[228]
Multiple	DGCr5	Promote	miR-330-5p	↑	[229]
	ITGB1		Snail		[230]
	SNHG12		miR-299-3p		[231]
	SOX21-AS1		p57		[232]
	TUSC-7	Inhibit	miR-146	↓	[233]
	FENDRR		HuR		[234]
	MBNL1-AS1		miR-301b-3p		[235]
Crizotinib	HOTAIR	Promote	ULK1	↑	[236]
	ROR		ALK		[237]
EGFR-TKIs	UCA1	Promote	Akt/mTOR	↑	[238]
	LINC00460		miR-149-5p		[239]

Table 6.
LncRNAs related to drug resistance in NSCLC (adapted from Zhou et al. [212]).

3. The role of ncRNAs in small cell lung cancer

Small-cell lung cancer makes up 15% of all lung cancer incidences with 250,000 new cases and at least 200,000 annual death rates globally [240]. Carcinogens present in tobacco are responsible for the initiation of SCLC with accompanying inactivation of tumor suppressors p53 and RB in the majority of SCLC patients [241]. Amplification of MYC family members and frequent mutations of chromatin modeling proteins (EP300, CREBBP and MLL2) and Notch family members were also observed in SCLC patients [241, 242]. The ability of ncRNAs to modulate gene expression at transcriptional, post-transcriptional and epigenetic levels makes them significant factors, with clinical implications and functional roles in SCLC.

3.1 Role of miRNAs in SCLC

The miR-335 is downregulated in multi-drug resistant human SCLC cell lines. When overexpressed, miR-335 leads to the sensitization of the human SCLC cell lines to chemotherapy and radiotherapy by targeting PARP-1 (Poly [ADP-ribose] polymerase 1) gene. On top of that, overexpression of miR-335 promoted cell apoptosis, inhibited cell migration ability in vitro, and inhibited tumor growth in vivo [243]. In a similar fashion, the noncoding miR-22 was found to enhance the radiosensitivity in human SCLC cell line by targeting WRNIP1, promoting apoptosis and inhibiting cell migration when overexpressed [244]. Another noteworthy observation is that methylation in SCLC cell lines reduced the expression of miR-34 family members, which are known tumor suppressive miRNAS. The transfection of miR-34b/c to SCLC cell lines (H1048 and SBC5) resulted in significantly decreased cell growth, migration, and invasion [245]. The circulating miR-141 from plasm exosomes and serum of SCLC patients was found to be upregulated when compared to healthy volunteers. The ability of miR-141 to promote angiogenesis by targeting KLF12 (Kruppel-like factor 12) was demonstrated [246]. Earlier, miR-126 was found to inhibit SCLC cells proliferation by targeting SLC7A5, whereas the miR-217 was reported to inhibit proliferation and to promote apoptosis in SCLC cells by targeting PCDH8 [247, 248]. The miR-195 promoted SCLC apoptosis by inhibiting Rap2C protein-dependent MAPK signal transduction [249]. Similarly, the miR-26b was reported to promote apoptosis and suppress tumorigenicity by targeting myeloid cell leukemia 1 protein [250]. In another study, miR-485-5p was found to suppress the proliferation, migration, and invasion of SCLC cells by targeting flotillin-2 [251].

3.2 Role of lncRNAs in SCLC

There are five lncRNAs that are known to be involved in SCLC: HOTTIP, HOTAIR, TUG1, CCAT2 and PVT1 [252]. The lncRNA HOTTIP is upregulated in SCLC, is associated with chemoresistance and shorter survival. The HOTTIP acts through HOTTIP/miR-574-5p/EZH1 and HOTTIP/miR-216a/BCL-2 axes [253, 254]. The lncRNA HOTAIR, same as in NSCLC, is upregulated in SCLC, and is associated with lymphatic invasion and chemoresistance in SCLC [255, 256]. The ncRNAs TUG1 and CCAT2 are also upregulated in SCLC, where TUG1 is associated with chemoresistance, clinical stage and shorter survival, whereas CCAT2 is associated with malignant status and poor prognosis [257, 258]. Similarly, the lncRNA PVT1 is upregulated in SCLC patients and is associated with lymph node metastasis and clinical stage [259]. Recently, Linc00173 was reported to modulate glucose metabolism and multidrug chemoresistance in SCLC [260].

4. Conclusion

Lung cancer remains to be a leading cause of cancer death. The past two decades have witnessed an unprecedented growth in cancer research, and new findings have continuously supported and expanded the notion that ncRNAs play a significant part in all aspects of lung cancer. Future advancements in molecular technology will help researchers answer more complicated questions about this disease, including uncovering the additional ncRNAs and the mechanisms by which these regulated lung cancer development, progression, and response to therapy. The heterogeneity of lung cancer subtypes, variation in mutational burden, sex differences, and different stages of cancer further necessitate a combination of individualized therapies, such as platinum-based doublet chemotherapy, immunotherapy, and targeted therapy to combat lung cancer effects on human health. The relative success of combined therapies underlines the need to further investigate the roles and functions of ncRNAs within cancer processes. A better understanding of tumorigenesis mechanisms and identification of ncRNAs and other participants will play an important role in improving lung cancer diagnosis, prognosis, prevention, and therapy.

Acknowledgements

This work was supported by NIH grant HL159764 (PS).

Conflict of interest

The authors declare no conflict of interest.

Author details

Maksat Babayev and Patricia Silveyra*
Indiana University School of Public Health, Bloomington, IN, USA

*Address all correspondence to: psilveyr@iu.edu

References

[1] Siegel RL et al. Cancer statistics, 2021. CA: A Cancer Journal for Clinicians. 2021;**71**(1):7-33

[2] Sung H et al. Global cancer statistics 2020: GLOBOCAN estimates of incidence and mortality worldwide for 36 cancers in 185 countries. CA: A Cancer Journal for Clinicians. 2021; **71**(3):209-249

[3] Cheng L et al. Molecular pathology of lung cancer: Key to personalized medicine. Modern Pathology. 2012; **25**(3):347-369

[4] Durham AL, Adcock IM. The relationship between COPD and lung cancer. Lung Cancer. 2015;**90**(2):121-127

[5] Rudin CM et al. Small-cell lung cancer. Nature Reviews. Disease Primers. 2021;**7**(1):3

[6] Duma N, Santana-Davila R, Molina JR. Non-small cell lung cancer: Epidemiology, screening, diagnosis, and treatment. Mayo Clinic Proceedings. 2019;**94**(8):1623-1640

[7] Nicholson AG et al. The 2021 WHO classification of lung tumors: impact of advances since 2015. Journal of Thoracic Oncology. 2022;**17**(3):362-387

[8] Brosnan CA, Voinnet O. The long and the short of noncoding RNAs. Current Opinion in Cell Biology. 2009;**21**(3): 416-425

[9] Boon RA et al. Long noncoding RNAs: From clinical genetics to therapeutic targets? Journal of the American College of Cardiology. 2016;**67**(10):1214-1226

[10] Napoli S. LncRNAs and available databases. In: Navarro A, editor. Long Non-coding RNAs in Cancer. New York, USA: Springer Nature; 2021. pp. 3-6

[11] Travis William D. Pathology of Lung Cancer. Clinics in Chest Medicine. 2011; **32**(4):669-692

[12] Li C, Lu H. Adenosquamous carcinoma of the lung. Oncotargets and Therapy. 2018;**11**:4829-4835

[13] Hanahan D, Weinberg RA. The hallmarks of cancer. Cell. 2000;**100**(1): 57-70

[14] Hanahan D. Hallmarks of cancer: New dimensions. Cancer Discovery. 2022;**12**(1):31-46

[15] Wu KL et al. The roles of MicroRNA in lung cancer. International Journal of Molecular Sciences. 2019;**20**(7):1611

[16] Yang N et al. Hepatocellular carcinoma and microRNA: New perspectives on therapeutics and diagnostics. Advanced Drug Delivery Reviews. 2015;**81**:62-74

[17] Brambilla E, Gazdar A. Pathogenesis of lung cancer signalling pathways: Roadmap for therapies. The European Respiratory Journal. 2009;**33**(6): 1485-1497

[18] Van Roosbroeck K, Calin GA. Cancer hallmarks and MicroRNAs: The therapeutic connection. Advances in Cancer Research. 2017;**135**:119-149

[19] Chan LW, Wang FF, Cho WC. Genomic sequence analysis of EGFR regulation by microRNAs in lung cancer. Current Topics in Medicinal Chemistry. 2012;**12**(8):920-926

[20] Qin Q et al. miR-134 inhibits non-small cell lung cancer growth by targeting the epidermal growth factor receptor. Journal of Cellular and

Molecular Medicine. 2016;**20**(10): 1974-1983

[21] Zhu K et al. Tumor-suppressive miR-218-5p inhibits cancer cell proliferation and migration via EGFR in non-small cell lung cancer. Oncotarget. 2016;**7**(19): 28075-28085

[22] Vishwamitra D et al. MicroRNA 96 is a post-transcriptional suppressor of anaplastic lymphoma kinase expression. The American Journal of Pathology. 2012;**180**(5):1772-1780

[23] Davies KD, Doebele RC. Molecular pathways: ROS1 fusion proteins in cancer. Clinical Cancer Research. 2013; **19**(15):4040-4045

[24] Yan C et al. MiR-760 suppresses non-small cell lung cancer proliferation and metastasis by targeting ROS1. Environmental Science and Pollution Research International. 2018;**25**(19): 18385-18391

[25] Friday BB, Adjei AA. K-ras as a target for cancer therapy. Biochimica et Biophysica Acta. 2005;**1756**(2):127-144

[26] Kopp F, Wagner E, Roidl A. The proto-oncogene KRAS is targeted by miR-200c. Oncotarget. 2014;**5**(1): 185-195

[27] Seviour EG et al. Targeting KRas-dependent tumour growth, circulating tumour cells and metastasis in vivo by clinically significant miR-193a-3p. Oncogene. 2017;**36**(10):1339-1350

[28] Ma Z et al. MiR-181a-5p inhibits cell proliferation and migration by targeting Kras in non-small cell lung cancer A549 cells. Acta Biochim Biophys Sin (Shanghai). 2015;**47**(8):630-638

[29] Xie Q et al. microRNA-148a-3p inhibited the proliferation and epithelial-mesenchymal transition progression of non-small-cell lung cancer via modulating Ras/MAPK/Erk signaling. Journal of Cellular Physiology. 2019; **234**(8):12786-12799

[30] Jiang W et al. MicroRNA-1258 suppresses tumour progression via GRB2/Ras/Erk pathway in non-small-cell lung cancer. Cell Proliferation. 2018; **51**(6):e12502

[31] Lv X et al. MicroRNA-520a-3p inhibits cell growth and metastasis of non-small cell lung cancer through PI3K/AKT/mTOR signaling pathway. European Review for Medical and Pharmacological Sciences. 2018;**22**(8): 2321-2327

[32] Bandi N et al. miR-15a and miR-16 are implicated in cell cycle regulation in a Rb-dependent manner and are frequently deleted or down-regulated in non-small cell lung cancer. Cancer Research. 2009;**69**(13):5553-5559

[33] Ren XS et al. Tumor-suppressive microRNA-449a induces growth arrest and senescence by targeting E2F3 in human lung cancer cells. Cancer Letters. 2014;**344**(2):195-203

[34] Kong Q et al. miR-641 functions as a tumor suppressor by targeting MDM2 in human lung cancer. Oncology Research. 2018;**26**(5):735-741

[35] Fortunato O et al. Mir-660 is downregulated in lung cancer patients and its replacement inhibits lung tumorigenesis by targeting MDM2-p53 interaction. Cell Death & Disease. 2014; **5**:e1564

[36] Fabbri M et al. MicroRNA-29 family reverts aberrant methylation in lung cancer by targeting DNA methyltransferases 3A and 3B. Proceedings of the National Academy of

Sciences of the United States of America. 2007;**104**(40):15805-15810

[37] Yang T et al. MicroRNA-15a induces cell apoptosis and inhibits metastasis by targeting BCL2L2 in non-small cell lung cancer. Tumour Biology. 2015;**36**(6): 4357-4365

[38] Wu SG et al. MicroRNA in lung cancer metastasis. Cancers (Basel). 2019;**11**:2

[39] Jia Z et al. miR-126 suppresses epithelial-to-mesenchymal transition and metastasis by targeting PI3K/AKT/Snail signaling of lung cancer cells. Oncology Letters. 2018;**15**(5):7369-7375

[40] Sun CC et al. MicroRNA-346 facilitates cell growth and metastasis, and suppresses cell apoptosis in human non-small cell lung cancer by regulation of XPC/ERK/Snail/E-cadherin pathway. Aging (Albany NY). 2016;**8**(10): 2509-2524

[41] Kumarswamy R et al. MicroRNA-30a inhibits epithelial-to-mesenchymal transition by targeting Snai1 and is downregulated in non-small cell lung cancer. International Journal of Cancer. 2012;**130**(9):2044-2053

[42] Zhang K et al. MiR-22 inhibits lung cancer cell EMT and invasion through targeting snail. European Review for Medical and Pharmacological Sciences. 2017;**21**(16):3598-3604

[43] Fan MJ et al. MiR-30 suppresses lung cancer cell 95D epithelial mesenchymal transition and invasion through targeted regulating Snail. European Review for Medical and Pharmacological Sciences. 2017;**21**(11):2642-2649

[44] Choi YC et al. Regulation of vascular endothelial growth factor signaling by miR-200b. Molecules and Cells. 2011; **32**(1):77-82

[45] Pecot CV et al. Tumour angiogenesis regulation by the miR-200 family. Nature Communications. 2013;**4**:2427

[46] Hu J et al. microRNA-128 plays a critical role in human non-small cell lung cancer tumourigenesis, angiogenesis and lymphangiogenesis by directly targeting vascular endothelial growth factor-C. European Journal of Cancer. 2014; **50**(13):2336-2350

[47] Liu B et al. MiR-126 restoration down-regulate VEGF and inhibit the growth of lung cancer cell lines in vitro and in vivo. Lung Cancer. 2009;**66**(2): 169-175

[48] Zhao WY et al. Downregulation of miR-497 promotes tumor growth and angiogenesis by targeting HDGF in non-small cell lung cancer. Biochemical and Biophysical Research Communications. 2013;**435**(3):466-471

[49] Mao G et al. Tumor-derived microRNA-494 promotes angiogenesis in non-small cell lung cancer. Angiogenesis. 2015;**18**(3):373-382

[50] Hsu YL et al. Hypoxic lung cancer-secreted exosomal miR-23a increased angiogenesis and vascular permeability by targeting prolyl hydroxylase and tight junction protein ZO-1. Oncogene. 2017; **36**(34):4929-4942

[51] Hanahan D, Weinberg RA. Hallmarks of cancer: The next generation. Cell. 2011;**144**(5):646-674

[52] Xiong S et al. MicroRNA-7 inhibits the growth of human non-small cell lung cancer A549 cells through targeting BCL-2. International Journal of Biological Sciences. 2011;**7**(6):805-814

[53] Wang H et al. Effect of miR-335 upregulation on the apoptosis and invasion of lung cancer cell A549 and

H1299. Tumour Biology. 2013;**34**(5): 3101-3109

[54] Othman N et al. Bcl-xL silencing induces alterations in hsa-miR-608 expression and subsequent cell death in A549 and SK-LU1 human lung adenocarcinoma cells. PLoS One. 2013; **8**(12):e81735

[55] Feng S et al. MicroRNA-192 targeting retinoblastoma 1 inhibits cell proliferation and induces cell apoptosis in lung cancer cells. Nucleic Acids Research. 2011;**39**(15):6669-6678

[56] Tian J et al. MicroRNA-130b promotes lung cancer progression via PPARgamma/VEGF-A/BCL-2-mediated suppression of apoptosis. Journal of Experimental & Clinical Cancer Research. 2016;**35**(1):105

[57] Salim H et al. miRNA-214 modulates radiotherapy response of non-small cell lung cancer cells through regulation of p38MAPK, apoptosis and senescence. British Journal of Cancer. 2012;**107**(8): 1361-1373

[58] Fiori ME et al. Antitumor effect of miR-197 targeting in p53 wild-type lung cancer. Cell Death and Differentiation. 2014;**21**(5):774-782

[59] Hatley ME et al. Modulation of K-Ras-dependent lung tumorigenesis by MicroRNA-21. Cancer Cell. 2010;**18**(3): 282-293

[60] Liu M et al. Downregulating microRNA-144 mediates a metabolic shift in lung cancer cells by regulating GLUT1 expression. Oncology Letters. 2016;**11**(6):3772-3776

[61] Zhai S et al. Downregulation of miR-33b promotes non-small cell lung cancer cell growth through reprogramming glucose metabolism miR-33b regulates non-small cell lung cancer cell growth. Journal of Cellular Biochemistry. 2019; **120**(4):6651-6660

[62] Ding G et al. MiR-199a suppresses the hypoxia-induced proliferation of non-small cell lung cancer cells through targeting HIF1alpha. Molecular and Cellular Biochemistry. 2013;**384**(1–2): 173-180

[63] Zhu B et al. MicroRNA-31-5p enhances the Warburg effect via targeting FIH. The FASEB Journal. 2019; **33**(1):545-556

[64] Cabili MN et al. Integrative annotation of human large intergenic noncoding RNAs reveals global properties and specific subclasses. Genes & Development. 2011;**25**(18):1915-1927

[65] Marchese FP, Raimondi I, Huarte M. The multidimensional mechanisms of long noncoding RNA function. Genome Biology. 2017;**18**(1):206

[66] Li S et al. The lncRNA MALAT1 contributes to non-small cell lung cancer development via modulating miR-124/ STAT3 axis. Journal of Cellular Physiology. 2018;**233**(9):6679-6688

[67] Li J et al. LncRNA MALAT1 exerts oncogenic functions in lung adenocarcinoma by targeting miR-204. American Journal of Cancer Research. 2016;**6**(5):1099-1107

[68] Liu J et al. Downregulation of LncRNA-XIST inhibited development of non-small cell lung cancer by activating miR-335/SOD2/ROS signal pathway mediated pyroptotic cell death. Aging (Albany NY). 2019;**11**(18):7830-7846

[69] Wang H et al. The long non-coding RNA XIST controls non-small cell lung Cancer proliferation and invasion by modulating miR-186-5p. Cellular

Physiology and Biochemistry. 2017; **41**(6):2221-2229

[70] Zhang YL et al. The lncRNA XIST exhibits oncogenic properties via regulation of miR-449a and Bcl-2 in human non-small cell lung cancer. Acta Pharmacologica Sinica. 2017;**38**(3): 371-381

[71] Liu XH et al. The long non-coding RNA HOTAIR indicates a poor prognosis and promotes metastasis in non-small cell lung cancer. BMC Cancer. 2013;**13**: 464

[72] Osato N et al. Transcriptional interferences in cis natural antisense transcripts of humans and mice. Genetics. 2007;**176**(2):1299-1306

[73] Balbin OA et al. The landscape of antisense gene expression in human cancers. Genome Research. 2015;**25**(7): 1068-1079

[74] Yuan XS et al. Clinical, cellular, and bioinformatic analyses reveal involvement of WRAP53 overexpression in carcinogenesis of lung adenocarcinoma. Tumour Biology. 2017; **39**(3):1010428317694309

[75] Shi R et al. Long noncoding antisense RNA FAM83A-AS1 promotes lung cancer cell progression by increasing FAM83A. Journal of Cellular Biochemistry. 2019;**120**(6):10505-10512

[76] He J et al. Long non-coding RNA AFAP1-AS1 plays an oncogenic role in promoting cell migration in non-small cell lung cancer. Cellular and Molecular Life Sciences. 2018;**75**(24):4667-4681

[77] Sun M et al. The pseudogene DUXAP8 promotes non-small-cell lung cancer cell proliferation and invasion by epigenetically silencing EGR1 and RHOB. Molecular Therapy. 2017;**25**(3): 739-751

[78] Wei CC et al. The pseudogene DUXAP10 promotes an aggressive phenotype through binding with LSD1 and repressing LATS2 and RRAD in non small cell lung cancer. Oncotarget. 2017; **8**(3):5233-5246

[79] Zhang H et al. The pseudogene-derived long noncoding RNA SFTA1P is down-regulated and suppresses cell migration and invasion in lung adenocarcinoma. Tumour Biology. 2017; **39**(2):1010428317691418

[80] Gao X et al. Knockdown of long noncoding RNA uc.338 by siRNA inhibits cellular migration and invasion in human lung cancer cells. Oncology Research. 2016;**24**(5):337-343

[81] Vannini I et al. Transcribed ultraconserved region 339 promotes carcinogenesis by modulating tumor suppressor microRNAs. Nature Communications. 2017;**8**(1):1801

[82] Zhou J et al. Uc.454 inhibited growth by targeting heat shock protein family a member 12B in non-small-cell lung cancer. Molecular Therapy Nucleic Acids. 2018;**12**:174-183

[83] Kristensen LS et al. The biogenesis, biology and characterization of circular RNAs. Nature Reviews. Genetics. 2019; **20**(11):675-691

[84] Braicu C et al. The function of non-coding RNAs in lung cancer tumorigenesis. Cancers (Basel). 2019;**11**(5):605

[85] Han W et al. Circular RNA circ-RAD23B promotes cell growth and invasion by miR-593-3p/CCND2 and miR-653-5p/TIAM1 pathways in non-small cell lung cancer. Biochemical and

Biophysical Research Communications. 2019;**510**(3):462-466

[86] Chen L et al. Circular RNA 100146 functions as an oncogene through direct binding to miR-361-3p and miR-615-5p in non-small cell lung cancer. Molecular Cancer. 2019;**18**(1):13

[87] Qin S et al. Circular RNA PVT1 acts as a competing endogenous RNA for miR-497 in promoting non-small cell lung cancer progression. Biomedicine & Pharmacotherapy. 2019; **111**:244-250

[88] Zhu X et al. hsa_circ_0013958: A circular RNA and potential novel biomarker for lung adenocarcinoma. The FEBS Journal. 2017;**284**(14): 2170-2182

[89] Li W et al. Enhanced expression of circ_0000735 forecasts clinical severity in NSCLC and promotes cell progression via sponging miR-1179 and miR-1182. Biochemical and Biophysical Research Communications. 2019;**510**(3):467-471

[90] Li X et al. Circular RNA circPVT1 promotes proliferation and invasion through sponging miR-125b and activating E2F2 signaling in non-small cell lung cancer. Cellular Physiology and Biochemistry. 2018;**51**(5):2324-2340

[91] Qiu BQ et al. CircRNA fibroblast growth factor receptor 3 promotes tumor progression in non-small cell lung cancer by regulating Galectin-1-AKT/ERK1/2 signaling. Journal of Cellular Physiology. 2019;**234**(7):11256-11264

[92] Zhou Y et al. Circular RNA hsa_circ_0004015 regulates the proliferation, invasion, and TKI drug resistance of non-small cell lung cancer by miR-1183/PDPK1 signaling pathway. Biochemical and Biophysical Research Communications. 2019;**508**(2):527-535

[93] Chen J et al. CircPUM1 promotes the malignant behavior of lung adenocarcinoma by regulating miR-326. Biochemical and Biophysical Research Communications. 2019;**508**(3): 844-849

[94] Li L et al. FLI1 Exonic circular RNAs as a novel oncogenic driver to promote tumor metastasis in small cell lung cancer. Clinical Cancer Research. 2019; **25**(4):1302-1317

[95] Tian X et al. CircABCB10 promotes nonsmall cell lung cancer cell proliferation and migration by regulating the miR-1252/FOXR2 axis. Journal of Cellular Biochemistry. 2019;**120**(3): 3765-3772

[96] Yu H, Chen Y, Jiang P. Circular RNA HIPK3 exerts oncogenic properties through suppression of miR-124 in lung cancer. Biochemical and Biophysical Research Communications. 2018;**506**(3): 455-462

[97] Wan L et al. Circular RNA-ITCH suppresses lung cancer proliferation via inhibiting the Wnt/beta-catenin pathway. BioMed Research International. 2016;**2016**:1579490

[98] Giege R. Toward a more complete view of tRNA biology. Nature Structural & Molecular Biology. 2008;**15**(10): 1007-1014

[99] Huang SQ et al. The dysregulation of tRNAs and tRNA derivatives in cancer. Journal of Experimental & Clinical Cancer Research. 2018;**37**(1):101

[100] Pekarsky Y et al. Dysregulation of a family of short noncoding RNAs, tsRNAs, in human cancer. Proceedings of the National Academy of Sciences of the United States of America. 2016; **113**(18):5071-5076

[101] Balatti V et al. tsRNA signatures in cancer. Proceedings of the National Academy of Sciences of the United States of America. 2017;**114**(30): 8071-8076

[102] Shao Y et al. tRF-leu-CAG promotes cell proliferation and cell cycle in non-small cell lung cancer. Chemical Biology & Drug Design. 2017;**90**(5):730-738

[103] Zhong F et al. A SnoRNA-derived piRNA interacts with human interleukin-4 pre-mRNA and induces its decay in nuclear exosomes. Nucleic Acids Research. 2015;**43**(21): 10474-10491

[104] Nogueira Jorge NA et al. snoRNA and piRNA expression levels modified by tobacco use in women with lung adenocarcinoma. PLoS One. 2017;**12**(8): e0183410

[105] Zheng D et al. Small nucleolar RNA 78 promotes the tumorigenesis in non-small cell lung cancer. Journal of Experimental & Clinical Cancer Research. 2015;**34**:49

[106] Mannoor K et al. Small nucleolar RNA signatures of lung tumor-initiating cells. Molecular Cancer. 2014;**13**:104

[107] Cox DN, Chao A, Lin H. Piwi encodes a nucleoplasmic factor whose activity modulates the number and division rate of germline stem cells. Development. 2000;**127**(3):503-514

[108] Reeves ME et al. Identification and characterization of RASSF1C piRNA target genes in lung cancer cells. Oncotarget. 2017;**8**(21):34268-34282

[109] Mei Y et al. A piRNA-like small RNA interacts with and modulates p-ERM proteins in human somatic cells. Nature Communications. 2015;**6**:7316

[110] Li C et al. Characterization and selective incorporation of small non-coding RNAs in non-small cell lung cancer extracellular vesicles. Cell & Bioscience. 2018;**8**:2

[111] Gao L et al. Genome-wide small nucleolar RNA expression analysis of lung cancer by next-generation deep sequencing. International Journal of Cancer. 2015;**136**(6):E623-E629

[112] Liao J et al. Small nucleolar RNA signatures as biomarkers for non-small-cell lung cancer. Molecular Cancer. 2010; **9**:198

[113] Siomi MC et al. PIWI-interacting small RNAs: The vanguard of genome defence. Nature Reviews. Molecular Cell Biology. 2011;**12**(4):246-258

[114] Dorner S et al. Delving into the diversity of silencing pathways. Symposium on MicroRNAs and siRNAs: Biological functions and mechanisms. EMBO Reports. 2007;**8**(8):723-729

[115] Han YN et al. PIWI proteins and PIWI-interacting RNA: Emerging roles in cancer. Cellular Physiology and Biochemistry. 2017;**44**(1):1-20

[116] Lebanony D et al. Diagnostic assay based on hsa-miR-205 expression distinguishes squamous from nonsquamous non-small-cell lung carcinoma. Journal of Clinical Oncology. 2009;**27**(12):2030-2037

[117] Bishop JA et al. Accurate classification of non-small cell lung carcinoma using a novel microRNA-based approach. Clinical Cancer Research. 2010;**16**(2):610-619

[118] Zhang YK et al. miRNAs expression profiling to distinguish lung squamous-cell carcinoma from adenocarcinoma subtypes. Journal of Cancer Research

and Clinical Oncology. 2012;**138**(10): 1641-1650

[119] Barshack I et al. MicroRNA expression differentiates between primary lung tumors and metastases to the lung. Pathology, Research and Practice. 2010;**206**(8):578-584

[120] Kim HK et al. miR-592 and miR-552 can distinguish between primary lung adenocarcinoma and colorectal cancer metastases in the lung. Anticancer Research. 2014;**34**(5):2297-2302

[121] Montani F et al. miR-test: A blood test for lung cancer early detection. Journal of the National Cancer Institute. 2015;**107**(6):djv063

[122] Sozzi G et al. Clinical utility of a plasma-based miRNA signature classifier within computed tomography lung cancer screening: A correlative MILD trial study. Journal of Clinical Oncology. 2014;**32**(8):768-773

[123] Takamizawa J et al. Reduced expression of the let-7 microRNAs in human lung cancers in association with shortened postoperative survival. Cancer Research. 2004;**64**(11):3753-3756

[124] Yang M et al. High expression of miR-21 and miR-155 predicts recurrence and unfavourable survival in non-small cell lung cancer. European Journal of Cancer. 2013;**49**(3):604-615

[125] Ji P et al. MALAT-1, a novel noncoding RNA, and thymosin beta4 predict metastasis and survival in early-stage non-small cell lung cancer. Oncogene. 2003;**22**(39):8031-8041

[126] Cui D et al. Long non-coding RNA PVT1 as a novel biomarker for diagnosis and prognosis of non-small cell lung cancer. Tumour Biology. 2016;**37**(3): 4127-4134

[127] Osielska MA, Jagodzinski PP. Long non-coding RNA as potential biomarkers in non-small-cell lung cancer: What do we know so far? Biomedicine & Pharmacotherapy. 2018;**101**:322-333

[128] Sun M et al. EZH2-mediated epigenetic suppression of long noncoding RNA SPRY4-IT1 promotes NSCLC cell proliferation and metastasis by affecting the epithelial-mesenchymal transition. Cell Death & Disease. 2014;**5**: e1298

[129] Lin L et al. Increased expression of the long non-coding RNA ANRIL promotes lung cancer cell metastasis and correlates with poor prognosis. Diagnostic Pathology. 2015;**10**:14

[130] Qiu M et al. CCAT2 is a lung adenocarcinoma-specific long non-coding RNA and promotes invasion of non-small cell lung cancer. Tumour Biology. 2014;**35**(6):5375-5380

[131] Guan Y et al. Amplification of PVT1 contributes to the pathophysiology of ovarian and breast cancer. Clinical Cancer Research. 2007;**13**(19): 5745-5755

[132] Sun J et al. A novel antisense long noncoding RNA within the IGF1R gene locus is imprinted in hematopoietic malignancies. Nucleic Acids Research. 2014;**42**(15):9588-9601

[133] White NM et al. Transcriptome sequencing reveals altered long intergenic non-coding RNAs in lung cancer. Genome Biology. 2014;**15**(8):429

[134] Hou Z et al. A long noncoding RNA Sox2ot regulates lung cancer cell proliferation and is a prognostic indicator of poor survival. The International Journal of Biochemistry & Cell Biology. 2014;**53**:380-388

[135] Zeng Z et al. AFAP1-AS1, a long noncoding RNA upregulated in lung cancer and promotes invasion and metastasis. Tumour Biology. 2016;**37**(1):729-737

[136] Zequn N et al. The role and potential mechanisms of LncRNA-TATDN1 on metastasis and invasion of non-small cell lung cancer. Oncotarget. 2016;**7**(14):18219-18228

[137] Rong L, Zhao R, Lu J. Highly expressed long non-coding RNA FOXD2-AS1 promotes non-small cell lung cancer progression via Wnt/beta-catenin signaling. Biochemical and Biophysical Research Communications. 2017;**484**(3):586-591

[138] Cui Y et al. Upregulated lncRNA SNHG1 contributes to progression of non-small cell lung cancer through inhibition of miR-101-3p and activation of Wnt/beta-catenin signaling pathway. Oncotarget. 2017;**8**(11):17785-17794

[139] Deng X et al. PM2.5 exposure-induced autophagy is mediated by lncRNA loc146880 which also promotes the migration and invasion of lung cancer cells. Biochimica et Biophysica Acta - General Subjects. 2017;**1861**(2):112-125

[140] Nie W et al. LncRNA-UCA1 exerts oncogenic functions in non-small cell lung cancer by targeting miR-193a-3p. Cancer Letters. 2016;**371**(1):99-106

[141] Wang HM et al. Upregulated lncRNA-UCA1 contributes to progression of lung cancer and is closely related to clinical diagnosis as a predictive biomarker in plasma. International Journal of Clinical and Experimental Medicine. 2015;**8**(7):11824-11830

[142] Chen JH et al. Overexpression of lncRNA HOXA11-AS promotes cell epithelial-mesenchymal transition by repressing miR-200b in non-small cell lung cancer. Cancer Cell International. 2017;**17**:64

[143] Chen Z et al. cAMP/CREB-regulated LINC00473 marks LKB1-inactivated lung cancer and mediates tumor growth. The Journal of Clinical Investigation. 2016;**126**(6):2267-2279

[144] Lu W et al. Long non-coding RNA linc00673 regulated non-small cell lung cancer proliferation, migration, invasion and epithelial mesenchymal transition by sponging miR-150-5p. Molecular Cancer. 2017;**16**(1):118

[145] Pan H et al. Long non-coding RNA BC087858 induces non-T790M mutation acquired resistance to EGFR-TKIs by activating PI3K/AKT and MEK/ERK pathways and EMT in non-small-cell lung cancer. Oncotarget. 2016;**7**(31):49948-49960

[146] Hanna N et al. Systemic therapy for stage IV non-small-cell lung cancer: American Society of Clinical Oncology clinical practice guideline update. Journal of Clinical Oncology. 2017;**35**(30):3484-3515

[147] Hirsch FR et al. Lung cancer: Current therapies and new targeted treatments. Lancet. 2017;**389**(10066):299-311

[148] Goldstraw P et al. The IASLC lung cancer staging project: Proposals for revision of the TNM stage groupings in the forthcoming (eighth) edition of the TNM classification for lung cancer. Journal of Thoracic Oncology. 2016;**11**(1):39-51

[149] Lu J et al. MicroRNAs associated with therapy of non-small cell lung cancer. International Journal of Biological Sciences. 2018;**14**(4):390-397

[150] Yu S et al. MicroRNA-106b-5p regulates cisplatin chemosensitivity by targeting polycystic kidney disease-2 in non-small-cell lung cancer. Anti-Cancer Drugs. 2017;**28**(8):852-860

[151] Wu Y et al. The reversing and molecular mechanisms of miR-503 on the drug-resistance to cisplatin in A549/DDP cells. Zhongguo Fei Ai Za Zhi. 2014;**17**(1):1-7

[152] Li JH et al. Inhibition of microRNA-196a might reverse cisplatin resistance of A549/DDP non-small-cell lung cancer cell line. Tumour Biology. 2016;**37**(2): 2387-2394

[153] Cortez MA et al. Therapeutic delivery of miR-200c enhances radiosensitivity in lung cancer. Molecular Therapy. 2014;**22**(8): 1494-1503

[154] Yang H et al. Up-regulation of microRNA-138 induce radiosensitization in lung cancer cells. Tumour Biology. 2014;**35**(7):6557-6565

[155] He Z et al. miR-25 modulates NSCLC cell radio-sensitivity through directly inhibiting BTG2 expression. Biochemical and Biophysical Research Communications. 2015;**457**(3):235-241

[156] Garofalo M et al. EGFR and MET receptor tyrosine kinase-altered microRNA expression induces tumorigenesis and gefitinib resistance in lung cancers. Nature Medicine. 2011; **18**(1):74-82

[157] Shen H et al. Alteration in Mir-21/PTEN expression modulates gefitinib resistance in non-small cell lung cancer. PLoS One. 2014;**9**(7):e103305

[158] Yun MR et al. Enhancer remodeling and microRNA alterations are associated with acquired resistance to ALK inhibitors. Cancer Research. 2018; **78**(12):3350-3362

[159] Beg MS et al. Phase I study of MRX34, a liposomal miR-34a mimic, administered twice weekly in patients with advanced solid tumors. Investigational New Drugs. 2017;**35**(2):180-188

[160] Yin J et al. Disturbance of the let-7/LIN28 double-negative feedback loop is associated with radio- and chemo-resistance in non-small cell lung cancer. PLoS One. 2017;**12**(2):e0172787

[161] Zhao Z et al. miR-15b regulates cisplatin resistance and metastasis by targeting PEBP4 in human lung adenocarcinoma cells. Cancer Gene Therapy. 2015;**22**(3):108-114

[162] Liu R et al. MicroRNA-7 sensitizes non-small cell lung cancer cells to paclitaxel. Oncology Letters. 2014;**8**(5): 2193-2200

[163] Bica-Pop C et al. Overview upon miR-21 in lung cancer: Focus on NSCLC. Cellular and Molecular Life Sciences. 2018;**75**(19):3539-3551

[164] Lin L et al. MicroRNA-21 regulates non-small cell lung cancer cell invasion and chemo-sensitivity through SMAD7. Cellular Physiology and Biochemistry. 2016;**38**(6):2152-2162

[165] Jiang Z et al. MiRNA 17 family regulates cisplatin-resistant and metastasis by targeting TGFbetaR2 in NSCLC. PLoS One. 2014;**9**(4):e94639

[166] Zhao J et al. The regulatory and predictive functions of miR-17 and miR-92 families on cisplatin resistance of non-small cell lung cancer. BMC Cancer. 2015;**15**:731

[167] Li J et al. miR-27a regulates cisplatin resistance and metastasis by targeting

RKIP in human lung adenocarcinoma cells. Molecular Cancer. 2014;**13**:193

[168] Yu G et al. Downregulation of PEBP4, a target of miR-34a, sensitizes drug-resistant lung cancer cells. Tumour Biology. 2014;**35**(10):10341-10349

[169] Ren P et al. MicroRNA-92a promotes growth, metastasis, and chemoresistance in non-small cell lung cancer cells by targeting PTEN. Tumour Biology. 2016;**37**(3):3215-3225

[170] Ye Z et al. Downregulation of miR-101 contributes to epithelial-mesenchymal transition in cisplatin resistance of NSCLC cells by targeting ROCK2. Oncotarget. 2016;**7**(25): 37524-37535

[171] Tian Y et al. Clinical significance of miRNA—106a in non-small cell lung cancer patients who received cisplatin combined with gemcitabine chemotherapy. Cancer Biology & Medicine. 2018;**15**(2):157-164

[172] Su W et al. miR-135b reverses chemoresistance of non-small cell lung cancer cells by downregulation of FZD1. Biomedicine & Pharmacotherapy. 2016; **84**:123-129

[173] Zhang H et al. miR-181c contributes to cisplatin resistance in non-small cell lung cancer cells by targeting Wnt inhibition factor 1. Cancer Chemotherapy and Pharmacology. 2017; **80**(5):973-984

[174] Shen H et al. MicroRNA-137 inhibits tumor growth and sensitizes chemosensitivity to paclitaxel and cisplatin in lung cancer. Oncotarget. 2016;**7**(15):20728-20742

[175] Jin Z et al. MicroRNA-138 regulates chemoresistance in human non-small cell lung cancer via epithelial mesenchymal transition. European Review for Medical and Pharmacological Sciences. 2016;**20**(6):1080-1086

[176] Shi L et al. Up-regulation of miR-146a increases the sensitivity of non-small cell lung cancer to DDP by downregulating cyclin. Journal of BMC Cancer. 2017;**17**(1):138

[177] Wang X et al. MiR-181b regulates cisplatin chemosensitivity and metastasis by targeting TGFbetaR1/Smad signaling pathway in NSCLC. Scientific Reports. 2015;**5**:17618

[178] Lei L, Huang Y, Gong W. miR-205 promotes the growth, metastasis and chemoresistance of NSCLC cells by targeting PTEN. Oncology Reports. 2013;**30**(6):2897-2902

[179] Zarogoulidis P et al. MiR-205 and miR-218 expression is associated with carboplatin chemoresistance and regulation of apoptosis via Mcl-1 and Survivin in lung cancer cells. Cellular Signalling. 2015;**27**(8):1576-1588

[180] Tung MC et al. Reduction of microRNA-184 by E6 oncoprotein confers cisplatin resistance in lung cancer via increasing Bcl-2. Oncotarget. 2016;**7**(22):32362-32374

[181] Fang C et al. MiR-488 inhibits proliferation and cisplatin sensibility in non-small-cell lung cancer (NSCLC) cells by activating the eIF3a-mediated NER signaling pathway. Scientific Reports. 2017;**7**:40384

[182] Xie J et al. MicroRNA-218 regulates cisplatin (DPP) chemosensitivity in non-small cell lung cancer by targeting RUNX2. Tumour Biology. 2016;**37**(1): 1197-1204

[183] Luo W et al. miRNA-296-3p modulates chemosensitivity of lung

cancer cells by targeting CX3CR1. American Journal of Translational Research. 2016;**8**(4):1848-1856

[184] Hao GJ et al. Suppression of EIF4G2 by miR-379 potentiates the cisplatin chemosensitivity in nonsmall cell lung cancer cells. FEBS Letters. 2017;**591**(4): 636-645

[185] Wang R et al. Acquisition of radioresistance in docetaxel-resistant human lung adenocarcinoma cells is linked with dysregulation of miR-451/c-Myc-survivin/rad-51 signaling. Oncotarget. 2014;**5**(15):6113-6129

[186] Sun CC et al. The novel miR-9600 suppresses tumor progression and promotes paclitaxel sensitivity in non-small-cell lung Cancer through altering STAT3 expression. Molecular Therapy Nucleic Acids. 2016;**5**(11):e387

[187] Arechaga-Ocampo E et al. Tumor suppressor miR-29c regulates radioresistance in lung cancer cells. Tumour Biology. 2017;**39**(3): 1010428317695010

[188] Jiang S et al. MicroRNA-21 modulates radiation resistance through upregulation of hypoxia-inducible factor-1alpha-promoted glycolysis in non-small cell lung cancer cells. Molecular Medicine Reports. 2016;**13**(5): 4101-4107

[189] Grosso S et al. MiR-210 promotes a hypoxic phenotype and increases radioresistance in human lung cancer cell lines. Cell Death & Disease. 2013;**4**:e544

[190] Ma W et al. Up- regulation of miR-328-3p sensitizes non-small cell lung cancer to radiotherapy. Scientific Reports. 2016;**6**:31651

[191] Li Y et al. Knockdown of microRNA-1323 restores sensitivity to radiation by suppression of PRKDC activity in radiation-resistant lung cancer cells. Oncology Reports. 2015; **33**(6):2821-2828

[192] Liu YJ et al. MicroRNA-449a enhances radiosensitivity in CL1-0 lung adenocarcinoma cells. PLoS One. 2013; **8**(4):e62383

[193] Zhong M et al. MicroRNAs reduce tumor growth and contribute to enhance cytotoxicity induced by gefitinib in non-small cell lung cancer. Chemico-Biological Interactions. 2010;**184**(3): 431-438

[194] Li B et al. MiR-21 overexpression is associated with acquired resistance of EGFR-TKI in non-small cell lung cancer. Lung Cancer. 2014;**83**(2):146-153

[195] Kitamura K et al. MiR-134/487b/655 cluster regulates TGF-beta-induced epithelial-mesenchymal transition and drug resistance to gefitinib by targeting MAGI2 in lung adenocarcinoma cells. Molecular Cancer Therapeutics. 2014; **13**(2):444-453

[196] Han Z et al. Inhibition of miR-23a increases the sensitivity of lung cancer stem cells to erlotinib through PTEN/PI3K/Akt pathway. Oncology Reports. 2017;**38**(5):3064-3070

[197] Zhou G et al. miR-200c enhances sensitivity of drug-resistant non-small cell lung cancer to gefitinib by suppression of PI3K/Akt signaling pathway and inhibites cell migration via targeting ZEB1. Biomedicine & Pharmacotherapy. 2017;**85**:113-119

[198] Chan LW et al. MiR-30 family potentially targeting PI3K-SIAH2 predicted interaction network represents a novel putative theranostic panel in non-small cell lung cancer. Frontiers in Genetics. 2017;**8**:8

[199] Han J et al. miR-223 reverses the resistance of EGFR-TKIs through IGF1R/PI3K/Akt signaling pathway. International Journal of Oncology. 2016; **48**(5):1855-1867

[200] Wang YS et al. MicroRNA-214 regulates the acquired resistance to gefitinib via the PTEN/AKT pathway in EGFR-mutant cell lines. Asian Pacific Journal of Cancer Prevention. 2012; **13**(1):255-260

[201] Yue J et al. Epigenetic silencing of miR-483-3p promotes acquired gefitinib resistance and EMT in EGFR-mutant NSCLC by targeting integrin beta3. Oncogene. 2018;**37**(31):4300-4312

[202] Gao HX et al. miR-200c regulates crizotinib-resistant ALK-positive lung cancer cells by reversing epithelial-mesenchymal transition via targeting ZEB1. Molecular Medicine Reports. 2016;**14**(5):4135-4143

[203] Gutschner T et al. The noncoding RNA MALAT1 is a critical regulator of the metastasis phenotype of lung cancer cells. Cancer Research. 2013;**73**(3): 1180-1189

[204] Fang Z et al. LncRNA-MALAT1 contributes to the cisplatin-resistance of lung cancer by upregulating MRP1 and MDR1 via STAT3 activation. Biomedicine & Pharmacotherapy. 2018; **101**:536-542

[205] Ji L et al. The novel Triazolonaphthalimide derivative LSS-11 synergizes the anti-proliferative effect of paclitaxel via STAT3-dependent MDR1 and MRP1 downregulation in chemoresistant lung cancer cells. Molecules. 2017;**22**(11):1822

[206] Ren K et al. Knockdown of long non-coding RNA KCNQ1OT1 depressed chemoresistance to paclitaxel in lung adenocarcinoma. Cancer Chemotherapy and Pharmacology. 2017;**80**(2):243-250

[207] Tian LJ et al. Upregulation of long noncoding RNA (lncRNA) X inactive specific transcript (XIST) is associated with cisplatin resistance in non-small cell lung Cancer (NSCLC) by downregulating MicroRNA-144-3p. Medical Science Monitor. 2019;**25**: 8095-8104

[208] Xu L et al. LncRNA SNHG14 regulates the DDP-resistance of non-small cell lung cancer cell through miR-133a/HOXB13 pathway. BMC Pulmonary Medicine. 2020;**20**(1):266

[209] Ma G et al. Long noncoding RNA LINC00460 promotes the gefitinib resistance of nonsmall cell lung cancer through epidermal growth factor receptor by sponging miR-769-5p. DNA and Cell Biology. 2019;**38**(2):176-183

[210] Hu B et al. LncRNA CCAT1/miR-130a-3p axis increases cisplatin resistance in non-small-cell lung cancer cell line by targeting SOX4. Cancer Biology & Therapy. 2017;**18**(12):974-983

[211] Chen K et al. SNHG7 mediates cisplatin-resistance in non-small cell lung cancer by activating PI3K/AKT pathway. European Review for Medical and Pharmacological Sciences. 2019; **23**(16):6935-6943

[212] Zhou H et al. The functional role of long non-coding RNAs and their underlying mechanisms in drug resistance of non-small cell lung cancer. Life Sciences. 2020;**261**:118362

[213] Wang P et al. LncRNA SNHG12 contributes to multidrug resistance through activating the MAPK/Slug pathway by sponging miR-181a in non-small cell lung cancer. Oncotarget. 2017; **8**(48):84086-84101

[214] Zhang XL et al. Tumorspheres derived from HCC cells are enriched with cancer stem cell-like cells and present high chemoresistance dependent on the Akt pathway. Anti-Cancer Agents in Medicinal Chemistry. 2015;**15**(6):755-763

[215] Mitsuya K et al. LIT1, an imprinted antisense RNA in the human KvLQT1 locus identified by screening for differentially expressed transcripts using monochromosomal hybrids. Human Molecular Genetics. 1999;**8**(7):1209-1217

[216] Gao L et al. CCR7 high expression leads to cetuximab resistance by cross-talking with EGFR pathway in PI3K/AKT signals in colorectal cancer. American Journal of Cancer Research. 2019;**9**(11):2531-2543

[217] Liu J et al. The long noncoding RNA MEG3 contributes to cisplatin resistance of human lung adenocarcinoma. PLoS One. 2015;**10**(5):e0114586

[218] Zheng T et al. Long noncoding RNA NBAT1 inhibits autophagy via suppression of ATG7 in non-small cell lung cancer. American Journal of Cancer Research. 2018;**8**(9):1801-1811

[219] Zhang EB et al. P53-regulated long non-coding RNA TUG1 affects cell proliferation in human non-small cell lung cancer, partly through epigenetically regulating HOXB7 expression. Cell Death & Disease. 2014;**5**:e1243

[220] Yang MH et al. Bmi1 is essential in Twist1-induced epithelial-mesenchymal transition. Nature Cell Biology. 2010;**12**(10):982-992

[221] Nakano Y et al. Clinical importance of long noncoding RNA LINC00460 expression in EGFRmutant lung adenocarcinoma. International Journal of Oncology. 2020;**56**(1):243-257

[222] Yang Y et al. Silencing of LncRNA-HOTAIR decreases drug resistance of non-small cell lung cancer cells by inactivating autophagy via suppressing the phosphorylation of ULK1. Biochemical and Biophysical Research Communications. 2018;**497**(4):1003-1010

[223] Zheng HC. The molecular mechanisms of chemoresistance in cancers. Oncotarget. 2017;**8**(35):59950-59964

[224] Chen L et al. The PVT1/miR-216b/Beclin-1 regulates cisplatin sensitivity of NSCLC cells via modulating autophagy and apoptosis. Cancer Chemotherapy and Pharmacology. 2019;**83**(5):921-931

[225] Ikner A, Ashkenazi A. TWEAK induces apoptosis through a death-signaling complex comprising receptor-interacting protein 1 (RIP1), Fas-associated death domain (FADD), and caspase-8. The Journal of Biological Chemistry. 2011;**286**(24):21546-21554

[226] Kimura T et al. Chloroquine in cancer therapy: A double-edged sword of autophagy. Cancer Research. 2013;**73**(1):3-7

[227] Yang F et al. Long noncoding RNA CCAT1, which could be activated by c-Myc, promotes the progression of gastric carcinoma. Journal of Cancer Research and Clinical Oncology. 2013;**139**(3):437-445

[228] Lan T et al. KIAA1429 contributes to liver cancer progression through N6-methyladenosine-dependent post-transcriptional modification of GATA3. Molecular Cancer. 2019;**18**(1):186

[229] Yang Y et al. lincROR influences the stemness and crizotinib resistance in EML-ALK(+) non-small-cell lung cancer cells. Oncotargets and Therapy. 2018;**11**:3649-3657

[230] Li P et al. microRNA-301b-3p downregulation underlies a novel inhibitory role of long non-coding RNA MBNL1-AS1 in non-small cell lung cancer. Stem Cell Research & Therapy. 2019;**10**(1):144

[231] Lu X et al. A novel long non-coding RNA, SOX21-AS1, indicates a poor prognosis and promotes lung adenocarcinoma proliferation. Cellular Physiology and Biochemistry. 2017; **42**(5):1857-1869

[232] Li X et al. The lncRNA RHPN1-AS1 downregulation promotes gefitinib resistance by targeting miR-299-3p/ TNFSF12 pathway in NSCLC. Cell Cycle. 2018;**17**(14):1772-1783

[233] Taylor MA, Das BC, Ray SK. Targeting autophagy for combating chemoresistance and radioresistance in glioblastoma. Apoptosis. 2018;**23**(11–12): 563-575

[234] Gong F et al. Long non-coding RNA FENDRR attenuates the stemness of non-small cell lung cancer cells via decreasing multidrug resistance gene 1 (MDR1) expression through competitively binding with RNA binding protein HuR. European Journal of Pharmacology. 2019;**853**:345-352

[235] Huang G et al. TUSC7 suppression of notch activation through sponging MiR-146 recapitulated the asymmetric cell division in lung adenocarcinoma stem cells. Life Sciences. 2019;**232**:116630

[236] Guo S et al. Long non-coding RNA TUG1 enhances chemosensitivity in non-small cell lung cancer by impairing microRNA-221-dependent PTEN inhibition. Aging (Albany NY). 2019; **11**(18):7553-7569

[237] Zhao Y et al. Long non-coding RNA MEG3 regulates migration and invasion of lung cancer stem cells via miR-650/ SLC34A2 axis. Biomedicine & Pharmacotherapy. 2019;**120**:109457

[238] Hao Y, Baker D, Ten Dijke P. TGF-beta-mediated epithelial-mesenchymal transition and Cancer metastasis. International Journal of Molecular Sciences. 2019;**20**(11):2767

[239] Wellner U et al. The EMT-activator ZEB1 promotes tumorigenicity by repressing stemness-inhibiting microRNAs. Nature Cell Biology. 2009; **11**(12):1487-1495

[240] Cancer I.A.f.R.o. Cancer Incidence in Five Continents. Vol. X. Geneva, Switzerland: IARC; 2014

[241] George J et al. Comprehensive genomic profiles of small cell lung cancer. Nature. 2015;**524**(7563):47-53

[242] Rudin CM et al. Comprehensive genomic analysis identifies SOX2 as a frequently amplified gene in small-cell lung cancer. Nature Genetics. 2012; **44**(10):1111-1116

[243] Luo Y et al. MiR-335 regulates the chemo-radioresistance of small cell lung cancer cells by targeting PARP-1. Gene. 2017;**600**:9-15

[244] Jiang W et al. miR-22 enhances the radiosensitivity of small-cell lung cancer by targeting the WRNIP1. Journal of Cellular Biochemistry. 2019;**120**(10): 17650-17661

[245] Tanaka N et al. Frequent methylation and oncogenic role of microRNA-34b/c in small-cell lung cancer. Lung Cancer. 2012;**76**(1):32-38

[246] Mao S et al. Exosomal miR-141 promotes tumor angiogenesis via KLF12 in small cell lung cancer. Journal of

Experimental & Clinical Cancer Research. 2020;**39**(1):193

[247] Wang B et al. MicroRNA-217 inhibits proliferation and promotes apoptosis of small cell lung cancer cells via targeting PCDH8. Panminerva Medica. 2021;**63**(1):95-96

[248] Miko E et al. miR-126 inhibits proliferation of small cell lung cancer cells by targeting SLC7A5. FEBS Letters. 2011;**585**(8):1191-1196

[249] Tong J et al. microRNA-195 promotes small cell lung cancer cell apoptosis via inhibiting Rap2C protein-dependent MAPK signal transduction. Technology in Cancer Research & Treatment. 2020;**19**: 1533033820977546

[250] Yu JG, Ji CH, Shi MH. MicroRNA-26b suppresses tumorigenicity and promotes apoptosis in small cell lung cancer cells by targeting myeloid cell leukemia 1 protein. The Kaohsiung Journal of Medical Sciences. 2018;**34**(11): 593-605

[251] Gao F et al. MicroRNA-485-5p suppresses the proliferation, migration and invasion of small cell lung cancer cells by targeting flotillin-2. Bioengineered. 2019;**10**(1):1-12

[252] Li TT et al. Long noncoding RNAs in small cell lung cancer: A potential opening to combat the disease (review). Oncology Reports. 2018;**40**(4): 1831-1842

[253] Sun Y et al. A long non-coding RNA HOTTIP expression is associated with disease progression and predicts outcome in small cell lung cancer patients. Molecular Cancer. 2017; **16**(1):162

[254] Sun Y et al. Long non-coding RNA HOTTIP promotes BCL-2 expression and induces chemoresistance in small cell lung cancer by sponging miR-216a. Cell Death & Disease. 2018;**9**(2):85

[255] Ono H et al. Long noncoding RNA HOTAIR is relevant to cellular proliferation, invasiveness, and clinical relapse in small-cell lung cancer. Cancer Medicine. 2014;**3**(3):632-642

[256] Fang S et al. Long noncoding RNA-HOTAIR affects chemoresistance by regulating HOXA1 methylation in small cell lung cancer cells. Laboratory Investigation. 2016;**96**(1):60-68

[257] Niu Y et al. Long non-coding RNA TUG1 is involved in cell growth and chemoresistance of small cell lung cancer by regulating LIMK2b via EZH2. Molecular Cancer. 2017;**16**(1):5

[258] Chen S et al. LncRNA CCAT2 predicts poor prognosis and regulates growth and metastasis in small cell lung cancer. Biomedicine & Pharmacotherapy. 2016;**82**:583-588

[259] Huang C et al. LncRNA PVT1 overexpression is a poor prognostic biomarker and regulates migration and invasion in small cell lung cancer. American Journal of Translational Research. 2016;**8**(11):5025-5034

[260] Wang S et al. lncRNA Linc00173 modulates glucosemetabolism and multidrug chemoresistancein SCLC: Potential molecular panel for therapy. Molecular Therapy. 2022;**30**(4):1787

Chapter 5

MicroRNAs and Pancreatic ß Cell Functional Modulation

Shahzad Irfan, Farhat Jabeen and Haseeb Anwar

Abstract

Recent reports of diabetes susceptibility loci located on the non-coding regions of the genome highlight the importance of epigenetic control in health and disease. Specifically, microRNAs have shown to have an important regulatory role in pancreatic ß cell physiology. Human studies implicated that ß cell mass and function are regulated by microRNAs in health and disease. Further, the microRNAs are also implicated in ensuing diabetic complications. Delineating the peculiar role of microRNAs in ß cell physiology and pathophysiology will fill the missing gaps in our current knowledge and help to devise better treatment regimens for diabetes. This chapter will discuss multiple effects of different microRNAs on the ß cell physiology in the context of maintenance and function in Type 2 diabetes mellitus.

Keywords: microRNA, beta-cell, insulin, diabetes mellitus

1. Introduction

MicroRNAs (miRNAs/miRs) are pertinent genetic regulators of embryonic development and differentiation, postnatal growth, and metabolism [1]. Initially discovered in *C. Elegans*, miRNAs are now considered a universal phenomenon for the gene expression regulation from multicellular organisms to mammals [2–6]. The mammalian genome has been reported to encode more than 500 known microRNA genes. microRNA binds with the mRNA (3′ untranslated region 3'UTR) and result either in the translational repression of that specific gene or in the total degradation of the mRNA [6–9]. Apart from 3'UTR, miRNA has been reported to interact with 5'UTR and gene promoters and enhancers [10]. miRNAs are critical for normal animal development. As expression pattern of numerous genes important for the embryonic development and subsequent cellular differentiation have been shown to be regulated by microRNAs [11].

The pathological importance of miRNAs is highlighted by the substantial reports of the association of aberrant expression of miRNAs in many human diseases [12, 13]. As miRNAs are also present in the extracellular fluids and act as a signaling molecule for cell communication, their diagnostic importance as a biomarker in different lethal diseases has also been reported [14, 15] Biogenesis of miRNAs and the mechanisms through which they regulate gene expression and their tissue distribution has been previously discussed in detail [1, 10, 16–18]. The transcriptional activity of miRNA sequences is solely dependent upon RNA polymerase II/III activity [19, 20]. The transcribed miRNA can act through canonical as well as non-canonical pathways [20, 21]. A complementary match either exact or partial between microRNA and the 3'-UTR (conserved) site of the mRNA will result in either the subsequent degradation of the mRNA or moderate reduction in the mRNA levels resulting in translation repression [22, 23]. The degradation of mRNA will result in complete blockage of protein expression. Whereas specific translation repression results in a reduction in the protein formation from the target genes. This fine-tuning of gene expression and subsequent protein formation by microRNAs is important for normal physiological responses. A single miRNA can target hundreds of different genes and mRNAs thus exhibiting multiple levels of complementarity. It is estimated that more than 60% of protein-coding genes are microRNA targets.

In the canonical pathway of microRNA generation (explained in more detail in [24]) events start with the transcription of microRNA sequence by the RNA polymerase II or III, the microRNA transcript is spliced, capped and polyadenylated in the nucleus and is called pri-microRNA. The nuclear pri-microRNA is cleaved by a nuclear protein complex called microprocessor complex and includes Drosha and DGRC8 proteins. After this cleavage event, the pri-microRNA is exported to the cytoplasm by the help of a protein called exportin 5 (Exp 5). Cytoplasmic pre-microRNA is further cleaved by another protein called Dicer and converting the pri-microRNA into a microRNA duplex of around 22 nucleotides. These duplex molecules are loaded onto another protein called Argonaute (AGO). Duplex microRNAs are unwinded and the passenger strand is removed while the guide microRNA strand remains with the AGO proteins and forms the mature effector complex called RNA-induced silencing complex (RISC). RISC complex is guided by the microRNA complementarity to bind with mRNA targets and 3'end de-adenylation occurs resulting in the mRNA degradation of the translation arrest on mRNA. Interestingly deletion of the components of this canonical pathway like DICER or AGO proteins leads to β cells functional impairment in terms of glucose-induced insulin secretion and dedifferentiation into a progenitor-like state [25–28]. The current chapter will focus on the physiology and pathophysiology of the β cells focusing on the insulin signaling responsible for glucose homeostasis and the influence and interplay of different microRNAs onβ cells functionality in Type 2 diabetes (T2DM).

2. β cells, insulin and macronutrient metabolism

Insulin is the primary endogenous protein responsible for the physiological regulation of metabolism [29]. The regulated secretion of insulin from the pancreas helps to maintain glucose homeostasis in distinct physiological conditions [30, 31]. Endocrine cells that secret specific hormones for the maintenance of glucose levels are present in specialized closed zones in the pancreas called Islets of Langerhans [31–33]. Islets of Langerhans contain numerous cell types with an appropriate amount of vascular and nervous innervation [31]. Four different types of endocrine cells populated Islets of Langerhans namely: alpha (α) cells, beta (ß) cells, delta (δ) cells, and pancreatic polypeptide (PP) cells. ß cells secrete insulin and initiate postprandial glucose metabolism and control the rising blood glucose levels and α cells secrete of glucagon which enhances blood glucose levels during fasting [34, 35]. Insulin is also responsible for lipid and protein metabolism [36–38]. The release of insulin from ß cells is initiated by glucose uptake, a phenomenon known as glucose-stimulated insulin secretion (GSIS) [39–41]. At physiological postprandial levels, glucose initiates insulin gene transcription by recruiting specific transcription factors (PDX-1, MafA, and NeuroD) and post-transcriptionally improves the insulin mRNA stability thus acting as a major physiologic regulator of insulin [42–44]. Glucose-specific channels/gates are present on the ß cell membrane which are commonly known as glucose transporters (GLUT) [30, 41]. Many types of glucose transporters are present throughout the body [45]. Specifically, GLUT2 is abundant in the pancreas and liver whereas GLUT4 is abundant in skeletal and cardiac muscles as well as adipocytes [45, 46].

Insulin initiates carbohydrate metabolism through phosphorylation of glucose and subsequent formation of glucose-6-phosphate [47, 48]. Insulin phosphorylates glucose through the hexokinase enzyme in muscles and glucokinase (GCK) in ß cells and hepatocytes [49–52]. Insulin binds to the cell surface insulin receptors commonly present in different tissues [53]. The insulin-insulin receptor binding activates cytoplasmic adaptor proteins called insulin receptor substrates (e.g., IRS1, IRS2) [54]. IRS proteins activate phosphoinositide2-kinase enzyme (PI3K) and convert tyrosine phosphorylation signal into the lipid kinase. Activated PI3K recruits ATP molecules which initiates the AKT activation (serine and threonine kinase) [55]. Activation of AKT by insulin proved landmark and explained the conversion of tyrosine phosphorylation into serine/threonine phosphorylation signal. Insulin-induced AKT activation also helped to describe the insulin-induced regulation of key steps in insulin signaling (a) glucose uptake by glucose transporter, (b) phosphorylation and subsequent inactivation of glycogen synthase kinase 3 (GSK3), (c) activation of the mechanistic target of rapamycin (mTOR) and subsequent synthesis of protein and fats, (d) Transcriptional control of gene expression by forkhead family box O (FOXO) transcription factor proteins. Insulin increases glucose uptake via GLUT4 in muscle and adipose tissue thus enhancing the postprandial rate of glucose transport, insulin also inactivates GSK3 and stimulates glycogen synthesis in these tissues [56]. Insulin prevents hepatic glucose synthesis by inhibiting glycogenolysis and gluconeogenesis. Insulin via AKT inhibits FoxO1 which results in the decreased expression of phosphoenolpyruvate carboxykinase (PEPCK) and glucose –6-phosphatase (G6PC) genes [57–59]. Insulin regulates lipid and protein metabolism also through AKT. Insulin via AKT induced an increase in mTOR and a decrease in FoxO1 and sterol regulatory element-binding protein (SREBP) inhibits adipocyte lipolysis and helps to lower the plasma fatty acid levels by promoting lipogenesis and enhancing the hepatic formation of very-low-density lipoprotein (VLDL) [60–65]. Insulin increases the protein synthesis in skeletal muscles and the liver by enhancing the amino acid transport inside the cells, accelerating mRNA translation, and reducing protein degradation and urea formation via AKT activated mTOR [37, 66–71].

3. Glucose homeostasis: α and β interplay

β cells exhibit a remarkable degree of plasticity in terms of insulin production. The α and ß cells work in conjunction to stabilize glucose levels in feeding and fasting conditions through the periodic release of insulin and glucagon respectively thus achieving glucose homeostasis [30, 49, 72]. Rising plasma glucose levels after feeding require immediate systemic activation of glucose metabolism. Delayed or decreased activation of glucose metabolism results in abnormally high glucose levels known as hyperglycemia. Higher-than-normal concentrations of glucose incite glucotoxic reactions inside the cells. ß cells are triggered by rising postprandial glucose levels to synthesize and secrete insulin. The resulting increasing insulin levels activate enzymes that help to metabolize glucose. Glucokinase and hexokinase initiate glucose phosphorylation primarily in hepatocytes and muscle cells respectively. The post-prandial rise in the insulin declines over time because of the decline in the glucose level, a feature of GSIS [39]. Interestingly insulin negatively impacts glucagon secretion [73–76]. Plasma glucose levels decline under fasting conditions. As glucose is the primary cellular source to generate ATP, a minimum threshold of plasma glucose levels must be maintained to avoid hypoglycemia. Glucagon maintains plasma glucose levels, to avoid hypoglycemia during fasting, by initiating hepatic gluconeogenesis/glucogenolysis [34, 77–81].

4. Diabetes mellitus

Diabetes mellitus is metabolic dysfunction that results in a significant decline in the cellular ability to metabolize glucose either because of the lack of insulin or insulin inactivity (insulin resistance) or both [82, 83]. Diabetes mellitus is estimated to affect 700 million people worldwide by the year 2040 [84]. The inability of the cells to metabolize glucose cause an abnormal increase in the cellular and plasma levels of glucose (hyperglycemia). Hyperglycemia causes cellular damage via multiple mechanisms including (a) the increased influx of glucose through the polyol pathway, (b) increased formation of advanced glycation end products (AGEs), and (c) subsequent increased expression of AGE receptors and their ligand [85, 86]. Hyperglycemia initiates the reactive oxygen species (ROS) formation via activated glycation reactions and mitochondrial electron transport chain where ROS acts as the main trigger for the initiation of the polyol pathway, formation of AGEs, and subsequent increased AGE receptor expression [87].

Diabetes mellitus has been categorized in two primary forms: Type 1 Diabetes Mellitus (T1DM) and Type 2 Diabetes Mellitus (T2DM). T1DM has been characterized by a mutation in the insulin gene or immune cell-mediated destruction of ß cell resulting in either the synthesis of abnormal insulin protein that fails to activate insulin receptors or a complete lack of endogenous insulin secretion [88]. T1DM patients are usually diagnosed early in their life. The only possible medical treatment referred to these patients is the multiple daily doses of synthetic insulin. T2DM on the other hand is much more complicated and requires a thorough diagnostic approach [82, 89–91]. T2DM is considered one of the most common metabolic disorders globally. Major risk factors for T2DM include a sedentary lifestyle, lack of exercise, excessive use of a high-carb and high-fat diet, overweight, and obesity [92]. Poor lifestyle and dietary habits have been attributed to the global incidence of Type 2 diabetes in the last 2 decades. Obesity, visceral fat deposition and increased body mass index (BMI) play a central role in the pathophysiology of Type 2 diabetic patients [82].

5. Pathophysiology of Type 2 diabetes mellitus (T2DM)

The development of T2DM is mainly attributed to the progressive decline in insulin secretion over time from ß cells and the progressive inability of insulin-responsive tissues (muscles, fat, and liver) to respond to insulin over time, resulting in hyperinsulinemia and subsequent insulin resistance [93–96]. The inability of the insulin hormone to activate insulin receptors at the cellular level has been attributed to be the major cause of hyperinsulinemia and insulin resistance [97, 98]. *Ex vivo* analysis of pancreatic islets from T2DM donors in terms of GSIS exhibit disproportional insulin levels where increased glucose concentration fails to elicit appropriate ß cells response in terms of insulin [99–101]. Insulin binding to insulin receptors at the plasma membrane activates a signaling cascade that initiates glucose metabolism inside the cells. Insulin-bound insulin receptors or activated insulin receptors go through internalization at the plasma membrane, a phenomenon known as insulin receptor endocytosis [29, 102]. Following the activation, the endocytosis of the insulin receptor is the primary physiological mechanism through which the duration and intensity of insulin signaling are controlled. Hyperinsulinemia accelerates insulin receptor endocytosis and affects the presence of adequate functional insulin receptors at the plasma membrane resulting in insulin resistance [103]. Apart from accelerated insulin receptor endocytosis, insulin-stimulated insulin receptor kinase activity is also decreased in diabetic patients [104].

Compromised insulin signaling in T2DM fails to activate glucose metabolic enzymes like glucokinase and hexokinase resulting in hyperglycemia. The expression levels of GCK and GLUT2 were found to be lower in human T2D islets as compared to healthy control [105]. As high plasma glucose levels initiate glucose-stimulated insulin secretory (GSIS) response from ß cells resulting in the rise of plasma insulin levels. The rising insulin levels should be normalized over time because of the renal insulin clearance mechanism. But compromised renal insulin clearance rate in diabetic subjects results in abnormally high plasma levels of insulin (hyperinsulinemia) [106, 107]. Hyperinsulinemia and hyperglycemia in theory cannot trigger alpha cells to secrete glucagon. But it has been observed that T2DM patients with insulin resistance, hyperinsulinemia, and hyperglycemia also have abnormally high plasma levels of glucagon [108]. Hinting toward the disturbance in the α and β cell interplay through the inability of the insulin to block glucagon gene transcription [109].

T2D has also been attributed to altering the gene expression of key proteins participating in the processes of insulin secretion and function. Specifically, the insulin receptor gene (*IR*) and genes involved in Ca^{2+} influx (*SUR1*, *TMEM37*), and mitochondrial metabolism (*GPD2, PCK1, FXYD2*) [110–113]. The compromised mitochondrial activity in the T2D β cells through reduced ATP/ADP ratio fails to close the K_{ATP} channels and subsequently impacts Ca^{2+} influx and exocytosis of insulin. ATP also enhances insulin granular priming prior to the exocytosis and thus regulates insulin quantity by initiating the modification of proinsulin into insulin inside the insulin granule. Substantial β cell loss has been considered the hallmark of T2DM which even starts during the prediabetic stage [114]. Up to ~50% loss in the β cell mass has been reported in T2DM patients [115–118]. Apoptosis and dedifferentiation have been attributed as the main reasons for this substantial decline in the β mass. Hyperinsulinemia has been attributed to the activation of caspases, formation of H_2O_2 increased expression of nitric oxide synthase (iNOS) in the β cells resulting in their substantial loss [119–121]. Hyperglycemia-induced production of AGE products and the subsequent activation of AGE receptors further promote the release of cytochrome and caspase activation [122]. Hyperglycemia along with increased levels of free fatty acids (glucolipotoxicity) has also been shown to induce β apoptosis and reduction in their overall mass in T2DM [123, 124]. Over accumulation of lipids and over-activation of lipid signaling pathways inβ cells are of pathological significance as it contributes to β cell loss and further lead to the significant decline in insulin secretion and the onset of T2DM. Glucolipotoxicity induces a cascade of events that starts from mitochondrial dysfunction leading to oxidative stress (ROS) which further leads to ER stress which results in improper protein unfolding response and results in the loss of GSIS and inflammation and activated autophagy. These above-mentioned cascades of events represent altered cell signaling pathways, lipogenic and pro-apoptotic genes, and proteins, increased expression of cytokines, and accumulation of lipids molecules like di and triacylglycerols, cholesterol, and cholesterol esters.

Apart from the above-mentioned mechanisms, β cell dedifferentiation has recently been shown to be another important contributing factor in the progressive decline in the β mass in T2DM [116, 125, 126]. Dedifferentiation is defined as the ability of a cell to revert to its progenitor-like stage (developmental stage). Interestingly it has been observed that dedifferentiation in β cells not only resulted in progenitor-like cells but an increase in other islets cells type has been observed. Implying the possibility that dedifferentiated β cells have further converted into α and δ cells, which interestingly involves the removal of epigenetic brake on glucagon and somatostatin genes for their expression in the functional β cells. This also explains the abnormally high levels of glucagon observed in T2D patients with hyperglycemia, where glucose fails to down-regulate the glucagon gene expression. The transition or dedifferentiation of β cells is characterized by the downregulation of β specific genes and upregulation of pluripotent genes [127–131]. β cell identity genes like *MafA, Nkx6.1,* and *FoxO1* were shown to be downregulated. Whereas pluripotent genes like *Ngn3, Oct4, Nanog,* and *L-Myc* were upregulated. In fact, it has been shown in T2DM patients that glucagon (α) and somatostatin (δ) positive cells have inactivated (cytoplasmic) FOXO1 and NKX6.1 proteins supporting the notion that trans-differentiation of β cells into other endocrine islet cell types [125].

6. Epigenetic regulation of β cell-specific gene expression profile

Epigenetic mechanisms resulting in the alteration of gene expression have been attributed to the regulation or dysregulation of proper β cell function in health and disease [132–137]. DNA methylation, chromatin modifications, and post-translational modifications of histones have been implicated as the main epigenetic mechanisms. Alteration in the expression pattern of Non-coding RNA sequences like microRNA (miRNA/miR) and long non-coding RNA (lncRNA) has also been shown to regulate the β cell function as well as its cellular identity [138–151].

7. MicroRNAs and β cell regulation

MicroRNA (miRNA/miR) sequences are typically small around ~22 nucleotide non-protein-coding transcripts. Activation of their transcriptional activity results in the formation of miRNAs. Formation or presence of miRNAs has been shown to regulate the expression of a network of genes involved in β cell development, function, and pathogenesis [152–158]. microRNAs have been shown to play a vital role in the compensation process of β cells during pregnancy, obesity and T2D [158–161]. MicroRNAs mediate mRNA silencing and posttranscriptional regulation of gene expression in different physiological states of β cells. These miRNAs induced fine tunned changes in β cell gene expression are considered vital in health and disease. As the inability of microRNAs to fine-tune the gene expression levels lead to β cells decompensation which results in abnormal insulin secretion and ultimately the development of diabetes. β cell decompensation is referred to as two main pathological conditions: (1) impaired (reduced) β cell function in terms of glucose sensitivity and insulin secretion (Reduced GSIS), and (2) reduced β cell number/mass due to dedifferentiation or apoptosis. Impaired β cell function involves molecular defects in insulin biosynthesis, glucose uptake, and exocytosis of insulin granules. β cell maintenance is regulated by microRNAs through the downregulation of non-β cell specific genes and upregulation of the β cells specific genes thus avoiding the β cell dedifferentiation process which is impaired in T2DM patients [162, 163]. As discussed earlier, different molecular components are involved in the secretion of insulin in response to the rising blood glucose levels. Failure of either one of these molecular components results in the failure of β cells to respond to the systemic demands of insulin for macronutrient metabolism. MicroRNAs are involved in the fine-tuned adjustments of β cells and regulate multiple aspects of glucose homeostasis via insulin secretion.

8. MicroRNAs and insulin synthesis and signaling

The insulin gene transcription results in the generation of mRNA which is translated in preproinsulin and cleaved into proinsulin in the endoplasmic reticulum [164–167]. Cleavage of proinsulin into insulin and C-peptide requires activation of convertase enzymes (PC1/3, PC1) through the change in the granular pH into acidic pH. Insulin gene (*ins1*) expression has been found to be compromised after the deletion or inactivation of *Dicer1* gene [27, 28]. Reduced insulin gene promoter activity and decreased insulin content was observed in isolated islets and cultured β cells after the experimental knock-down of a set of microRNAs including miRNA-24, miRNA-26, miRNA-148 and miRNA-181 [168]. A positive correlation in the insulin mRNA levels and negative correlation in terms of GSIS response and the expression profile of miRNA-127-3p and miRNA-184 was observed in the islets isolated from healthy subjects. Interestingly these correlations were found to be absent in the isolated islets of glucose-intolerant (diabetic) donors [169]. *In vitro* expansion of β cells from adult pancreatic islets were found to be dedifferentiated after the proliferation and levels of miRNA-375 (an islet-specific microRNA) were found to be significantly reduced [170] Experimental overexpression of miRNA-375 in dedifferentiated β cells lead to the activation of the β cell specific gene expression profile. MafA, a key β cell specific transcription factor regulating insulin gene expression, has been shown to be directly targeted by the miRNA-204 [171]. Thioredoxin-interacting protein (TXNIP), a redox regulator intracellular protein, has been found to be upregulated in diabetes and its deficiency protect β cells from diabetes-associated apoptosis. TXNIP induces the expression of miRNA-204 by inhibiting STAT3 activity. miRNA-204 thus blocks insulin production in diabetes by downregulating MafA. microRNA-181c-5p has been shown to induce the expression of INS1, PDX1, NKX6.1, and MafA in human induced pluripotent stem cells (hiPSCs) [172]. microRNA-124a has been shown to be highly expressed in islets of T2DM patients [173]. microRNA-124a has shown to be a negative regulator of insulin by targeting 3'UTR regions of mRNAs of Akt, Sirt1, NeuroD, and Foxa2 proteins. All these proteins are vital in the insulin gene transcriptional activity as well as the insulin signaling via insulin receptors. microRNA-7 has been shown to influence insulin signaling by down-regulating insulin receptor substrate protein genes (IRS1, IRS2) in gestational diabetes in humans [174]. Glucagon-like peptide 1 receptors (GLP1R) are present in the β cells and activation of these receptors by GLP-1 induces GSIS response from β cells [175, 176]. GLP1 receptor expression has shown to be downregulated by microRNA-204 in rat ins-1 cell line and primary mouse and human islets cells by targeting the 3'UTR region of GLP1R mRNA [177].

This is particularly important as GLP-1 receptor agonists are primary drugs used by T2DM patients to increase insulin levels.

9. MicroRNAs and insulin secretion

Several microRNAs have been shown to impact glucose uptake and metabolism by the β cells and the exocytotic process of insulin secretion. As GSIS regulates the key components of the process of β cell insulin release. Islets isolated from T2DM patients have shown decreased expression of proteins involved in K_{ATP} and Ca^{2+} channel regulation, metabolism, and exocytosis of insulin resulting in hyperglycemia [178]. Islets from T2DM patients show increased levels of microRNA-130a, microRNA-130b, and microRNA-152 and were found to be glucose-induced [179]. microRNA-130a, microRNA-130b, and microRNA-152 target *Gck* gene and downregulates ATP synthesis by reducing glucose metabolism in β cells thus affecting insulin exocytosis by not only blocking the closure of K_{ATP} channels but also affecting the insulin granule priming. microRNA-29a, microRNA-29b and microRNA-124 have been shown to suppress the gene expression of a β cell disallowed mitochondrial protein called monocarboxylate transporter (MCT-1) [180]. MCT-1 inhibition allows the β cells to only consume glucose for metabolism. Thus microRNA-29a, microRNA-29b, and microRNA-124 help in preserving the cell-specific identity. Human and mouse islets incubated with high glucose (hyperglycemic conditions) exhibit an increased expression of microRNA-29 in β cells [181]. microRNA-29 has been shown to positively impact the expression of a transcription factor called Onecut2. This transcription factor upregulates the granuphilin protein gene expression. Granuphilin protein blocks the exocytosis of secretory granules in endocrine cells. Apart from Onecut2-granuphilin mediated blocking of exocytosis, microRNA-29 also influences exocytotic protein genes like Syntaxin1A and SNAP25 (members of SNARE complex: a family of proteins involved in membrane fusion during exocytosis) [182].

10. MicroRNAs and lipid accumulation in β cells

The characteristic hallmark of T2D is the dysregulation of lipid metabolism and subsequent obesity. Excess amounts of fats present in the bloodstream of T2D patients have been attributed to β cell mass reduction and decreased insulin secretion. MicroRNA sequences have been shown to be manipulated by the exposure of β cells to circulating fats in T2D patients [183]. β cell-specific genes which encode proteins that are involved in lipid metabolism and subsequent cholesterol homeostasis have been found to be under miRNA control [184]. miRNA-33 has been reported to control cholesterol homeostasis through modulating the expression of sterol regulatory binding protein (SREBP) genes [185] miRNA-34a has been shown to induce β cell lipotoxicity through multiple mechanisms after the *in vitro* and *in vivo* exposure to saturated fatty acids [186–189]. Increased β cell influx of fatty acids through di/triacylglycerol and esterified cholesterol pathways including targeting sirtuin1 (SIRT1). Importantly SIRT1 (NAD^+-dependent deacetylase) regulates the expression of multiple genes encoding proteins like tumor suppressor protein p53 and DNA repair factor ku70 and transcription factor protein including nuclear factor κB (NF-κB) and FOXO family. Exposure of β cells to saturated fatty acids alters the expression profile of important miRNAs which might contribute to β cell lipotoxicity. These miRNAs include miRNA-146 [184], miRNA-182-5p [190], miRNA-297b-5p [191], and miRNA375 [192]. miRNA-146 target genes which are involved with the inflammatory response (Toll-like receptors) [193]. It has been demonstrated that in cultured human islets, the miRNA-146 level increased after the exposure to pro-inflammatory cytokines and decreased exposure to high glucose concentrations but interestingly miRNA-146 levels were unchanged after the palmitate exposure [194]. miRNA-146 along with miRNA 182-5p have been shown to protect against high-fat diet-induced steatohepatitis in a mice model by decreasing in the expression of IL-1 receptor-associated kinase (IRAK1) and tumor necrosis factor (TNF) receptor-associated factor 6 (TRAF6) which results in the reduced cytoplasmic lipid accumulation and inflammation [195]. miRNA-182-5p was found to be increased in INS-1 cells incubated with palmitate and significantly decreased the cell viability and increased palmitate-induced apoptosis. When INS-1 cells were supplemented with miRNA-182-5p inhibitors a significant increase in the cellular viability and palmitate-induced apoptosis was observed [190]. C57BL/6 mouse and β-TC6 cell line exposed to stearic acid and palmitic acid lowers the expression of miRNA-297b-5p. Upregulation of miRNA-297b-5p reduced the stearic acid-induced apoptosis but decreased insulin secretion in β-TC6 cells by inhibiting large-tumor-suppressor kinase 2 (LATS-2) [191] miRNA-375 has been shown to block high-fat diet-induced insulin resistance and obesity in mice by promoting hepatic expression of insulin-responsive genes [196].

11. Conclusion

The important role of epigenetics in the functional regulation of β cells in health and disease has been supported by the increasing number of high levels studies on human and rodent models. Excellent research efforts in the last decades have established that microRNAs help to define the β cell identity and dysregulation of β cell microRNA expression acts as a key event in the pathogenesis of T2DM. As the mechanisms involved in the biogenesis of microRNAs are well understood, it is plausible to assume that microRNAs represent attractive therapeutic targets. Selective inhibition of Dicer molecules by using specific siRNAs or pharmacological tools and selective modulation of a single microRNA. Specific microRNAs involved in diabetes represent a new class of specialized biomarkers for the early detection of diabetes. As microRNAs are biochemically quite stable in the extracellular fluid like blood, they represent a very good biomarker for diagnostics. Further in-depth studies are needed to assess the predictive value of serum levels of microRNAs in relation to the disease progression. Novel therapeutic approaches need to be devised for the prevention and treatment of metabolic disorders.

Author details

Shahzad Irfan[1*], Farhat Jabeen[2] and Haseeb Anwar[1]

1 Department of Physiology, G.C. University Faisalabad, Faisalabad, Pakistan

2 Department of Zoology, G.C. University Faisalabad, Faisalabad, Pakistan

*Address all correspondence to: shahzadirfan@gcuf.edu.pk

References

[1] O'Brien J, Hayder H, Zayed Y, Peng C. Overview of microRNA biogenesis, mechanisms of actions, and circulation. Frontiers in Endocrinology. 2018;**9**(Aug):402

[2] Lee RC, Feinbaum RL, Ambros V. The C. elegans heterochronic gene lin-4 encodes small RNAs with antisense complementarity to lin-14. Cell. 1993;**75**(5):843-854

[3] Friedländer MR, Lizano E, Houben AJS, Bezdan D, Báñez-Coronel M, Kudla G, et al. Evidence for the biogenesis of more than 1,000 novel human microRNAs. Genome Biology. 2014;**15**(4):R57

[4] Li SC, Chan WC, Hu LY, Lai CH, Hsu CN, Lin W, et al. Identification of homologous microRNAs in 56 animal genomes. Genomics. 2010;**96**(1):1-9

[5] de Rie D, Abugessaisa I, Alam T, Arner E, Arner P, Ashoor H, et al. An integrated expression atlas of miRNAs and their promoters in human and mouse. Nature Biotechnology. 2017;**35**(9):872-878

[6] Wightman B, Ha I, Ruvkun G. Posttranscriptional regulation of the heterochronic gene lin-14 by lin-4 mediates temporal pattern formation in C. elegans. Cell. 1993;**75**(5):855-862

[7] Bartel DP. MicroRNAs: Genomics, biogenesis, mechanism, and function. Cell. 2004;**116**(2):281-297

[8] Pasquinelli AE, Hunter S, Bracht J. MicroRNAs: A developing story. Current Opinion in Genetics & Development. 2005;**15**(2):200-205

[9] Giraldez AJ, Mishima Y, Rihel J, Grocock RJ, van Dongen S, Inoue K, et al. Zebrafish MiR-430 promotes deadenylation and clearance of maternal mRNAs. Science. 2006;**312**(5770):75-79

[10] Vasudevan S. Posttranscriptional upregulation by MicroRNAs. Wiley Interdisciplinary Reviews: RNA. 2012;**3**(3):311-330. DOI: 10.1002/wrna.121

[11] Fu G, Brkić J, Hayder H, Peng C. MicroRNAs in human placental development and pregnancy complications. International Journal of Molecular Sciences. 2013;**14**:5519-5544

[12] Paul P, Chakraborty A, Sarkar D, Langthasa M, Rahman M, Bari M, et al. Interplay between miRNAs and human diseases. Journal of Cellular Physiology. 2018;**233**(3):2007-2018. DOI: 10.1002/jcp.25854

[13] Tüfekci KU, Öner MG, Meuwissen RLJ, Genç Ş. The role of MicroRNAs in human diseases. Methods in Molecular Biology. 2014;**1107**:33-50. DOI: 10.1007/978-1-62703-748-8_3

[14] Huang W. MicroRNAs: Biomarkers, diagnostics, and therapeutics. Methods in Molecular Biology. 2017;**1617**:57-67. DOI: 10.1007/978-1-4939-7046-9_4

[15] Wang J, Chen J, Sen S. MicroRNA as biomarkers and diagnostics. Journal of Cellular Physiology. 2016;**231**(1):25-30. DOI: 10.1002/jcp.25056

[16] Hartig SM, Hamilton MP, Bader DA, McGuire SE. The miRNA Interactome in metabolic homeostasis. Trends in Endocrinology and Metabolism. 2015;**26**(12):733-745

[17] Jeon T, il, Osborne TF. miRNA and cholesterol homeostasis.

Biochimica et Biophysica Acta—Molecular and cell biology of. Lipids. 2016;**1861**(12):2041-2046

[18] Brandao BB, Lino M, Kahn CR. Extracellular miRNAs as mediators of obesity-associated disease. Journal of Physiology. 2022;**600**(5):1155-1169

[19] Borchert GM, Lanier W, Davidson BL. RNA polymerase III transcribes human microRNAs. Nature Structural & Molecular Biology. 2006;**13**(12):1097-1101

[20] Lee Y, Kim M, Han J, Yeom KH, Lee S, Baek SH, et al. MicroRNA genes are transcribed by RNA polymerase II. The EMBO Journal. 2004;**23**(20):4051-4060

[21] Abdelfattah AM, Park C, Choi MY. Update on non-canonical microRNAs. Biomolecular Concepts. 2014;**5**(4):275-287

[22] Grimson A, Farh KKH, Johnston WK, Garrett-Engele P, Lim LP, Bartel DP. MicroRNA targeting specificity in mammals: Determinants beyond seed pairing. Molecular Cell. 2007;**27**(1):91-105

[23] Moore MJ, Scheel TKH, Luna JM, Park CY, Fak JJ, Nishiuchi E, et al. miRNA-target chimeras reveal miRNA 3′-end pairing as a major determinant of Argonaute target specificity. Nature Communications. 2015;**6**

[24] Ha M, Kim VN. Regulation of microRNA biogenesis. Nature Reviews Molecular Cell Biology. 2014;**15**(8):509-524

[25] Mandelbaum AD, Melkman-Zehavi T, Oren R, Kredo-Russo S, Nir T, Dor Y, et al. Dysregulation of Dicer1 in beta cells impairs islet architecture and glucose metabolism. Experimental Diabetes Research. 2012;**2012**

[26] Tattikota SG, Rathjen T, McAnulty SJ, Wessels HH, Akerman I, van de Bunt M, et al. Argonaute2 mediates compensatory expansion of the pancreatic β cell. Cell Metabolism. 2013;**19**(1):122-134

[27] Martinez-Sanchez A, Nguyen-Tu MS, Rutter GA. DICER inactivation identifies pancreatic β-cell “disallowed” genes targeted by MicroRNAs. Molecular Endocrinology (Baltimore, Md). 2015;**29**(7):1067-1079

[28] Kalis M, Bolmeson C, Esguerra JLS, Gupta S, Edlund A, Tormo-Badia N, et al. Beta-cell specific deletion of Dicer1 leads to defective insulin secretion and diabetes mellitus. PLoS One. 2011;**6**(12):e29166-e29166

[29] Petersen MC, Shulman GI. Mechanisms of insulin action and insulin resistance. Physiological Reviews. 2018;**98**(4):2133-2223

[30] Thorens B. GLUT2, glucose sensing and glucose homeostasis. Diabetologia. 2015;**58**:221-232

[31] Atkinson MA, Campbell-Thompson M, Kusmartseva I, Kaestner KH. Organisation of the human pancreas in health and in diabetes. Diabetologia. 2020;**63**:1966-1973

[32] Tengholm A, Gylfe E. cAMP signalling in insulin and glucagon secretion. Diabetes, Obesity and Metabolism. 2017;**19**:42-53

[33] Rutter GA, Hodson DJ. Minireview: Intraislet regulation of insulin secretion in humans. Molecular Endocrinology. 2013;**27**:1984-1995

[34] Yu Q, Shuai H, Ahooghalandari P, Gylfe E, Tengholm A. Glucose

controls glucagon secretion by directly modulating cAMP in alpha cells. Diabetologia. 2019;**62**(7):1212-1224

[35] Kim MK, Shin HM, Jung HS, Lee EJ, Kim TK, Kim TN, et al. Comparison of pancreatic beta cells and alpha cells under hyperglycemia: Inverse coupling in pAkt-FoxO1. Diabetes Research and Clinical Practice. 2017;**131**:1-11

[36] Lee S, Dong HH. FoxO integration of insulin signaling with glucose and lipid metabolism. Journal of Endocrinology. 2017;**233**:R67-R79

[37] Tessari P. Changes in protein, carbohydrate, and fat metabolism with aging: Possible role of insulin. Nutrition Reviews. 2000;**58**(1):11-19

[38] Tessari P. Role of insulin in age-related changes in macronutrient metabolism. European Journal of Clinical Nutrition. 2000;**54**(Suppl 3): S126-S130

[39] Komatsu M, Takei M, Ishii H, Sato Y. Glucose-stimulated insulin secretion: A newer perspective. Journal of Diabetes Investigation. 2013;**4**(6):511-516

[40] Straub SG, Sharp GWG. Glucose-stimulated signaling pathways in biphasic insulin secretion. Diabetes/Metabolism Research and Reviews. 2002;**18**(6):451-463

[41] Wang J, Gu W, Chen C. Knocking down insulin receptor in pancreatic beta cell lines with lentiviral-small hairpin RNA reduces glucose-stimulated insulin secretion via decreasing the gene expression of insulin, GLUT2 and Pdx1. International Journal of Molecular Sciences. 2018;**19**(4):985

[42] Poitout V, Hagman D, Stein R, Artner I, Robertson RP, Harmon JS. Regulation of the insulin gene by glucose and fatty acids. The Journal of Nutrition. 2006;**136**(4):873-876

[43] Tillmar L, Carlsson C, Welsh N. Control of insulin mRNA stability in rat pancreatic islets. Regulatory role of a 3′-untranslated region pyrimidine-rich sequence. The Journal of Biological Chemistry. 2002;**277**(2):1099-1106

[44] Tillmar L, Welsh N. Glucose-induced binding of the polypyrimidine tract-binding protein (PTB) to the 3′-untranslated region of the insulin mRNA (ins-PRS) is inhibited by rapamycin. Molecular and Cellular Biochemistry. 2004;**260**(1):85-90

[45] Thorens B, Mueckler M. Glucose transporters in the 21st century. American Journal of Physiology. Endocrinology and Metabolism. 2010;**298**:141-145

[46] Mueckler M, Thorens B. The SLC2 (GLUT) family of membrane transporters. Molecular Aspects of Medicine. 2013;**34**(2-3):121-138

[47] Posner BI. Insulin signalling: The inside story. Canadian Journal of Diabetes. 2017;**41**(1):108

[48] Newsholme EA, Dimitriadis G. Integration of biochemical and physiologic effects of insulin on glucose metabolism. Experimental and Clinical Endocrinology and Diabetes. 2001;**109**(Suppl 2):S122-S134. DOI: 10.1055/s-2001-18575

[49] Matschinsky FM, Wilson DF. The central role of glucokinase in glucose homeostasis: A perspective 50 years after demonstrating the presence of the enzyme in islets of Langerhans. Frontiers in Physiology. 2019;**10**:148

[50] Massa ML, Gagliardino JJ, Francini F. Liver glucokinase: An overview on the

regulatorymechanisms of its activity. IUBMB Life. 2011;**63**:1-6

[51] Iynedjian PB. Molecular physiology of mammalian glucokinase. Cellular and Molecular Life Sciences. 2009;**66**:27-42

[52] Matschinsky FM. Regulation of pancreatic-cell glucokinase from basics to therapeutics. Diabetes. 2002;**51**(Suppl 3):S394-S404

[53] Haeusler RA, TE MG, Accili D. Metabolic Signalling: Biochemical and cellular properties of insulin receptor signalling. Nature Reviews Molecular Cell Biology. 2018;**19**:31-44

[54] White MF. IRS proteins and the common path to diabetes. American Journal of Physiology—Endocrinology and Metabolism. 2002;**283**(3):E413-E422

[55] Kohn AD, Kovacina KS, Roth RA. Insulin stimulates the kinase activity of RAC-PK, a pleckstrin homology domain containing ser/thr kinase. The EMBO Journal. 1995;**14**(17):4288-4295. DOI: 10.1002/j.1460-2075.1995.tb00103.x

[56] Zorzano A, Palacín M, Gumà A. Mechanisms regulating GLUT4 glucose transporter expression and glucose transport in skeletal muscle. Acta Physiologica Scandinavica. 2005;**183**(1):43-58

[57] Wang L, Liu Q, Kitamoto T, Hou J, Qin J, Accili D. Identification of insulin-responsive transcription factors that regulate glucose production by hepatocytes. Diabetes. 2019;**68**(6):1156-1167

[58] den Boer MAM, Voshol PJ, Kuipers F, Romijn JA, Havekes LM. Hepatic glucose production is more sensitive to insulin-mediated inhibition than hepatic VLDL-triglyceride production. American Journal of Physiology. Endocrinology and Metabolism. 2006;**291**:1360-1364

[59] Hatting M, Tavares CDJ, Sharabi K, Rines AK, Puigserver P. Insulin regulation of gluconeogenesis. Annals of the New York Academy of Sciences. 2018;**1411**:21-35

[60] Kamagate A, Dong HH. FoxO1 integrates insulin signaling to VLDL production NIH public access. Cell Cycle. 2008;**7**(20):3162-3170

[61] Kamagate A, Qu S, Perdomo G, Su D, Dae HK, Slusher S, et al. FoxO1 mediates insulin-dependent regulation of hepatic VLDL production in mice. Journal of Clinical Investigation. 2008;**118**(6):2347-2364

[62] Kim DH, Zhang T, Lee S, Calabuig-Navarro V, Yamauchi J, Piccirillo A, et al. FoxO6 integrates insulin signaling with MTP for regulating VLDL production in the liver. Endocrinology. 2014;**155**(4):1255-1267

[63] Scherer T, OHare J, Diggs-Andrews K, Schweiger M, Cheng B, Lindtner C, et al. Brain insulin controls adipose tissue lipolysis and lipogenesis. Cell Metabolism. 2011;**13**(2):183-194

[64] Iwen KA, Scherer T, Heni M, Sayk F, Wellnitz T, Machleidt F, et al. Intranasal insulin suppresses systemic but not subcutaneous lipolysis in healthy humans. Journal of Clinical Endocrinology and Metabolism. 2014;**99**(2)

[65] Saltiel AR. Insulin signaling in the control of glucose and lipid homeostasis. Handbook of Experimental Pharmacology. 2016;**233**:51-71

[66] Charlton M, Nair KS. Protein metabolism in insulin-dependent

diabetes mellitus. The Journal of Nutrition. 1998;**128**(2):323S-327S

[67] Fukagawa NK, Minaker KL, Rowe JW, Goodman MN, Matthews DE, Bier DM, et al. Insulin-mediated reduction of whole body protein breakdown. Dose-response effects on leucine metabolism in postabsorptive men. Journal of Clinical Investigation. 1985;**76**(6):2306-2311

[68] Newgard CB, An J, Bain JR, Muehlbauer MJ, Stevens RD, Lien LF, et al. A branched-chain amino acid-related metabolic signature that differentiates obese and lean humans and contributes to insulin resistance. Cell Metabolism. 2009;**9**(4):311-326

[69] Tessari P, Nosadini R, Trevisan R, de Kreutzenberg SV, Inchiostro S, Duner E, et al. Defective suppression by insulin of leucine-carbon appearance and oxidation in type 1, insulin-dependent diabetes mellitus. Evidence for insulin resistance involving glucose and amino acid metabolism. Journal of Clinical Investigation. 1986;**77**(6):1797-1804

[70] Yoon MS. The emerging role of branched-chain amino acids in insulin resistance and metabolism. Nutrients. 2016;**8**(7)

[71] Asghari G, Farhadnejad H, Teymoori F, Mirmiran P, Tohidi M, Azizi F. High dietary intake of branched-chain amino acids is associated with an increased risk of insulin resistance in adults. Journal of Diabetes. 2018;**10**(5):357-364

[72] Holst JJ, Holland W, Gromada J, Lee Y, Unger RH, Yan H, et al. Insulin and glucagon: Partners for life. Endocrinology. 2017;**158**(4):696-701

[73] Vergari E, Knudsen JG, Ramracheya R, Salehi A, Zhang Q, Adam J, et al. Insulin inhibits glucagon release by SGLT2-induced stimulation of somatostatin secretion. Nature. Communications. 2019;**10**(1):139

[74] Wan CKN, Giacca A, Matsuhisa M, El-Bahrani B, Lam L, Rodgers C, et al. Increased responses of glucagon and glucose production to hypoglycemia with intraperitoneal versus subcutaneous insulin treatment. Metabolism: Clinical and Experimental. 2000;**49**(8):984-989

[75] Ito K, Maruyama H, Hirose H, Kido K, Koyama K, Kataoka K, et al. Exogenous insulin dose-dependently suppresses glucopenia-induced glucagon secretion from perfused rat pancreas. Metabolism. 1995;**44**(3):358-362

[76] Göbl C, Morettini M, Salvatori B, Alsalim W, Kahleova H, Ahrén B, et al. Temporal patterns of glucagon and its relationships with glucose and insulin following ingestion of different classes of macronutrients. Nutrients. 2011;**14**(2):376

[77] Walker JN, Ramracheya R, Zhang Q, Johnson PRV, Braun M, Rorsman P. Regulation of glucagon secretion by glucose: Paracrine, intrinsic or both? Diabetes, Obesity and Metabolism. 2011;**13**(Suppl 1):95-105. DOI: 10.1111/j.1463-1326.2011.01450.x

[78] Onyango AN. Mechanisms of the regulation and dysregulation of glucagon secretion. Oxidative Medicine and Cellular Longevity. 2020;**2020**:3089139

[79] Barthel A, Schmoll D. Novel Concepts in Insulin Regulation of Hepatic Gluconeogenesis. 2003. Available from: http://www.ajpendo.org

[80] Cooperberg BA, Cryer PE. Insulin reciprocally regulates glucagon secretion in humans. Diabetes. 2010;**59**(11):2936-2940

[81] Bansal P, Wang Q. Insulin as a physiological modulator of glucagon secretion. American Journal of Physiology—Endocrinology and Metabolism. 2008;**295**(4)

[82] Galicia-Garcia U, Benito-Vicente A, Jebari S, Larrea-Sebal A, Siddiqi H, Uribe KB, et al. Pathophysiology of type 2 diabetes mellitus. International Journal of Molecular Sciences. MDPI AG. 2020;**21**:1-34

[83] Harrison LC. The dark side of insulin: A primary autoantigen and instrument of self-destruction in type 1 diabetes. Molecular Metabolism. 2021;**52**

[84] Maiese K. New insights for oxidative stress and diabetes mellitus. Oxidative Medicine and Cellular Longevity. 2015;**2015**:875961

[85] Brownlee M. The pathobiology of diabetic complications a unifying mechanism. Diabetes. 2005;**54**(6):1615-1625

[86] Giacco F, Brownlee M. Oxidative stress and diabetic complications. Circulation Research. 2010;**107**:1058-1070

[87] Pi J, Zhang Q, Fu J, Woods CG, Hou Y, Corkey BE, et al. ROS signaling, oxidative stress and Nrf2 in pancreatic beta-cell function. Toxicology and Applied Pharmacology. 2010;**244**:77-83

[88] Harrison LC. The dark side of insulin: A primary autoantigen and instrument of self-destruction in type 1 diabetes. Molecular Metabolism. 2021;**52**:101288

[89] Hanley SC, Austin E, Assouline-Thomas B, Kapeluto J, Blaichman J, Moosavi M, et al. β-Cell mass dynamics and islet cell plasticity in human type 2 diabetes. Endocrinology. 2010;**151**(4):1462-1472

[90] Satin LS, Butler PC, Ha J, Sherman AS. Pulsatile insulin secretion, impaired glucose tolerance and type 2 diabetes. Molecular Aspects of Medicine. 2015;**42**:61-77

[91] Moin ASM, Dhawan S, Cory M, Butler PC, Rizza RA, Butler AE. Increased frequency of hormone negative and polyhormonal endocrine cells in lean individuals with type 2 diabetes. Journal of Clinical Endocrinology and Metabolism. 2016;**101**(10):3628-3636

[92] Roden M, Shulman GI. The integrative biology of type 2 diabetes. Nature. 2019;**576**(7785):51-60

[93] Zick Y. Insulin resistance: A phosphorylation-based uncoupling of insulin signaling. Trends in Cell Biology. 2001;**11**(11):437-441

[94] Chatterjee S, Khunti K, Davies MJ. Type 2 diabetes. The Lancet. 2017;**389**(10085):2239-2251

[95] Lewis GF, Carpentier A, Vranic M, Giacca A. Resistance to insulin's acute direct hepatic effect in suppressing steady-state glucose production in individuals with type 2 diabetes. Diabetes. 1999;**48**(3):570-576

[96] Weyer C, Bogardus C, Mott DM, Pratley RE. The natural history of insulin secretory dysfunction and insulin resistance in the pathophysiology of type diabetes mellitus. Journal of Clinical Investigation. 1999;**104**(6):787-794

[97] RA Haeusler TMDA. Biochemical and cellular properties of insulin receptor signalling. Nature Reviews. Molecular Cell Biology. 2018;**19**:31-44

[98] Boucher J, Kleinridders A, Ronald KC. Insulin receptor signaling in normal and insulin-resistant states. Cold

Spring Harbor Perspectives in Biology. 2014;**6**(1)

[99] Solimena M, Schulte AM, Marselli L, Ehehalt F, Richter D, Kleeberg M, et al. Systems biology of the IMIDIA biobank from organ donors and pancreatectomised patients defines a novel transcriptomic signature of islets from individuals with type 2 diabetes. Diabetologia. 2018;**61**(3):641-657

[100] Lyon J, Manning Fox JE, Spigelman AF, Kim R, Smith N, O'Gorman D, et al. Research-focused isolation of human islets from donors with and without diabetes at the Alberta diabetes institute IsletCore. Endocrinology. 2016;**157**(2):560-569

[101] Deng S, Vatamaniuk M, Huang X, Doliba N, Lian MM, Frank A, et al. Structural and functional abnormalities in the islets isolated from type 2 diabetic subjects. Diabetes. 2004;**53**(3):624-632

[102] Kaksonen M, Roux A. Mechanisms of clathrin-mediated endocytosis. Nature Reviews. Molecular Cell Biology. 2018;**19**(5):313-326

[103] Hall C, Yu H, Choi E. Insulin receptor endocytosis in the pathophysiology of insulin resistance. Experimental & Molecular Medicine. 2020;**52**(6):911-920

[104] Caro JF, Ittoop O, Pories WJ, Meelheim D, Flickinger EG, Thomas F, et al. Studies on the mechanism of insulin resistance in the liver from humans with noninsulin-dependent diabetes. Insulin action and binding in isolated hepatocytes, insulin receptor structure, and kinase activity. The Journal of Clinical Investigation. 1986;**78**(1):249-258

[105] Gunton JE, Kulkarni RN, Yim SH, Okada T, Hawthorne WJ, Tseng YH, et al. Loss of ARNT/HIF1beta mediates altered gene expression and pancreatic-islet dysfunction in human type 2 diabetes. Cell. 2005;**122**(3):337-349

[106] Thomas DD, Corkey BE, Istfan NW, Apovian CM. Hyperinsulinemia: An early indicator of metabolic dysfunction. Journal of the Endocrine Society. 2019;**3**(9):1727

[107] Kurauti MA, Ferreira SM, Soares GM, Vettorazzi JF, Carneiro EM, Boschero AC, et al. Hyperinsulinemia is associated with increasing insulin secretion but not with decreasing insulin clearance in an age-related metabolic dysfunction mice model. Journal of Cellular Physiology. 2019;**234**(6):9802-9809

[108] D'alessio D. The role of dysregulated glucagon secretion in type 2 diabetes. Diabetes, Obesity and Metabolism. 2011;**13**(Suppl 1):126-132

[109] Philippe J, Knepel W, Waeber G. Insulin regulation of the glucagon gene is mediated by an insulin-responsive DNA element. Proceedings of the National Academy of Sciences of the United States of America. 1991;**88**(16):7224

[110] Ottosson-Laakso E, Krus U, Storm P, Prasad RB, Oskolkov N, Ahlqvist E, et al. Glucose-induced changes in gene expression in human pancreatic islets: Causes or consequences of chronic hyperglycemia. Diabetes. 2017;**66**(12):3013-3028

[111] Segerstolpe Å, Palasantza A, Eliasson P, Andersson EM, Andréasson AC, Sun X, et al. Single-cell transcriptome profiling of human pancreatic islets in health and type 2 diabetes. Cell Metabolism. 2016;**24**(4):593-607

[112] Marselli L, Piron A, Suleiman M, Colli ML, Yi X, Khamis A, et al.

Persistent or transient human β cell dysfunction induced by metabolic stress: Specific signatures and shared gene expression with type 2 diabetes. Cell Reports. 2020;**33**(9):108466

[113] Marselli L, Thorne J, Dahiya S, Sgroi DC, Sharma A, Bonner-Weir S, et al. Gene expression profiles of Beta-cell enriched tissue obtained by laser capture microdissection from subjects with type 2 diabetes. PLoS One. 2010;**5**(7):e11499

[114] Weir GC, Bonner-Weir S. Five of stages of evolving β-cell dysfunction during progression to diabetes. Diabetes. 2004;**53**(Suppl 3):S16-S21

[115] Khin PP, Lee JH, Jun HS. A brief review of the mechanisms of β-cell dedifferentiation in type 2 diabetes. Nutrients. 2021;**13**(5):1593

[116] Bensellam M, Jonas JC, Laybutt DR. Mechanisms of β;-cell dedifferentiation in diabetes: Recent findings and future research directions. Journal of Endocrinology. 2018;**236**(2):R109-R143

[117] Sun T, Han X. Death versus dedifferentiation: The molecular bases of beta cell mass reduction in type 2 diabetes. Seminars in Cell & Developmental Biology. 2020;**103**:76-82

[118] Marrif HI, Al-Sunousi SI. Pancreatic β cell mass death. Frontiers in Pharmacology. 2016;**7**:83

[119] Rachdaoui N, Polo-Parada L, Ismail-Beigi F. Prolonged exposure to insulin inactivates Akt and Erk 1/2 and increases pancreatic islet and INS1E β-cell apoptosis. Journal of the Endocrine Society. 2018;**3**(1):69-90

[120] Bucris E, Beck A, Boura-Halfon S, Isaac R, Vinik Y, Rosenzweig T, et al. Prolonged insulin treatment sensitizes apoptosis pathways in pancreatic β cells. The Journal of Endocrinology. 2016;**230**(3):291-307

[121] Sampson SR, Bucris E, Horovitz-Fried M, Parnas A, Kahana S, Abitbol G, et al. Insulin increases H2O2-induced pancreatic beta cell death. Apoptosis. 2010;**15**(10):1165-1176

[122] Zhu Y, Shu T, Lin Y, Wang H, Yang J, Shi Y, et al. Inhibition of the receptor for advanced glycation endproducts (RAGE) protects pancreatic β-cells. Biochemical and Biophysical Research Communications. 2011;**404**(1):159-165

[123] Imai Y, Cousins RS, Liu S, Phelps BM, Promes JA. Connecting pancreatic islet lipid metabolism with insulin secretion and the development of type 2 diabetes. Annals of the New York Academy of Sciences. 2020;**1461**(1):53-72

[124] Lytrivi M, Castell AL, Poitout V, Cnop M. Recent insights into mechanisms of β-cell lipo- and glucolipotoxicity in type 2 diabetes. Journal of Molecular Biology. 2020;**432**(5):1514-1534

[125] Hunter CS, Stein RW. Evidence for loss in identity, de-differentiation, and trans-differentiation of islet β-cells in type 2 diabetes. Frontiers in Genetics. 2017;**8**:35

[126] Cinti F, Bouchi R, Kim-Muller JY, Ohmura Y, Sandoval PR, Masini M, et al. Evidence of β-cell dedifferentiation in human type 2 diabetes. The Journal of Clinical Endocrinology and Metabolism. 2016;**101**(3):1044-1054

[127] Brereton MF, Iberl M, Shimomura K, Zhang Q, Adriaenssens AE, Proks P, et al. Reversible changes in pancreatic islet structure and function produced by elevated blood glucose. Nature Communications. 2014;**5**

[128] Wang Z, York NW, Nichols CG, Remedi MS. Pancreatic β cell dedifferentiation in diabetes and redifferentiation following insulin therapy. Cell Metabolism. 2014;**19**(5):872-882

[129] Neelankal John A, Ram R, Jiang FX. RNA-Seq analysis of islets to characterise the dedifferentiation in type 2 diabetes model mice db/db. Endocrine Pathology. 2018;**29**(3):207-221

[130] Talchai C, Xuan S, Lin H, v., Sussel L, Accili D. Pancreatic β cell dedifferentiation as a mechanism of diabetic β cell failure. Cell. 2012;**150**(6):1223-1234

[131] Spijker HS, Ravelli RBG, Mommaas-Kienhuis AM, van Apeldoorn AA, Engelse MA, Zaldumbide A, et al. Conversion of mature human β-cells into glucagon-producing α-cells. Diabetes. 2013;**62**(7):2471-2480

[132] Schuit F. Epigenetic programming of glucose-regulated insulin release. The Journal of Clinical Investigation. 2015;**125**(7):2565-2568

[133] Dhawan S, Tschen SI, Zeng C, Guo T, Hebrok M, Matveyenko A, et al. DNA methylation directs functional maturation of pancreatic β cells. Journal of Clinical Investigation. 2015;**125**(7):2851-2860

[134] Spaeth JM, Walker EM, Stein R. Impact of Pdx1-associated chromatin modifiers on islet β-cells. Diabetes, Obesity & Metabolism. 2016;**18**(Suppl 1):123-127

[135] Dayeh T, Ling C. Does epigenetic dysregulation of pancreatic islets contribute to impaired insulin secretion and type 2 diabetes? Biochemistry and Cell Biology. 2015;**93**(5):511-521

[136] Campbell SA, Hoffman BG. Chromatin regulators in pancreas development and diabetes. Trends in Endocrinology and Metabolism. 2016;**27**(3):142-152

[137] Astro V, Adamo A. Epigenetic control of endocrine pancreas differentiation in vitro: Current knowledge and future perspectives. Frontiers in Cell and Developmental Biology. 2018;**6**:141

[138] Akerman I, Tu Z, Beucher A, Rolando DMY, Sauty-Colace C, Benazra M, et al. Human pancreatic β cell lncRNAs control cell-specific regulatory networks. Cell Metabolism. 2017;**25**(2):400-411

[139] Brodnicki TC. A role for lncRNAs in regulating inflammatory and autoimmune responses underlying type 1 diabetes. Advances in Experimental Medicine and Biology. 2022;**1363**:97-118

[140] Ruan Y, Lin N, Ma Q, Chen R, Zhang Z, Wen W, et al. Circulating LncRNAs analysis in patients with type 2 diabetes reveals novel genes influencing glucose metabolism and islet β-cell function. Cellular Physiology and Biochemistry. 2018;**46**(1):335-350

[141] Motterle A, Sanchez-Parra C, Regazzi R. Role of long non-coding RNAs in the determination of β-cell identity. Diabetes, Obesity and Metabolism. 2016;**18**:41-50

[142] Wilson ME, Pullen TJ. The role of long non-coding RNAs in the regulation of pancreatic beta cell identity. Biochemical Society Transactions. 2021;**49**(5):2153-2161

[143] López-Noriega L, Rutter GA. Long non-coding RNAs as key modulators of pancreatic β-cell mass and function. Front Endocrinol (Lausanne). 2021;**11**:610213

[144] Motterle A, Gattesco S, Peyot ML, Esguerra JLS, Gomez-Ruiz A, Laybutt DR, et al. Identification of islet-enriched long non-coding RNAs contributing to β-cell failure in type 2 diabetes. Molecular Metabolism. 2017;**6**(11):1407-1418

[145] Latreille M, Hausser J, Stützer I, Zhang Q, Hastoy B, Gargani S, et al. MicroRNA-7a regulates pancreatic β cell function. The Journal of Clinical Investigation. 2014;**124**(6):2722-2735

[146] Dumortier O, Fabris G, Pisani DF, Casamento V, Gautier N, Hinault C, et al. microRNA-375 regulates glucose metabolism-related signaling for insulin secretion. Journal of Endocrinology. 2020;**244**(1):189-200

[147] Wan S, Zhang J, Chen X, Lang J, Li L, Chen F, et al. MicroRNA-17-92 regulates beta-cell restoration after streptozotocin treatment. Frontiers in Endocrinology. 2020;**11**:9

[148] Rodríguez-Comas J, Moreno-Asso A, Moreno-Vedia J, Martín M, Castaño C, Marzà-Florensa A, et al. Stress-induced microrna-708 impairs b-cell function and growth. Diabetes. 2017;**66**(12):3029-3040

[149] Fu X, Dong B, Tian Y, Lefebvre P, Meng Z, Wang X, et al. MicroRNA-26a regulates insulin sensitivity and metabolism of glucose and lipids. Journal of Clinical Investigation. 2015;**125**(6):2497-2509

[150] Baroukh N, Ravier MA, Loder MK, Hill EV, Bounacer A, Scharfmann R, et al. MicroRNA-124a regulates foxa2 expression and intracellular signaling in pancreatic β-cell lines. Journal of Biological Chemistry. 2007;**282**(27):19575-19588

[151] Xu Y, Huang Y, Guo Y, Xiong Y, Zhu S, Xu L, et al. MicroRNA-690 regulates induced pluripotent stem cells (iPSCs) differentiation into insulin-producing cells by targeting Sox9. Stem Cell Research and Therapy. 2019;**10**(1):59

[152] Filios SR, Shalev A. β-Cell MicroRNAs: Small but powerful. Diabetes. 2015;**64**(11):3631-3644

[153] Fernández-Hernando C, Ramírez CM, Goedeke L, Suárez Y. MicroRNAs in metabolic disease. Arteriosclerosis, Thrombosis, and Vascular Biology. 2013;**33**(2):178-185

[154] Esguerra JLS, Nagao M, Ofori JK, Wendt A, Eliasson L. MicroRNAs in islet hormone secretion. Diabetes, Obesity and Metabolism. 2018;**20**:11-19

[155] Kim KH, Hartig SM. Contributions of microRNAs to peripheral insulin sensitivity. Endocrinology. 2022;**163**(2):bqab250

[156] Özcan S. Minireview: MicroRNA function in pancreatic β cells. Molecular Endocrinology. 2014;**28**(12):1922-1933

[157] Kaviani M, Azarpira N, Karimi MH, Al-Abdullah I. The role of microRNAs in islet β-cell development. Cell Biology International. 2016;**40**(12):1248-1255

[158] LaPierre MP, Stoffel M. MicroRNAs as stress regulators in pancreatic beta cells and diabetes. Molecular Metabolism. 2017;**6**(9):1010-1023

[159] Jacovetti C, Abderrahmani A, Parnaud G, Jonas JC, Peyot ML, Cornu M, et al. MicroRNAs contribute to compensatory β cell expansion during pregnancy and obesity. The Journal of Clinical Investigation. 2012;**122**(10):3541-3551

[160] Eliasson L, Esguerra JLS. Role of non-coding RNAs in pancreatic beta-cell development and physiology.

Acta Physiologica (Oxford, England). 2014;**211**(2):273-284

[161] Esguerra JLS, Mollet IG, Salunkhe VA, Wendt A, Eliasson L. Regulation of pancreatic Beta cell stimulus-secretion coupling by microRNAs. Genes (Basel). 2014;**5**(4):1018-1031

[162] Cerf ME. Beta cell dynamics: Beta cell replenishment, beta cell compensation and diabetes. Endocrine. 2013;**44**(2):303-311

[163] Geach T. Diabetes: Preventing β-cell apoptosis and T2DM with microRNAs—A role for MIR-200? Nature Reviews Endocrinology. 2015;**11**(8):444

[164] Liu M, Wright J, Guo H, Xiong Y, Arvan P. Proinsulin entry and transit through the endoplasmic reticulum in pancreatic beta cells. Vitamins and Hormones. 2014;**95**:35-62

[165] Liu M, Weiss MA, Arunagiri A, Yong J, Rege N, Sun J, et al. Biosynthesis, structure, and folding of the insulin precursor protein. Diabetes, Obesity and Metabolism. 2018;**20**:28-50

[166] Steiner DF. The proinsulin C-peptide—A multirole model. Experimental Diabesity Research. 2004;**5**(1):7-14

[167] Steiner DF. On the discovery of precursor processing. Methods in Molecular Biology. 2011;**768**:3-11

[168] Melkman-Zehavi T, Oren R, Kredo-Russo S, Shapira T, Mandelbaum AD, Rivkin N, et al. miRNAs control insulin content in pancreatic β-cells via downregulation of transcriptional repressors. The EMBO Journal. 2011;**30**(5):835-845

[169] Bolmeson C, Esguerra JLS, Salehi A, Speidel D, Eliasson L, Cilio CM. Differences in islet-enriched miRNAs in healthy and glucose intolerant human subjects. Biochemical and Biophysical Research Communications. 2010;**404**(1):16-22

[170] Nathan G, Kredo-Russo S, Geiger T, Lenz A, Kaspi H, Hornstein E, et al. MiR-375 promotes redifferentiation of adult human β cells expanded in vitro. PLoS One. 2015;**10**(4):e0122108-e0122108

[171] Xu G, Chen J, Jing G, Shalev A. Thioredoxin-interacting protein regulates insulin transcription through microRNA-204. Nature Medicine. 2013;**19**(9):1141-1146

[172] Li N, Jiang D, He Q, He F, Li Y, Deng C, et al. microRNA-181c-5p promotes the formation of insulin-producing cells from human induced pluripotent stem cells by targeting smad7 and TGIF2. Cell Death & Disease. 2020;**11**(6):1-12

[173] MicroRNA miR-124a, a negative regulator of insulin secretion, is hyperexpressed in human pancreatic islets of type 2 diabetic patients. RNA & DISEASE. 2015

[174] Bhushan R, Rani A, Gupta D, Akhtar A, Dubey PK. MicroRNA-7 regulates insulin signaling pathway by targeting IRS1, IRS2, and RAF1 genes in gestational diabetes mellitus. MicroRNA (Shariqah, United Arab Emirates). 2022;**11**

[175] Drucker DJ. Mechanisms of action and therapeutic application of glucagon-like peptide-1. Cell Metabolism. 2018;**27**(4):740-756

[176] Drucker DJ, Nauck MA. The incretin system: Glucagon-like peptide-1 receptor agonists and dipeptidyl peptidase-4

inhibitors in type 2 diabetes. Lancet. 2006;**368**(9548):1696-1705

[177] Jo SH, Chen J, Xu G, Grayson TB, Thielen LA, Shalev A. miR-204 controls glucagon-like peptide 1 receptor expression and agonist function. Diabetes. 2018;**67**(2):256-264

[178] Rorsman P, Ashcroft FM. Pancreatic β-cell electrical activity and insulin secretion: Of mice and men. Physiological Reviews. 2018;**98**(1):117-214

[179] Ofori JK, Salunkhe VA, Bagge A, Vishnu N, Nagao M, Mulder H, et al. Elevated miR-130a/miR130b/miR-152 expression reduces intracellular ATP levels in the pancreatic beta cell. Scientific Reports. 2017;**7**(1):1-15

[180] Pullen TJ, da Silva XG, Kelsey G, Rutter GA. miR-29a and miR-29b contribute to pancreatic β-cell-specific silencing of monocarboxylate transporter 1 (Mct1). Molecular and Cellular Biology. 2011;**31**(15):3182-3194

[181] Bagge A, Clausen TR, Larsen S, Ladefoged M, Rosenstierne MW, Larsen L, et al. MicroRNA-29a is up-regulated in beta-cells by glucose and decreases glucose-stimulated insulin secretion. Biochemical and Biophysical Research Communications. 2012;**426**(2):266-272

[182] Bagge A, Dahmcke CM, Dalgaard LT. Syntaxin-1a is a direct target of miR-29a in insulin-producing β-cells. Hormone and Metabolic Research. 2013;**45**(6):463-466

[183] Tarlton JMR, Patterson S, Graham A. MicroRNA sequences modulated by beta cell lipid metabolism: Implications for type 2 diabetes mellitus. Biology (Basel). 2021;**10**(6):534

[184] Lovis P, Roggli E, Laybutt DR, Gattesco S, Yang JY, Widmann C, et al. Alterations in microRNA expression contribute to fatty acid-induced pancreatic beta-cell dysfunction. Diabetes. 2008;**57**(10):2728-2736

[185] Najafi-Shoushtari SH, Kristo F, Li Y, Shioda T, Cohen DE, Gerszten RE, et al. MicroRNA-33 and the SREBP host genes cooperate to control cholesterol homeostasis. Science. 2010;**328**(5985):1566-1569

[186] Han YB, Wang MN, Li Q, Guo L, Yang YM, Li PJ, et al. MicroRNA-34a contributes to the protective effects of glucagon-like peptide-1 against lipotoxicity in INS-1 cells. Chinese Medical Journal. 2012;**125**(23):4202-4208

[187] Lu H, Hao L, Li S, Lin S, Lv L, Chen Y, et al. Elevated circulating stearic acid leads to a major lipotoxic effect on mouse pancreatic beta cells in hyperlipidaemia via a miR-34a-5p-mediated PERK/p53-dependent pathway. Diabetologia. 2016;**59**(6):1247-1257

[188] Kong X, Liu CX, Wang GD, Yang H, Yao XM, Hua Q, et al. LncRNA LEGLTBC functions as a ceRNA to antagonize the effects of miR-34a on the downregulation of SIRT1 in glucolipotoxicity-induced INS-1 Beta cell oxidative stress and apoptosis. Oxidative Medicine and Cellular Longevity. 2019;**2019**:4010764

[189] Lin X, Guan H, Huang Z, Liu J, Li H, Wei G, et al. Downregulation of Bcl-2 expression by miR-34a mediates palmitate-induced Min6 cells apoptosis. Journal Diabetes Research. 2014;**2014**:258695

[190] Liu Y, Dong J, Ren BO. MicroRNA-182-5p contributes to the protective effects of thrombospondin 1 against lipotoxicity in INS-1 cells.

Experimental and Therapeutic Medicine. 2018;**16**(6):5272-5279

[191] Guo R, Yu Y, Zhang Y, Li Y, Chu X, Lu H, et al. Overexpression of miR-297b-5p protects against stearic acid-induced pancreatic β-cell apoptosis by targeting LATS2. American Journal of Physiology. Endocrinology and Metabolism. 2020;**318**(3):E430-E439

[192] Li Y, Xu X, Liang Y, Liu S, Xiao H, Li F, et al. miR-375 enhances palmitate-induced lipoapoptosis in insulin-secreting NIT-1 cells by repressing myotrophin (V1) protein expression. International Journal of Clinical and Experimental Pathology. 2010;**3**(3):254

[193] Paterson MR, Kriegel AJ. MiR-146a/b: A family with shared seeds and different roots. Physiological Genomics. 2017;**49**(4):243-252

[194] Fred RG, Bang-Berthelsen CH, Mandrup-Poulsen T, Grunnet LG, Welsh N. High glucose suppresses human islet insulin biosynthesis by inducing miR-133a leading to decreased polypyrimidine tract binding protein-expression. PLoS One. 2010;**5**(5)

[195] Jiang W, Liu J, Dai Y, Zhou N, Ji C, Li X. MiR-146b attenuates high-fat diet-induced non-alcoholic steatohepatitis in mice. Journal of Gastroenterology and Hepatology. 2015;**30**(5):933-943

[196] Kumar A, Ren Y, Sundaram K, Mu J, Sriwastva MK, Dryden GW, et al. miR-375 prevents high-fat diet-induced insulin resistance and obesity by targeting the aryl hydrocarbon receptor and bacterial tryptophanase (tnaA) gene. Theranostics. 2021;**11**(9):4061-4077

Chapter 6

Predicting SNPs in Mature MicroRNAs Dysregulated in Breast Cancer

Thanh Thi Ngoc Nguyen, Thu Huynh Ngoc Nguyen, Luan Huu Huynh, Hoang Ngo Phan and Hue Thi Nguyen

Abstract

Breast cancer (BC) is the leading type of cancer among women. Findings have revolutionized current knowledge of microRNA (miRNA) in breast tumorigenesis. The seed region of miRNA regulates the process of gene expression negatively. The presence of SNPs in the seed regions of miRNA dramatically alters the mature miRNA function. Additionally, SNPs in the out-seed region of miRNAs have a significant impact on miRNA targeting. This study focuses on the *in silico* analysis procedure of mature miRNA SNPs and their impact on BC risk. The database annotated SNPs on mature miRNAs was used. Also, target gene alterations, miRNAs function in BC, and the interaction of miRNAs with targets were predicted. A list of 101 SNPs in 100 miRNAs with functional targets in BC was indicated. Under the SNPs allele variation, 10 miRNAs changed function, 6 miRNAs lost targets, 15 miRNAs gained targets, 48 onco-miRNAs remained unchanged, and 21 tumor suppressor miRNAs remained unchanged. At last, a list of 89 SNPs, which alter miRNA function and miRNA-mRNA interaction, were shown to be potentially associated with BC risk. This research theoretically generated a list of possible causative SNPs in the mature miRNA gene that might be used in future BC management studies.

Keywords: mature microRNA, SNP, breast cancer, bioinformatics, *in silico*

1. Introduction

Breast cancer (BC) is the most prevalent cancer among women across the world. The malignant growth begins in the ducts (85%) or lobules epithelium (15%) ("*in situ*"), where it typically causes no symptoms and has a minimal chance of spreading (metastasis). These *in situ* (stage 0) tumors may increase substantially, infiltrating neighboring breast tissue (invasive BC) and expanding to nearby lymph nodes (regional metastasis) or organs (distant metastasis). This cancer is generally deadly due to metastasis spread [1]. BC was diagnosed in 2.3 million women in 2020, with 685,000 fatalities worldwide [2]. This cancer was also found in 7.8 million women living in the last 5 years, making it the world's most frequent malignancy by the end of 2020 [2]. BC affects women at all ages following puberty in every country worldwide, with incidence increasing with age. Therefore, many researchers and clinicians are focused on the etiology of the disease to enhance current medications and discover novel treatments.

MicroRNAs (miRNAs), short non-coding RNAs of approximately 18–24 nucleotides in length, affect gene expression negatively by directly binding the 3′-untranslated region (UTR) of the target messenger RNA (mRNA) and diminishing its stability and translatability. Numerous miRNAs have roles in cell signaling, including proliferation, death, differentiation, and immunity [3]. It has been proposed that they have a role in the formation and development of human malignancies, making them important markers of cancer [4]. The involvement of microRNAs in complex diseases like BC has focused on recent studies [5]. Various miRNAs have been related to regulating genes that have a role in the development of BC. MiR-21, miR-26a, miR-155, miR-221/miR-222, and miR-495 are some of the onco-miRs involved in tumor proliferation and angiogenesis [6–12]. Various miRNAs (miR-100, miR-125b, miR-126, miR-145, miR-200c, miR-298, and miR-335) have been involved in cell cycle regulation, hypoxia and stress response, and apoptotic induction [13–22]. In addition, McAnena et al. [23] found that circulating miR-332 and miR-195 may be utilized to discriminate between local and metastatic BC. Meanwhile, Sathipati et al. [24] indicated that 34 miRNAs could be employed to classify the early and late stages of BC development. These findings support the concept that a small selection of miRNAs can be considered biomarkers for BC risk prediction or prognosis [25].

The seed region of miRNA, located between the second and eighth positions in miRNA, regulates gene expression negatively [26]. As miRNAs are small, even a single alteration in the mature sequence of miRNAs might impact the development of miRNAs, which leads to the production of new miRNA [27]. A novel repertoire of target genes is produced by the presence of SNPs in the seed regions of miRNA, which dramatically alters the biological activity of the miRNA [28]. Additionally, SNPs in the out-seed region of miRNAs significantly impact miRNA targeting enhancements [29].

Therefore, in this study, the functional effect of SNPs in miRNAs regulating the genes implicated in BC has been predicted by bioinformatics approaches, including (1) screening miRNAs that reveal SNPs in mature sequences, (2) identifying miRNAs' target genes related to BC, (3) predicting miRNAs function in BC, and (4) estimating the degree of interaction between miRNAs and target mRNAs. The results may be beneficial in determining potential SNPs to analyze further and investigate SNPs that are causative to BC. Furthermore, the findings may potentially help generate theories and evaluate therapies for BC.

2. Materials and methods

2.1 SNPs in miRNA mature sequences database

In this study, the list of SNPs in mature miRNA sequences was extracted from the "SNPs in pre-miRNAs" database provided by miRNASNP-v3 [30] (http://bioinfo.life.hust.edu.cn/miRNASNP#W/). Mature miRNA location, positioning, and sequences were obtained from miRbase (www.mirbase.org), release 22 [31]. SNP position were acquired from dbSNP [32] (MAF > 1%) (https://www.ncbi.nlm.nih.gov/projects/SNP/snp_summary.cgi).

2.2 *In silico* target prediction in BC pathways

The miRDB (http://mirdb.org/) was adapted to input both miRNA reference and SNP altered sequences for target prediction [33]. Target prediction was performed for all miRNAs containing reference and SNP alternative sequences. All predicted targets with prediction scores ≥80 that are most likely to be accurate [34], were collected and applied to conduct Kyoto encyclopedia of genes and genomes (KEGG) enrichment analyses for the identified target genes in the BC pathway (hsa05224). KEGG is a knowledge base for systematic analysis of gene functions [35] (https://www.genome.jp/pathway/hsa05224). MiRNAs that target genes in the BC pathway are considered to be involved in BC formation. The target with the highest predicted target score from miRDB is considered the gene most likely to affect BC via the miRNA regulation.

2.3 Function prediction of target genes and miRNAs in BC

The target genes with the highest target score from miRDB of each miRNA were further analyzed. The published expression level (Log2FC value) of genes in BC was collected from GENT2. GENT2 is a platform for exploring Gene Expression patterns across Normal and Tumor tissues [36] (http://gent2.appex.kr). From Log2FC value, target genes were considered as oncogenes (Log2FC > 0, $P < 0.05$) or tumor suppressors of BC (Log2FC < 0, $P < 0.05$).

MiRNAs may contribute to (onco-miRNAs) or repress (tumor suppressor miRNAs) the cancer phenotype by inhibiting the expression of tumor suppressor genes or oncogenes, respectively. Therefore, the role of miRNAs in BC can be predicted based on the role of target genes in BC. MiRNAs are considered oncogenic miRNAs when their target genes act as tumor suppressors. Furthermore, conversely, miRNAs were considered tumor-suppressive miRNAs when they target oncogenes. The presence of SNPs on the seed region can alter the target, thereby changing the role of miRNAs in BC.

2.4 Predicting the interaction between miRNAs and targets

The interaction between mature miRNA sequences, in both reference and alternative allele versions of the SNP, and their target genes were analyzed based on the number of seed binding sites of a miRNA at the 3'UTR by TargetScan 8.0 [37] and the Minimum Free Energy (MFE) of the whole mature miRNA sequence with the 3'UTR by RNAhybrid. The target sequences extracted from TargetScan 8.0 (http://www.targetscan.org/vert_80/). The miRNA sequences were further included in RNAhybrid (https://bibiserv.cebitec.uni-bielefeld.de/rnahybrid), a tool for finding the MFE hybridization of a long and a short RNA [38]. The MFE values should be between −10 and − 30 kcal/mole. The more negative the MFE value (closer to −30), the stronger the interaction of the mature miRNA sequence with the 3'UTR. A miRNA can bind at multiple sites on the 3'UTR of its target, and each interaction site has a corresponding MFE value. Therefore, the interaction between the 3'UTR and the whole mature sequence of miRNA was determined via the mean value of MFEs from all miRNA binding sites on 3'UTR (Mean MFE).

The level of miRNA inhibition on target genes could be influenced by the presence of an alternative allele SNP, which could be shown through the difference between the mean MFE value of the alternative and reference allele version (ΔG). A non-zero ΔG value means a difference in the interaction degree with the same target between miRNA reference and alteration, indicating the SNP is potentially associated with BC risk. A ΔG value of 0 indicates no change in the level of interaction between the miRNA reference and the miRNA variation with the same target, suggesting that the SNP is unlikely to relate to BC risk.

3. Results

3.1 SNPs in miRNA mature sequences

This study collected a list of 169 SNPs on mature sequences of 161 miRNAs from miRNASNP-v3. The mature reference sequences of 161 miRNAs were obtained from miRBase. The 169 alternative mature sequences of miRNAs corresponding to positional changes of 169 SNPs identified from dbSNP are described in Supplement 1.

3.2 In silico target prediction in BC pathways

After predicting the target genes of the reference and alternative sequences by miRDB (score $\geq$ 80) and comparing them in the list of genes on the BC pathway of KEGG, out of 161 miRNAs, there are 100 miRNAs with functional targets in BC (Supplement 2). Thirty-eight miRNAs with 38 in-seed SNPs had altered targets, and 62 with 63 out-seed SNPs did not change targets. The most likely target gene, which has the highest target score, of each miRNA was selected to analyze the possible effect on BC further.

3.3 Function prediction of target genes and miRNAs in BC

The functional target genes in BC were determined from the GENT2 database. Hence, the function of miRNAs in BC was also predicted. Of the 38 miRNAs with altered targets, the targets of 31 miRNAs were functionally altered in BC under the influence of SNPs (**Table 1**). Of these 31 miRNAs, 4 predicted onco-miRNAs were predicted to change to tumor suppressor miRNAs because of their new target working as oncogenes (hsa-miR-4257, hsa-miR-499a-3p, hsa-miR-501-3p, hsa-miR-593-5p), 5 predicted onco-miRNAs were predicted to lost targets in BC (hsa-miR-1178-5p, hsa-miR-4482-5p, hsa-miR-4661-3p, hsa-miR-5589-3p, hsa-miR-7854-3p), 6 predicted tumor suppressor miRNAs were predicted to change to onco-miRNAs because of their new target working as tumor suppressor genes (hsa-miR-1302, hsa-miR-2682-3p, hsa-miR-3117-3p, hsa-miR-4695-5p, hsa-miR-5692b, hsa-miR-6810-5p), 1 tumor suppressor miRNA was predicted to lost targets in BC (hsa-miR-627-5p), 10 miRNAs were predicted to gain onco-miRNAs (hsa-miR-4513, hsa-miR-4707-3p, hsa-miR-4741, hsa-miR-4781-3p, hsa-miR-4804-5p, hsa-miR-5090, hsa-miR-662, hsa-miR-6796-3p, hsa-miR-6826-5p, hsa-miR-6879-3p), and 5 miRNAs were predicted to gain tumor suppressor miRNAs (hsa-miR-1269b, hsa-miR-4467, hsa-miR-6717-5p, hsa-miR-6763-3p, hsa-miR-6777-5p). By altering the function of miRNAs, 31 in-seed SNPs on these miRNAs are likely to be associated with BC risk (**Table 1**).

The remaining 7 of 38 miRNAs with altered targets were predicted to remain functional despite the allele change of the SNPs (**Table 2**). Four (hsa-miR-146a-3p, hsa-miR-4284, hsa-miR-4731-3p, hsa-miR-557) and three miRNAs (hsa-miR-3622a-5p, hsa-miR-449c-3p, hsa-miR-548 t-3p) were predicted to be onco-miRNAs and tumor suppressor miRNAs, respectively.

miRNA	SNP			Reference					Alternative					
	ID	Position	Allele	Target				Role of miRNA	Allele	Target				Role of miRNA
				Gene	Log2FC	Expression trend	Category			Gene	Log2FC	Expression trend	Category	
hsa-miR-1178-5p	rs7311975	chr12:119713688	T	FGF9	−1.22	Down	Tumor suppressor genes	Onco-miRNA	C					
hsa-miR-1269b	rs7210937	chr17:12917329	G						C	DVL3	0.28	Up	Oncogenes	Tumor suppressor miRNA
hsa-miR-1302	rs74647838	chr12:112695096	G	ESR1	0.95	Up	Oncogenes	Tumor suppressor miRNA	A	CTNNB1	−0.40	Down	Tumor suppressor genes	Onco-miRNA
hsa-miR-2682-3p	rs74904371	chr1:98045291	C	TNFSF11	1.80	Up	Oncogenes	Tumor suppressor miRNA	T	SOS1	−0.43	Down	Tumor suppressor genes	Onco-miRNA
hsa-miR-3117-3p	rs12402181	chr1:66628488	G	KRAS	0.31	Up	Oncogenes	Tumor suppressor miRNA	A	SOS2	−0.37	Down	Tumor suppressor genes	Onco-miRNA
hsa-miR-4257	rs74743733	chr1:150551992	G	MAPK1	−0.09	Down	Tumor suppressor genes	Onco-miRNA	A	E2F2	1.20	Up	Oncogenes	Tumor suppressor miRNA
hsa-miR-4467	rs115101071	chr7:102471476	G						A	IGF1R	0.41	Up	Oncogenes	Tumor suppressor miRNA
hsa-miR-4482-5p	rs45596840	chr10:104268396	G	TCF7	−0.47	Down	Tumor suppressor genes	Onco-miRNA	A					
hsa-miR-4513	rs2168518	chr15:74788737	G						A	NCOA1	−0.21	Down	Tumor suppressor genes	Onco-miRNA
hsa-miR-4661-3p	rs12335005	chr8:91205534	G	NOTCH2	−0.60	Down	Tumor suppressor genes	Onco-miRNA	T					

miRNA	SNP		Reference						Alternative					
	ID	Position	Allele	Target				Role of miRNA	Allele	Target				Role of miRNA
				Gene	Log2FC	Expression trend	Category			Gene	Log2FC	Expression trend	Category	
hsa-miR-4695-5p	rs79637190	chr1:18883265	C	SHC1	0.21	Up	Oncogenes	Tumor suppressor miRNA	T	MAPK1	−0.09	Down	Tumor suppressor genes	Onco-miRNA
hsa-miR-4707-3p	rs2273626	chr14:22956973	C						A	FGF9	−1.22	Down	Tumor suppressor genes	Onco-miRNA
hsa-miR-4741	rs7227168	chr18:22933411	C						T	FZD8	−0.70	Down	Tumor suppressor genes	Onco-miRNA
hsa-miR-4781-3p	rs74085143	chr1:54054127	G						A	FGF2	−1.44	Down	Tumor suppressor genes	Onco-miRNA
hsa-miR-4804-5p	rs266435	chr5:72878605	C						G	WNT2B	−0.96	Down	Tumor suppressor genes	Onco-miRNA
hsa-miR-499a-3p	rs3746444	chr20:34990448	A	TCF7L2	−0.68	Down	Tumor suppressor genes	Onco-miRNA	G	WNT4	0.38	Up	Oncogenes	Tumor suppressor miRNA
hsa-miR-501-3p	rs149912461	chrX:50009773	A	HEY1	−0.39	Down	Tumor suppressor genes	Onco-miRNA	G	FGF4	0.30	Up	Oncogenes	Tumor suppressor miRNA
hsa-miR-5090	rs3823658	chr7:102465754	G						A	FZD4	−1.31	Down	Tumor suppressor genes	Onco-miRNA
hsa-miR-5589-3p	rs116796353	chr19:10038396	A	MAP2K1	−0.16	Down	Tumor suppressor genes	Onco-miRNA	G					
hsa-miR-5692b	rs451887	chr21:42951004	T	FGF18	0.34	Up	Oncogenes	Tumor suppressor miRNA	C	EGF	−0.71	Down	Tumor suppressor genes	Onco-miRNA

miRNA	SNP		Reference						Alternative					
	ID	Position	Allele	Target				Role of miRNA	Allele	Target				Role of miRNA
				Gene	Log2FC	Expression trend	Category			Gene	Log2FC	Expression trend	Category	
hsa-miR-593-5p	rs73721294	chr7:128081882	C	SP1	−0.29	Down	Tumor suppressor genes	Onco-miRNA	T	KRAS	0.31	Up	Oncogenes	Tumor suppressor miRNA
hsa-miR-627-5p	rs2620381	chr15:42199650	A	DVL3	0.28	Up	Oncogenes	Tumor suppressor miRNA	C					
hsa-miR-662	rs9745376	chr16:770249	G						A	IGF1	−1.13	Down	Tumor suppressor genes	Onco-miRNA
hsa-miR-6717-5p	rs117650137	chr14:21023373	G						A	SHC1	0.21	Up	Oncogenes	Tumor suppressor miRNA
hsa-miR-6763-3p	rs3751304	chr12:132582046	C						T	WNT4	0.38	Up	Oncogenes	Tumor suppressor miRNA
hsa-miR-6777-5p	rs56155608	chr17:17813539	G						A	CSNK1A1	0.13	Up	Oncogenes	Tumor suppressor miRNA
hsa-miR-6796-3p	rs3745198	chr19:40369893	C						G	CDK6	−0.67	Down	Tumor suppressor genes	Onco-miRNA
hsa-miR-6810-5p	rs62182086	chr2:218341922	A	CSNK1A1	0.13	Up	Oncogenes	Tumor suppressor miRNA	G	FGF19	−1.16	Down	Tumor suppressor genes	Onco-miRNA
hsa-miR-6826-5p	rs6771809	chr3:129272155	T						C	MTOR	−0.22	Down	Tumor suppressor genes	Onco-miRNA

miRNA	SNP		Reference						Alternative					
	ID	Position	Allele	Target				Role of miRNA	Allele	Target				Role of miRNA
				Gene	Log2FC	Expression trend	Category			Gene	Log2FC	Expression trend	Category	
hsa-miR-6879-3p	rs74814065	chr11:65018557	C						T	FGF9	−1.22	Down	Tumor suppressor genes	Onco-miRNA
hsa-miR-7854-3p	rs2925980	chr16:81533949	A	AKT3	−0.41	Down	Tumor suppressor genes	Onco-miRNA	G					

Ref = The allele in the reference genome. Alt = Any other allele found at that locus. Target gene with score ≥ 80. Log2FC = Log 2 Fold Change with $P < 0.05$.

Table 1.
Prediction of the effect of in-seed SNPs in 31 miRNAs on BC development.

MiRNA	ID	Position	Reference							Alternative							ΔG
			Allele	Target				Role of miRNA	Mean MFE	Allele	Target				Role of miRNA	Mean MFE	
				Gene	Log2FC	Expression trend	Category				Gene	Log2FC	Expression trend	Category			
has-miR-146a-3p	rs2910164	chr5:160485411	C	FZD4	−1.31	Down	Tumor suppressor genes	Onco-miRNA	−16.55	G	WNT9B	−0.40	Down	Tumor suppressor genes	Onco-miRNA	−18.2	−1.7
hsa-miR-3622a-5p	rs66683138	chr8:27701697	G	E2F3	0.25	Up	Oncogenes	Tumor suppressor miRNA	−22.6	A	SHC1	0.21	Up	Oncogenes	Tumor suppressor miRNA	−19.4	3.2
hsa-miR-4284	rs11973069	chr7:73711334	C	FZD4	−1.31	Down	Tumor suppressor genes	Onco-miRNA	−23.7	T	DLL1	−0.64	Down	Tumor suppressor genes	Onco-miRNA	−20.5	3.2
hsa-miR-449c-3p	rs35770269	chr5:55172296	A	KRAS	0.31	Up	Oncogenes	Tumor suppressor miRNA	−18.2	T	AKT2	0.05	Up	Oncogenes	Tumor suppressor miRNA	−17.6	0.6
hsa-miR-4731-3p	rs66507245	chr17:15251649	T	NOTCH2	−0.60	Down	Tumor suppressor genes	Onco-miRNA	−14.7	A	CTNNB1	−0.39	Down	Tumor suppressor genes	Onco-miRNA	−19.7	−5.0
hsa-miR-548 t-3p	rs73872515	chr4:173268209	A	NRAS	0.21	Up	Oncogenes	Tumor suppressor miRNA	−15.2	C	IGF1R	0.41	Up	Oncogenes	Tumor suppressor miRNA	−16.7	−1.5
hsa-miR-557	rs78825966	chr1:168375591	C	RPS6KB1	−0.05	Down	Tumor suppressor genes	Onco-miRNA	−18.8	T	PGR	−0.85	Down	Tumor suppressor genes	Onco-miRNA	−18.5	0.3

Log2FC = Log 2 Fold Change with $P < 0.05$.
MFE: Minimum Free Energy between miRNA and 3'UTR (kcal/mol).
ΔG: The difference of mean MFE between alterative allele and reference allele.

Table 2.
Prediction of the effect of in-seed SNPs in 7 miRNAs on the degree of miRNA role in BC.

For the 62 miRNAs with 63 out-seed SNPs, the targets were not changed because the seed sequence was preserved between the two alleles of the SNPs (**Table 3**). The result showed that 44 and 18 miRNAs were predicted to function as oncogene and tumor suppressors, respectively. The predictive results do not sufficiently demonstrate an association of these 70 SNPs with BC risk. Therefore, the next step is further to predict the interaction of 69 miRNAs and targets to elucidate the potential association of these 70 SNPs on BC risk.

3.4 Predicting the interaction between miRNAs and targets

Among the 69 miRNAs, the interaction of 12 miRNAs with their targets did not differ under the allele variation of the SNPs ($\Delta G = 0$) (**Table 3**), indicating 12 SNPs in these 12 miRNAs are not likely to be associated with BC risk. The remaining 57 miRNAs have different levels of interaction with their targets under the allele variation of the SNPs ($\Delta G \neq 0$) (**Tables 2** and **3**). It suggested that 58 SNPs in these miRNAs are potentially associated with BC risk (**Tables 2** and **3**).

4. Discussion

In knowledge and improvements in bioinformatics, computational predictions of causative factors are being used as a supplementary approach to support the practical assessment of multifactorial disorders. Although miRNA can modulate up to 92% of mammalian genes, only a few target pairings of miRNAs have been experimentally verified [39]. Numerous technical challenges, such as tissue selectivity, poor expression, 3' UTR selection, and miRNA preservation, make existing methodologies difficult for experimental confirmation of interactions between miRNAs and their mRNA targets [40]. Recognizing functional SNPs in genes and examining their impacts on phenotypes may allow for more in-depth knowledge of the possible consequences of making such changes. Biogenesis, expression level, and biological function are all influenced by SNPs in human miRNA genes. For identifying the possible impacts of SNPs, several useful bioinformatics tools have been developed. All mature microRNAs with SNPs implicated in BC and their target genes were obtained. In addition, bioinformatics strategies for predicting these functional SNPs were presented. All steps and results are summarized in **Figure 1**.

The results showed that 12 SNPs did not appear to be associated with BC risk. Thirty-one in-seed SNPs are likely to be strongly associated with disease risk by altering miRNA function in BC (**Table 1**). 58 SNPs appear to be moderately or weakly associated with BC risk by altering the degree of interaction between miRNAs and their targets (**Tables 2** and **3**). According to the most significant difference between Mean MFE values in the hsa-miR-4731-3p, the effect of T/A replacement can significantly increase the change of interaction ($\Delta G = -5$); thus, it increases the effect of SNP rs66507245 on the risk of BC (**Table 2**). It seems that the association of rs66507245 with BC risk was moderate among the group of 70 SNPs predicted based on the ΔG value. The most negligible difference occurs in hsa-miR-6077, hsa-miR-8060, hsa-miR-4704-3p, and hsa-miR-6868-3p, indicating the effect of the SNPs on BC risk were weak (**Table 3**).

These SNPs were not found in GWASs since GWAS is a whole-genome sequencing approach that does not determine SNPs in non-coding regions. Only four SNPs (rs3746444, rs2910164, rs11614913, and rs4919510) have been investigated for the

MiRNA	ID	Position	Allele Ref./Alt.	Target				Role of miRNA	Mean MFE		ΔG
				Gene	Log2FC	Expression trend	Category		Ref.	Alt.	
hsa-miR-449b-5p	rs10061133	chr5:55170716	A/G	DLL1	−0.64	Down	Tumor suppressor genes	Onco-miRNA	−25.8	−24.6	1.2
hsa-miR-6801-3p	rs10412196	chr19:52222085	T/C	AKT3	−0.41	Down	Tumor suppressor genes	Onco-miRNA	−20.8	−19.8	1.1
hsa-miR-548ae-5p	rs10461441	chr5:58530093	A/G	CDK6	−0.67	Down	Tumor suppressor genes	Onco-miRNA	−14.2	−12.9	1.3
hsa-miR-4700-3p	rs1055070	chr12:120723245	T/G	NCOA3	−0.01	Down	Tumor suppressor genes	Onco-miRNA	−18.1	−18.6	−0.5
hsa-miR-4302	rs11048315	chr12:25874055	G/A	CDK6	−0.67	Down	Tumor suppressor genes	Onco-miRNA	−19.4	−19.0	0.4
hsa-miR-5579-3p	rs11237828	chr11:79422176	T/C	JAG1	−0.21	Down	Tumor suppressor genes	Onco-miRNA	−18.6	−18.6	0.0
hsa-miR-501-3p	rs112489955	chrX:50009781	G/A	CDK6	−0.67	Down	Tumor suppressor genes	Onco-miRNA	−18.3	−18.3	0.0
hsa-miR-5691	rs112511786	chr11:9090358	G/C	MAPK1	−0.09	Down	Tumor suppressor genes	Onco-miRNA	−19.1	−19.7	−0.6
hsa-miR-4786-5p	rs115063401	chr2:239943064	G/A	AKT3	−0.41	Down	Tumor suppressor genes	Onco-miRNA	−23.7	−23.7	0.0
hsa-miR-580-5p	rs115089112	chr5:36147955	T/C	FZD3	0.31	Up	Oncogenes	Tumor suppressor miRNA	−13.4	−13.9	−0.5
hsa-miR-3124-3p	rs115160731	chr1:248826432	C/A	PGR	−0.86	Down	Tumor suppressor genes	Onco-miRNA	−16.0	−17.0	−1.0
hsa-miR-942-3p	rs115372145	chr1:117094703	C/T	SOS2	−0.37	Down	Tumor suppressor genes	Onco-miRNA	−18.3	−18.3	0.0
hsa-miR-4457	rs115769169	chr5:1309319	C/T	APC	−0.22	Down	Tumor suppressor genes	Onco-miRNA	−16.7	−16.1	0.6

MiRNA	ID	Position	Allele Ref./Alt.	Target				Role of miRNA	Mean MFE		ΔG
				Gene	Log2FC	Expression trend	Category		Ref.	Alt.	
hsa-miR-3130-3p	rs115772313	chr2:206783285	G/A	E2F3	0.25	Up	Oncogenes	Tumor suppressor miRNA	−17.3	−17.3	0.0
hsa-miR-4514	rs116034786	chr15:80997457	A/G	ESR1	0.95	Up	Oncogenes	Tumor suppressor miRNA	−22.1	−20.4	1.7
hsa-miR-196a-3p	rs11614913	chr12:53991815	C/T	JAG1	−0.21	Down	Tumor suppressor genes	Onco-miRNA	−19.9	−13.9	1.0
hsa-miR-548at-5p	rs11651671	chr17:42494785	G/A	PGR	−0.86	Down	Tumor suppressor genes	Onco-miRNA	−15.3	−13.8	1.5
hsa-miR-3192-3p	rs11907020	chr20:18470681	T/C	NCOA3	−0.01	Down	Tumor suppressor genes	Onco-miRNA	−14.0	−14.0	0.0
hsa-miR-5700	rs12314280	chr12:94561809	T/C	AXIN2	−0.51	Down	Tumor suppressor genes	Onco-miRNA	−12.9	−14.4	−1.5
hsa-miR-4433a-5p	rs12473206	chr2:64340782	C/G	KRAS	0.31	Up	Oncogenes	Tumor suppressor miRNA	−17.0	−16.6	0.4
hsa-miR-6077	rs1280409926	chr1:148388307	C/T	SP1	−0.29	Down	Tumor suppressor genes	Onco-miRNA	−21.7	−21.9	−0.2
hsa-miR-548 l	rs13447640	chr11:94466555	G/A	SP1	−0.29	Down	Tumor suppressor genes	Onco-miRNA	−14.5	−15.9	−1.5
hsa-miR-548ar-3p	rs141659366	chr13:114244551	G/A	FZD4	−1.31	Down	Tumor suppressor genes	Onco-miRNA	−14.4	−12.9	1.5
hsa-miR-4444	rs142357696	chr3:75214531	A/G	E2F1	1.18	Up	Oncogenes	Tumor suppressor miRNA	−24.7	−22.1	2.6
hsa-miR-888-5p	rs143634721	chrX:145994837	C/A	PGR	−0.86	Down	Tumor suppressor genes	Onco-miRNA	−16.2	−15.3	0.9
hsa-miR-892b	rs146806052	chrX:145997215	A/G	DLL1	−0.64	Down	Tumor suppressor genes	Onco-miRNA	−21.0	−24.2	−3.2

MiRNA	ID	Position	Allele Ref./ Alt.	Target				Role of miRNA	Mean MFE		ΔG
				Gene	Log2FC	Expression trend	Category		Ref.	Alt.	
hsa-miR-8060	rs1514422	chr3:96360020	G/A	KRAS	0.31	Up	Oncogenes	Tumor suppressor miRNA	−18.3	−18.5	−0.2
hsa-miR-6887-5p	rs1688017	chr19:35122719	G/A	PIK3R3	0.33	Up	Oncogenes	Tumor suppressor miRNA	−28.7	−25.2	3.5
hsa-miR-1304-3p	rs2155248	chr11:93733700	G/T	NOTCH2	−0.60	Down	Tumor suppressor genes	Onco-miRNA	−18.3	−18.6	−0.3
hsa-miR-3130-5p	rs2241347	chr2:206783257	C/T	TCF7	−0.47	Down	Tumor suppressor genes	Onco-miRNA	−22.3	−22.6	−0.4
hsa-miR-1343-5p	rs2986407	chr11:34941869	T/C	CSNK1A1	0.13	Up	Oncogenes	Tumor suppressor miRNA	−21.7	−20.9	0.8
hsa-miR-5087	rs2992458	chr1:148334528	A/G	GSK3B	0.14	Up	Oncogenes	Tumor suppressor miRNA	−17.2	−16.2	1.0
hsa-miR-5189-3p	rs35613341	chr16:88468999	C/G	JAG1	−0.21	Down	Tumor suppressor genes	Onco-miRNA	−25.6	−28.3	−2.7
hsa-miR-8084	rs404337	chr8:93029770	G/A	NOTCH1	−0.28	Down	Tumor suppressor genes	Onco-miRNA	−12.7	−13.4	−0.7
hsa-miR-548ap-5p	rs4414449	chr15:85825667	G/A	CDK6	−0.67	Down	Tumor suppressor genes	Onco-miRNA	−14.0	−13.0	0.9
hsa-miR-608	rs4919510	chr10:100975021	C/G	CDKN1A	−0.36	Down	Tumor suppressor genes	Onco-miRNA	−30.7	−31.2	−0.5
hsa-miR-7157-3p	rs56148568	chr2:140586631	T/C	EGFR	−1.44	Down	Tumor suppressor genes	Onco-miRNA	−19.1	−19.1	0.0
hsa-miR-6744-3p	rs56310773	chr11:1256664	C/T	PIK3R1	−0.81	Down	Tumor suppressor genes	Onco-miRNA	−32.5	−30.0	2.5
hsa-miR-6805-3p	rs56312243	chr19:55388234	C/T	MAPK1	−0.09	Down	Tumor suppressor genes	Onco-miRNA	−19.5	−19.7	−0.3

MiRNA	ID	Position	Allele Ref./ Alt.	Target				Role of miRNA	Mean MFE		ΔG
				Gene	Log2FC	Expression trend	Category		Ref.	Alt.	
hsa-miR-6071	rs56790095	chr2:85783659	C/G	WNT3	0.34	Up	Oncogenes	Tumor suppressor miRNA	−17.0	−17.0	0.0
hsa-miR-548ab	rs59323834	chr3:103524093	C/T	CDK6	−0.67	Down	Tumor suppressor genes	Onco-miRNA	−14.6	−12.1	2.5
hsa-miR-3928-5p	rs5997893	chr22:31160117	A/G	ESR1	0.95	Up	Oncogenes	Tumor suppressor miRNA	−17.7	−15.6	2.1
hsa-miR-596	rs61388742	chr8:1817259	T/C	PTEN	−0.26	Down	Tumor suppressor genes	Onco-miRNA	−19.7	−17.5	2.2
hsa-miR-3922-5p	rs61938575	chr12:104591665	G/A	SHC1	0.21	Up	Oncogenes	Tumor suppressor miRNA	−28.6	−27.3	1.4
hsa-miR-4772-5p	rs62154973	chr2:102432320	C/T	FOS	−1.17	Down	Tumor suppressor genes	Onco-miRNA	−20.3	−20.3	0.0
hsa-miR-646	rs6513497	chr20:60308547	T/G	PIK3R1	−0.81	Down	Tumor suppressor genes	Onco-miRNA	−23.4	−20.9	2.6
hsa-miR-8063	rs7162033	chr15:36972836	C/G	IGF1	−1.13	Down	Tumor suppressor genes	Onco-miRNA	−17.6	−15.9	1.7
hsa-miR-8063	rs7183051	chr15:36972838	G/A	IGF1	−1.13	Down	Tumor suppressor genes	Onco-miRNA	−17.6	−16.9	0.7
hsa-miR-6868-3p	rs7208391	chr17:76098024	C/G	AXIN2	−0.51	Down	Tumor suppressor genes	Onco-miRNA	−18.8	−18.5	0.2
hsa-miR-4679	rs72810954	chr10:89063382	G/A	WNT16	0.12	Up	Oncogenes	Tumor suppressor miRNA	−17.0	−17.0	0.0
hsa-miR-4799-5p	rs72955519	chr4:147782619	G/A	MAPK1	−0.09	Down	Tumor suppressor genes	Onco-miRNA	−18.8	−16.3	2.5
hsa-miR-4999-5p	rs72996752	chr19:8389352	A/G	CTNNB1	−0.40	Down	Tumor suppressor genes	Onco-miRNA	−18.5	−17.4	1.1
hsa-miR-624-3p	rs73251987	chr14:31014677	C/G	GSK3B	0.14	Up	Oncogenes	Tumor suppressor miRNA	−15.5	−13.7	1.9

MiRNA	ID	Position	Allele Ref./Alt.	Target				Role of miRNA	Mean MFE		ΔG
				Gene	Log2FC	Expression trend	Category		Ref.	Alt.	
hsa-miR-4727-5p	rs73295187	chr17:38825855	A/C	CDK6	−0.67	Down	Tumor suppressor genes	Onco-miRNA	−21.4	−19.6	1.8
hsa-miR-4739	rs73410309	chr17:79707227	G/C	BAK1	0.49	Up	Oncogenes	Tumor suppressor miRNA	−32.5	−31.6	0.9
hsa-miR-6504-5p	rs74469188	chr16:81611365	T/C	FZD5	−0.56	Down	Tumor suppressor genes	Onco-miRNA	−21.9	−21.5	0.4
hsa-miR-323b-5p	rs75330474	chr14:101056252	C/T	PIK3R3	0.33	Up	Oncogenes	Tumor suppressor miRNA	−18.5	−16.5	2.0
hsa-miR-6841-3p	rs76347846	chr8:24953808	A/G	GADD45A	−0.30	Down	Tumor suppressor genes	Onco-miRNA	−19.1	−15.2	3.9
hsa-miR-4704-3p	rs76595065	chr13:66218307	T/C	GSK3B	0.14	Up	Oncogenes	Tumor suppressor miRNA	−23.2	−23.4	−0.2
hsa-miR-6839-5p	rs7804972	chr7:64679085	G/A	CDK6	−0.67	Down	Tumor suppressor genes	Onco-miRNA	−19.4	−18.1	1.3
hsa-miR-6885-5p	rs78293125	chr19:6389688	A/G	TCF7L2	−0.68	Down	Tumor suppressor genes	Onco-miRNA	−24.4	−24.4	0.0
hsa-miR-4520-3p	rs8078913	chr17:6655449	C/G	GRB2	0.35	Up	Oncogenes	Tumor suppressor miRNA	−24.2	−21.2	3.0
hsa-miR-548 h-5p	rs9913045	chr17:13543607	G/A	CDK6	−0.67	Down	Tumor suppressor genes	Onco-miRNA	−13.8	−13.8	0.0

Ref = The allele in the reference genome. Alt = any other allele found at that locus.
Log2FC = Log 2 fold change with $P < 0.05$.
MFE: Minimum free energy between miRNA and 3'UTR (kcal/mol).
Mean MFE: the mean value of MFEs from all miRNA binding sites on 3'UTR.
ΔG: The difference of mean MFE between alterative allele and reference allele.

Table 3.
Prediction of the effect of 63 out-seed SNPs in 62 miRNAs on the degree of miRNA role in BC.

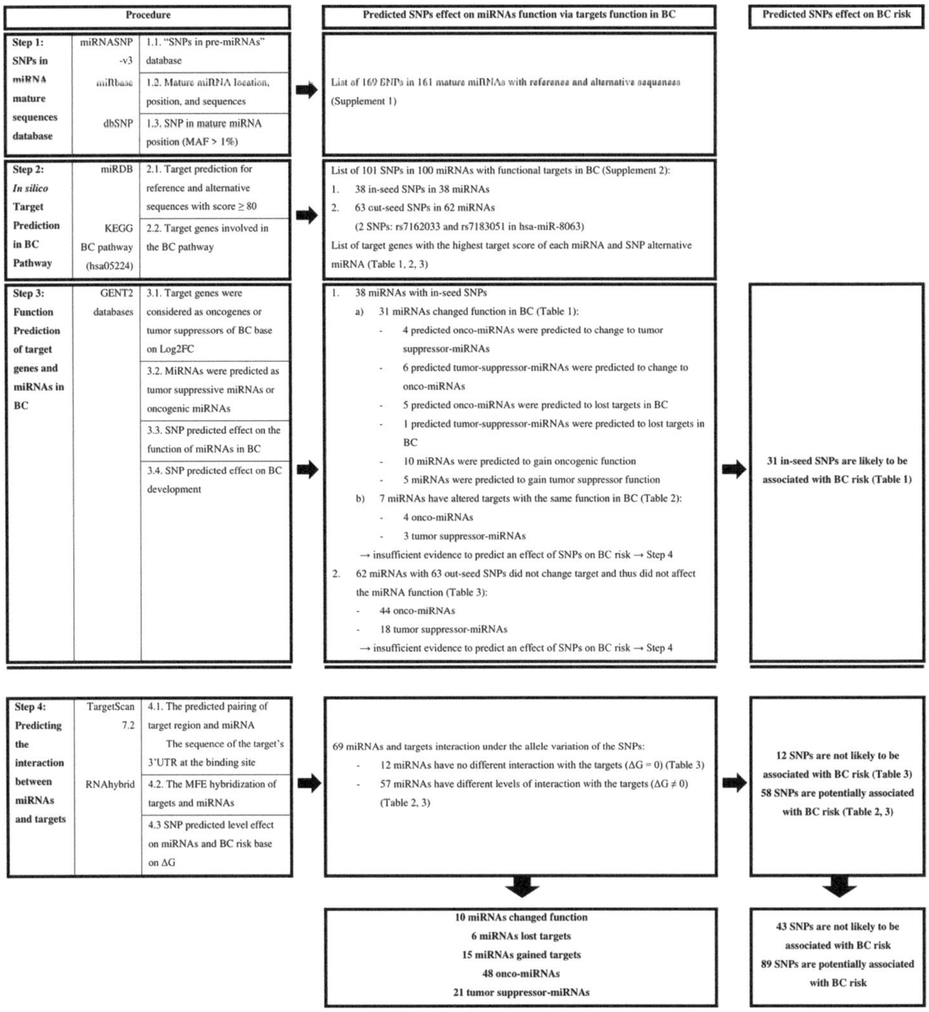

Figure 1.
The methodology and summary results of study.

association with BC risk in case–control studies. The presence of the C allele of rs2910164, an in-seed SNP, in hsa-miR-146a-3p was associated with an increased risk of BC (C vs. G: OR = 1.4, 95% CI = 1.03–1.85, p = 0.03) [41]. Allele C of rs11614913 in hsa-miR-196a-3p was found to be significantly associated with decreased risk of BC (C vs. T: OR = 0.64, 95%CI = 0.49–0.85, p = 0.0019) [42]. Allele G of rs3746444 in seed region of hsa-miR-499a-3p significantly increased BC susceptibility only among Asians (G vs. A: OR = 1.12, 95% CI = 1.00–1.26, P = 0.04) [43]. The G allele rs4919510 in hsa-miR-608 decreased the risk of BC (G vs. C: OR = 0.53, 95%CI 0.30–0.92, p = 0.024) [44]. The remaining 97 SNPs have not been identified for an association with BC risk in any association studies. However, 7 of these (rs7210937, rs12402181, rs2273626, rs2620381, rs35770269, rs10061133, and rs6513497) are associated with the risk of other cancers, including oral and pharyngeal squamous cell carcinoma [45], acute lymphoblastic leukemia [46], leukopenia [47], gastric cancer [48], colon cancer [49], esophageal squamous cell carcinoma [50], and hepatocellular carcinoma [51].

These shreds of evidence suggest that candidate SNPs in this study can be associated with risk in BC and other types of cancer.

At the level of investigating the role of miRNAs in BC, 31 miRNAs and 69 miRNAs were predicted to change and remain unchanged function in the presence of SNP allele changes, respectively. Among them, 7 miRNAs (miR-4513, miR-501-3p, miR-580-5p, miR-3130-3p, miR-196a-3p, miR-8084, and miR-3922-5p) had predicted roles in BC consistent with the results of previous functional studies. Hsa-miR-4513, has-miR-196a-3p, and has-miR-8084 suggested functions as an oncogene in the progression of BC [52–54] were also predicted as onco-miRNAs in this study (**Tables 1** and **3**). Hsa-miR-501-3p, has-miR-580-5p, has-miR-3130-3p, and has-miR-3922-5p indicated tumor suppressor function [55–58] were also predicted as tumor suppressor miRNAs (**Tables 1** and **3**).

Our work gives vital insights into the pathophysiology and progression of BC by presenting essential information on the likely influence of SNPs and distinct regulation patterns on miRNA production and function. Consequently, genetic variations appear to be the appropriate criterion for early diagnosis of BCs in future.

5. Conclusion

In brief, numerous resources were applied following a comprehensive screening of mature miRNAs, including SNPs that play a deciding role on BC to identify SNP's functional effect in the miRNA gene. We conducted a thorough investigation into the influence of the mined SNPs on miRNA function, including target prediction, miRNA-target interaction, and target expression level. Theoretically, this work revealed a list of possible causative SNPs in the mature miRNA gene that may be addressed for further practical research in BC management.

Acknowledgements

This research was funded by Vietnam National University, Ho Chi Minh City (VNU-HCM), under grant number 562-2020-2118-02.

Conflict of interest

The authors declare no potential conflicts of interest.

Credit authorship contribution statement

Thanh Thi Ngoc Nguyen was involved in conceptualization, methodology, formal analysis, data curation, software, writing—original draft, writing—editing, visualization, project administration, and funding acquisition. Thu Huynh Ngoc Nguyen was involved in investigation, validation, and writing—review. Luan Huu Huynh and Hoang Ngo Phan were involved in investigation and writing—review. Hue Thi Nguyen was involved in resources, conceptualization, methodology, supervision, writing—review, project administration, and funding acquisition.

Author details

Thanh Thi Ngoc Nguyen[1,2]*, Thu Huynh Ngoc Nguyen[2], Luan Huu Huynh[1,2], Hoang Ngo Phan[1,2] and Hue Thi Nguyen[1,2]

1 Faculty of Biology and Biotechnology, University of Science, Ho Chi Minh City, Vietnam

2 Vietnam National University, Ho Chi Minh City, Vietnam

*Address all correspondence to: ngtnthanh@hcmus.edu.vn

References

[1] Liu S, Clouthier SG, Wicha MS. Role of microRNAs in the regulation of breast cancer stem cells. Journal of Mammary Gland Biology and Neoplasia. 2012;**17**(1): 15-21

[2] Sung H, Ferlay J, Siegel RL, Laversanne M, Soerjomataram I, Jemal A, et al. Global cancer statistics 2020: GLOBOCAN estimates of incidence and mortality worldwide for 36 cancers in 185 countries. CA: a Cancer Journal for Clinicians. 2021;**71**(3):209-249

[3] Wahid F, Shehzad A, Khan T, Kim YY. MicroRNAs: Synthesis, mechanism, function, and recent clinical trials. Biochimica et Biophysica Acta. 2010;**1803**(11):1231-1243

[4] Galvão-Lima LJ, Morais AHF, Valentim RAM, Barreto EJSS. miRNAs as biomarkers for early cancer detection and their application in the development of new diagnostic tools. BioMedical Engineering OnLine. 2021;**20**(1):21

[5] Loh HY, Norman BP, Lai KS, Rahman N, Alitheen NBM, Osman MA. The regulatory role of MicroRNAs in breast cancer. International Journal of Molecular Sciences. 2019;**20**(19):4940

[6] Wang H, Tan Z, Hu H, Liu H, Wu T, Zheng C, et al. microRNA-21 promotes breast cancer proliferation and metastasis by targeting LZTFL1. BMC Cancer. 2019;**19**(1):738

[7] Li P, Guo Y, Bledsoe G, Yang Z, Chao L, Chao J. Kallistatin induces breast cancer cell apoptosis and autophagy by modulating Wnt signaling and microRNA synthesis. Experimental Cell Research. 2016;**340**(2):305-314

[8] Liu J, Li X, Wang M, Xiao G, Yang G, Wang H, et al. A miR-26a/E2F7 feedback loop contributes to tamoxifen resistance in ER-positive breast cancer. International Journal of Oncology. 2018; **53**(4):1601-1612

[9] Tormo E, Adam-Artigues A, Ballester S, Pineda B, Zazo S, Gonzalez-Alonso P, et al. The role of miR-26a and miR-30b in HER2+ breast cancer trastuzumab resistance and regulation of the CCNE2 gene. Scientific Reports. 2017;**7**:41309

[10] Dinami R, Ercolani C, Petti E, Piazza S, Ciani Y, Sestito R, et al. miR-155 drives telomere fragility in human breast cancer by targeting TRF1. Cancer Research. 2014;**74**(15):4145-4156

[11] Rao X, Di Leva G, Li M, Fang F, Devlin C, Hartman-Frey C, et al. MicroRNA-221/222 confers breast cancer fulvestrant resistance by regulating multiple signaling pathways. Oncogene. 2011;**30**(9):1082-1097

[12] Mishra S, Srivastava AK, Suman S, Kumar V, Shukla Y. Circulating miRNAs revealed as surrogate molecular signatures for the early detection of breast cancer. Cancer Letters. 2015; **369**(1):67-75

[13] Gong Y, He T, Yang L, Yang G, Chen Y, Zhang X. The role of miR-100 in regulating apoptosis of breast cancer cells. Scientific Reports. 2015;**5**:11650

[14] Pakravan K, Babashah S, Sadeghizadeh M, Mowla SJ, Mossahebi-Mohammadi M, Ataei F, et al. MicroRNA-100 shuttled by mesenchymal stem cell-derived exosomes suppresses in vitro angiogenesis through modulating the mTOR/HIF-1alpha/VEGF signaling axis in breast cancer cells. Cellular Oncology (Dordrecht). 2017;**40**(5):457-470

[15] Akhavantabasi S, Sapmaz A, Tuna S, Erson-Bensan AE. miR-125b targets ARID3B in breast cancer cells. Cell Structure and Function. 2012;**37**(1):27-38

[16] Chen J, Tian W, Cai H, He H, Deng Y. Down-regulation of microRNA-200c is associated with drug resistance in human breast cancer. Medical Oncology. 2012;**29**(4):2527-2534

[17] Alhasan L. MiR-126 modulates angiogenesis in breast cancer by targeting VEGF-A-mRNA. Asian Pacific Journal of Cancer Prevention. 2019; **20**(1):193-197

[18] Zou C, Xu Q, Mao F, Li D, Bian C, Liu LZ, et al. MiR-145 inhibits tumor angiogenesis and growth by N-RAS and VEGF. Cell Cycle. 2012;**11**(11):2137-2145

[19] Shi J, Zhang Y, Zheng W, Michailidou K, Ghoussaini M, Bolla MK, et al. Fine-scale mapping of 8q24 locus identifies multiple independent risk variants for breast cancer. International Journal of Cancer. 2016;**139**(6):1303-1317

[20] Bao L, Hazari S, Mehra S, Kaushal D, Moroz K, Dash S. Increased expression of P-glycoprotein and doxorubicin chemoresistance of metastatic breast cancer is regulated by miR-298. The American Journal of Pathology. 2012; **180**(6):2490-2503

[21] Meng Y, Zou Q, Liu T, Cai X, Huang Y, Pan J. microRNA-335 inhibits proliferation, cell-cycle progression, colony formation, and invasion via targeting PAX6 in breast cancer cells. Molecular Medicine Reports. 2015;**11**(1): 379-385

[22] Gao Y, Zeng F, Wu J-Y, Li H-Y, Fan J-J, Mai L, et al. MiR-335 inhibits migration of breast cancer cells through targeting oncoprotein c-met. Tumor Biology. 2015;**36**(4):2875-2883

[23] McAnena P, Tanriverdi K, Curran C, Gilligan K, Freedman JE, Brown JAL, et al. Circulating microRNAs miR-331 and miR-195 differentiate local luminal a from metastatic breast cancer. BMC Cancer. 2019;**19**(1):436

[24] Yerukala Sathipati S, Ho SY. Identifying a miRNA signature for predicting the stage of breast cancer. Scientific Reports. 2018;**8**(1):16138

[25] Farina NH, Ramsey JE, Cuke ME, Ahern TP, Shirley DJ, Stein JL, et al. Development of a predictive miRNA signature for breast cancer risk among high-risk women. Oncotarget. 2017; **8**(68):112170

[26] John B, Enright AJ, Aravin A, Tuschl T, Sander C, Marks DS. Human MicroRNA targets. PLoS Biology. 2004; **2**(11):e363

[27] Dong H, Lei J, Ding L, Wen Y, Ju H, Zhang X. MicroRNA: Function, detection, and bioanalysis. Chemical Reviews. 2013;**113**(8):6207-6233

[28] Ryan BM, Robles AI, Harris CC. Genetic variation in microRNA networks: The implications for cancer research. Nature Reviews. Cancer. 2010; **10**(6):389-402

[29] Grimson A, Farh KK, Johnston WK, Garrett-Engele P, Lim LP, Bartel DP. MicroRNA targeting specificity in mammals: Determinants beyond seed pairing. Molecular Cell. 2007;**27**(1):91-105

[30] Liu CJ, Fu X, Xia M, Zhang Q, Gu Z, Guo AY. miRNASNP-v3: A comprehensive database for SNPs and disease-related variations in miRNAs and miRNA targets. Nucleic Acids Research. 2021;**49**(D1):D1276-D1D81

[31] Kozomara A, Birgaoanu M, Griffiths-Jones S. miRBase: From

microRNA sequences to function. Nucleic Acids Research. 2019;**47**(D1): D155-DD62

[32] Sherry ST, Ward MH, Kholodov M, Baker J, Phan L, Smigielski EM, et al. dbSNP: The NCBI database of genetic variation. Nucleic Acids Research. 2001; **29**(1):308-311

[33] Chen Y, Wang X. miRDB: An online database for prediction of functional microRNA targets. Nucleic Acids Research. 2020;**48**(D1):D127-DD31

[34] Wong N, Wang X. miRDB: An online resource for microRNA target prediction and functional annotations. Nucleic Acids Research. 2015;**43** (Database issue):D146-D152

[35] Kanehisa M, Furumichi M, Tanabe M, Sato Y, Morishima K. KEGG: New perspectives on genomes, pathways, diseases and drugs. Nucleic Acids Research. 2017;**45**(D1):D353-DD61

[36] Park S-J, Yoon B-H, Kim S-K, Kim S-Y. GENT2: An updated gene expression database for normal and tumor tissues. BMC Medical Genomics. 2019;**12**(5):101

[37] McGeary SE, Lin KS, Shi CY, Pham TM, Bisaria N, Kelley GM, et al. The biochemical basis of microRNA targeting efficacy. Science (New York, NY). 2019;**366**(6472):eaav1741

[38] Rehmsmeier M, Steffen P, Hochsmann M, Giegerich R. Fast and effective prediction of microRNA/target duplexes. RNA. 2004;**10**(10):1507-1517

[39] Boissonneault V, Plante I, Rivest S, Provost P. MicroRNA-298 and microRNA-328 regulate expression of mouse beta-amyloid precursor protein-converting enzyme 1. The Journal of biological chemistry. 2009;**284**(4): 1971-81

[40] Andrés-León E, Cases I, Alonso S, Rojas AM. Novel miRNA-mRNA interactions conserved in essential cancer pathways. Scientific Reports. 2017;**7**(1):46101.

[41] Brincas HM, Augusto DG, Mathias C, Cavalli IJ, Lima RS, Kuroda F, et al. A genetic variant in microRNA-146a is associated with sporadic breast cancer in a southern Brazilian population. Genetics and Molecular Biology. 2020;**42**(4):e20190278

[42] Ahmad M, Shah AA. Predictive role of single nucleotide polymorphism (rs11614913) in the development of breast cancer in Pakistani population. Personalized Medicine. 2020;**17**(3):213-227

[43] Tan SC, Lim PY, Fang J, Mokhtar MFM, Hanif EAM, Jamal R. Association between MIR499A rs3746444 polymorphism and breast cancer susceptibility: A meta-analysis. Scientific Reports. 2020;**10**(1):3508

[44] Hashemi M, Sanaei S, Rezaei M, Bahari G, Hashemi SM, Mashhadi MA, et al. miR-608 rs4919510 C>G polymorphism decreased the risk of breast cancer in an Iranian subpopulation. Experimental Oncology. 2016;**38**(1):57-59

[45] Chen HC, Tseng YK, Chi CC, Chen YH, Yang CM, Huang SJ, et al. Genetic variants in microRNA-146a (C>G) and microRNA-1269b (G>C) are associated with the decreased risk of oral premalignant lesions, oral cancer, and pharyngeal cancer. Archives of Oral Biology. 2016;**72**:21-32

[46] Gutierrez-Camino A, Martin-Guerrero I, Dolzan V, Jazbec J, Carbone-Baneres A, Garcia de Andoin N, et al. Involvement of SNPs in miR-3117 and miR-3689d2 in childhood acute

lymphoblastic leukemia risk. Oncotarget. 2018;**9**(33):22907-22914

[47] Huang Y, Feng Y, Ren H, Zhang M, Li H, Qiao Y, et al. Associations of genetic variations in MicroRNA seed regions with acute adverse events and survival in patients with rectal cancer receiving postoperative Chemoradiation therapy. International Journal of Radiation Oncology, Biology, Physics. 2018;**100**(4):1026-1033

[48] Raad M, Salehi Z, Habibzaadeh Baalsini M, Mashayekhi F, Saeidi SH. Association of rs2620381 polymorphism in miR-627 and gastric cancer. British Journal of Biomedical Science. 2020; **77**(2):76-80

[49] Mao Y, Zou C, Meng F, Kong J, Wang W, Hua D. The SNPs in pre-miRNA are related to the response of capecitabine-based therapy in advanced colon cancer patients. Oncotarget. 2018; **9**(6):6793-6799

[50] Zhang P, Wang J, Lu T, Wang X, Zheng Y, Guo S, et al. miR-449b rs10061133 and miR-4293 rs12220909 polymorphisms are associated with decreased esophageal squamous cell carcinoma in a Chinese population. Tumour Biology. 2015;**36**(11):8789-8795

[51] Wang R, Zhang J, Jiang W, Ma Y, Li W, Jin B, et al. Association between a variant in microRNA-646 and the susceptibility to hepatocellular carcinoma in a large-scale population. ScientificWorldJournal. 2014;**2014**: 312704

[52] Li Y, Zhu H, Wang J, Qian X, Li N. miR-4513 promotes breast cancer progression through targeting TRIM3. American Journal of Translational Research. 2019;**11**(4):2431-2438

[53] Xiong M, Wang P, Pan B, Nie J, Wang S, He B. The diagnostic and prognostic values of microRNA-196a in cancer. Bioscience Reports. 2021;**41**(1): BSR20203559

[54] Gao Y, Ma H, Gao C, Lv Y, Chen X, Xu R, et al. Tumor-promoting properties of miR-8084 in breast cancer through enhancing proliferation, suppressing apoptosis and inducing epithelial-mesenchymal transition. Journal of Translational Medicine. 2018;**16**(1):38

[55] Hadavi R, Mohammadi-Yeganeh S, Razaviyan J, Koochaki A, Kokhaei P, Bandegi A. Expression of Bioinformatically candidate miRNAs including, miR-576-5p, miR-501-3p and miR-3143, targeting PI3K pathway in triple-negative breast cancer. Galen Medical Journal. 2019;**8**:e1646

[56] Zhan Y, Du J, Min Z, Ma L, Zhang W, Zhu W, et al. Carcinoma-associated fibroblasts derived exosomes modulate breast cancer cell stemness through exonic circHIF1A by miR-580-5p in hypoxic stress. Cell Death Discovery. 2021;**7**(1):141

[57] Wang GP, Mou ZL, Xu YY, Liu GX, Wang DM, Zhang HP. LINC01096 knockdown inhibits progression of triple-negative breast cancer by increasing miR-3130-3p. European Review for Medical and Pharmacological Sciences. 2019;**23**(17):7445-7456

[58] Shi SH, Jiang J, Zhang W, Sun L, Li XJ, Li C, et al. A novel lncRNA HOXC-AS3 acts as a miR-3922-5p sponge to promote breast cancer metastasis. Cancer Investigation. 2020;**38**(1):1-12

Chapter 7

Long Non-Coding RNA in Neural Stem Cells Self-Renewal, Neurogenesis, Gliogenesis and Synaptogenesis

Neetu Singh

Abstract

Evidence reports the key roles of lncRNAs in several regulatory mechanisms of neurons and other brain cells. Neuronal lncRNAs are crucial for NSCs mediated-neuronal developmental stages like neurogenesis, neuronal differentiation, and synaptogenesis. Moreover, multilineage properties of NSCs and their association to specific cell types render them to identify the commonly accepted biomarkers for the brain. It is important to delineate the correlation between lncRNAs and NSCs fate decisions during neuronal development stages. In this review, we will summarize how NSCs fabricate embryonic tissue architecture of the central nervous system (CNS) and act as residuum in subventricular zone (SVZ) nearby the lateral wall of the lateral ventricles and the subgranular zone (SGZ) of hippocampus dentate gyrus (DG) of the adult brain. Additionally, describe the roles and molecular mechanisms of lncRNAs involved in NSCs self-renewal, neurogenesis, gliogenesis and synaptogenesis over the course of neural development. This will help us to better understand neuronal physiology.

Keywords: long noncoding RNAs, neurons, neuronal development, neuronal differentiation, neurogenesis, synaptic activity, synaptic plasticity

1. Introduction

In the central nervous system (CNS), an efficient spatio-temporal regulatory mechanisms play an important role in neural stem cells (NSCs) for the development of neurons and other brain cells. The development and differentiation of the CNS is intricate in nature, and plethora of regulatory factors are involved and express ~40% of lncRNAs [1]. lncRNAs are involved in the early development/differentiation of the nervous system (NS) through NSCs to synaptogenesis [2–4]. Field et al. [5] constituted pluripotent stem cell (PSC)-derived cerebral cortex organoid (CO) cell cultures which recapitulate the cellular organization and gene expression events observed in fetal tissue. PAX6 (neural progenitors), CTIP2 and TBR1 express during early deep-layer neuron and TBR2 expression is in intermediate progenitors in Human COs at

IntechOpen

Human cell atlas		ARCHS4	
Week 2-GO-Term enrichment	**Week 5-GO-Term enrichment**	**Week 2-GO-Term enrichment**	**Week 5-GO-Term enrichment**
Fetal brain	Fetal brain	Motor neuron	Motor neuron
Prefrontal cortex	Prefrontal cortex	Prefrontal cortex	Prefrontal cortex
Amygdala	Amygdala	Neuronal epithelium	Spinal cord
Pineal night	Pineal night	Cerebellum	Spinal cord (bulk)
Pineal day	Pineal day	Spinal cord	Cerebellum
Smooth muscle	Cerebellum peduncle	Spinal cord (bulk)	Fetal brain
Occipital lobe	Whole brain	Mid brain	Cingulate gyrus
Uterus	Cardiac myocytes	Fetal brain cortex	Sensory neuron
Prostrate	Cerebellum	Fetal brain	Cerebral cortex
Cardiac myocytes	Occipital lobe	Sensory neuron	Brain (bulk)

Table 1.
The top 10 enriched GO terms from ARCHS4 [6]; based on publicly available RNA-seq data from human and mouse) and Human Cell Atlas ([7]; based on microarrays of human and mouse tissues) ranked by their combined enrichment score [5].

day 35. The ratio of human COs, pluripotency markers such as *OCT3/4* were down-regulated, while early neural stem cell markers, including *PAX6*, were up-regulated during the first week. Subsequently by 5th week *TBR1* were strongly expressed in Deep-layer neurons. Gene Ontology (GO) term analysis showed significant enrichment of lncRNA associated with neuronal development along with prefrontal cortex and foetus brain as described in **Table 1**. On assessing lncRNAs, previously described mammalian conserved lncRNAs *MALAT1*, *NEAT1*, *H19*, *PRWN1*, and *CRNDE* and 79 unannotated lncRNAs were observed among the 920 primate-conserved category. Markedly, in week 2 transient expression of lncRNAs (TREX) originated from *TREX2174* (RP11-314P15) which includes 19 bp insertion overlay at its transcription start site. Importantly, *TREX4039* (extends over AC011306 and *MIR217HG*) peaks at first or second week human COs and disappears by fifth week. At week 2 of human Cos gene expression specific single cells were processed for scRNA-seq libraries and TREX, which have potential roles in early cortical cell fate specifications were identified as depicted in **Table 2**. The clusters identified at week 2 (neuroepithelium (NE) cells-cluster of 1261 cells; early-forming Cajal-Retzius (CR) cells-cluster of 356 cells; the cortical radial glia (RG)-cluster of up 2593 cells were converted into clusters of early neurons (26%), intermediate progenitors (11%), mature radial glial (RG) (26%), immature RG (18%), dividing RG (12%), and cell doublets (8%) at week 5 of organoid cells.

The study showed the importance of cellular specificity of lncRNA function [8]; robust regulatory effects on distal genes upon activation/repression of these TREX lncRNAs was also observed (**Table 2**). In our recent review [9], we have already discussed the mechanisms to identify lncRNA, synthesize lncRNA, transcription of lncRNA and localized processing of lncRNA in nuclear and cellular portions, and their regulatory functions mediated by linking to chromatin alone or by constructing lncRNA-protein-chromatin complexes owing to chromatin modifications and genomic stability, hence influencing pluripotency. LncRNA are also involved in

Name of cells	Gene expression markers	Cluster of single cells	Enrichment of transiently expressed lncRNAs (TREX) at week 2	Activity of lncRNA in trans manner
Neuroepithelium (NE) cells	*HES3* and *NR2F1*	Cluster of 1261 cells	*TREX108* and *TREX8168*	Genes associated with whole brain, superior frontal gyrus, and cerebral cortex suggesting a role in general neural gene networks
Cajal-Retzius (CR) cells	*TBR1*, *EOMES*, *LHX9*, and *NHLH1*	Cluster of 356 cells	*TREX4039*	Induced genes enriched in the ARCHS4 neural epithelium gene set and repressed expression of those associated with superior frontal gyrus and astrocytes
Cortical radial glia (RG)	*SOX2*, *EMX2*, *NNAT*, *PTN*, and *TLE4*	Cluster of 2593cells	*TREX5008*	Induced genes enriched in the ARCHS4 neural epithelium gene set and repressed expression of those associated with superior frontal gyrus and astrocytes

Early-forming Cajal-Retzius (CR) cells expressed TBR1, EOMES, LHX9, and NHLH1, comprising a cluster of 356 cells. The largest cluster strongly expressed cortical radial glia (RG) markers SOX2, EMX2, NNAT, PTN, and TLE4, making up 2593 cells showed discovery of transiently expressed lncRNAs, which have potential roles in early cortical cell fate specifications [5].

Table 2.
10× Chromium 3′ end scRNA-seq on week 2 human COs gene expression based neuroepithelium (NE) cells, were identified by expression of HES3 and NR2F1, forming a cluster of 1261 cells.

transcriptional and post transcriptional regulation and serve as scaffolds, chromatin modifiers and miRNA sponges have also been explained in our recent review [9]. This review aims to explain the roles and molecular mechanisms of lncRNAs focusing on NSCs self-renewal, neurogenesis, gliogenesis and synaptic excitability over the course of neural development.

2. Role of NSCs in designing embryonic tissue architectonics of the central nervous system

Embryonically, the neurons of the brain are organized into layers (cortices) and clusters (nuclei), each having different function and interrelation with other neurons. The embryonic neural tube comprises single cell layer thick germinal neuroepithelium (GNE) which encompasses most proliferative neural stem cells. The GNE continues from the outer edge to the lumen of the neural tube [10], the nuclei of GNE exist at discrete levels, hence giving the impression of numerous cell layers in the neural tube. The nuclei move inside GNE as they move forward to different G0/G1, S and M phases of cell cycle. First and foremost, the S phase or DNA synthesis occurs when the nucleus is at the outer border of the neural tube, subsequently the nucleus moves towards lumen of the neural tube as the cell cycle proceeds.

However, after a certain time period some of the GNE-cells stop DNA synthesis and mitosis and migrate and differentiate into neuronal and glial cells outside the neural tube [11, 12]. The dividing cells of GNE have been found in the outer cortex of the adult brain, this was explained by radioactive thymidine studies. The published reports suggested neuroepithelial stem cells split "vertically" instead of "horizontally." After vertical division, the daughter cell besides the lumen of the neural tube remains affixed to the ventricular surface (and persists as stem cells in the ventricular zone), while the other daughter cell migrates away [13]. This ultimate vertical division is the terminal division and origination of a neuron happens. The cells which originate late move through GNE and form the most superficial regions of the cortex. Consecutive differentiation is based on the inhabitancy of the new neurons once outside the GNE [14, 15]. The process of division persists i.e., the cells next to the lumen sustain division and are exported outwards to the lumen. In such a manner they form a second layer and sequential addition of more cells derived from GNE thickens and widens the outermost layer and forms mantle (or intermediate zone). The GNE itself acts as a ventricular zone (later known as ependyma that embraces neural stem cells). Further, the cells of the mantle zone differentiates both in neurons and glia. The axons of neurons make connections and move away from the lumen while glial cells form sheath around axons and these are suggested as white matter. While the neuronal cell bodies represent the grey matter.

3. Spinal cord and medulla assembly

In the spinal cord and medulla, three-zone decorum first-ependymal, second-mantle, and third-marginal layers are maintained throughout development. The grey matter (mantle) is a butterfly-shaped structure and is surrounded by white matter; both grey and white matter are enclosed by the connective tissue. Further, on maturation the neural tube is divided into dorsal and ventral halves through a longitudinal groove, the sulcus limitans. The dorsal portion receives input from sensory neurons, whereas the ventral portion is intricated in performing various motor functions.

4. Cerebellar structure

In cerebellum the different neurons which migrate outside the GNE through cell migration, further undergoes differential neuronal proliferation, and selective cell death that creates modifications in the three-zone pattern (ependymal, mantle, and marginal layers).

In the cerebellum, a small quantity of neuronal precursors i.e., neuroblasts derived from GNE either enter the marginal zone to form clusters of neurons called nuclei or migrate to the outer surface of the neural tube to form a new germinal zone. Each single nucleus of the marginal zone works as an individual functional unit, and connects to the outer layers of the cerebellum and other parts of the brain. The new germinal zone forms the outer layer of the developing cerebellum and is also known as the external granule layer-EGL (two cells thick layer. The outer layer of the EGL is composed of dividing neuroblasts, while the inner layer of EGL comprises post-mitotic neuroblasts. The latter are the precursors of the preeminent neurons of the cerebellar cortex and the granule neurons. Granule neurons are the major component of the internal granule layer-IGL that migrates back to white matter of developing cerebellum. Concurrently, the ependymal layer (ventricular zone of GNE) differentiates into neurons and glial cells which include the unique Purkinje neurons. Purkinje neurons interact to form electrical synapses (unlike chemical synapses, there is direct interaction between presynaptic and postsynaptic neurons and also support granule neurons. These neurons secrete a specific morphogen Sonic hedgehog (SHH), which maintains the division of granule neuron precursors (neuroblasts) in the EGL [16].

Each Purkinje neuronal cell body is shaped like a flask and has a large, flat, highly branched thread like extensions creating a dendritic Arbor. This helps in forming hundreds of thousands connections (synapses) with other cells like Bergmann glial cells and granule cells. The axon of each Purkinje neuron connects to neurons in the deep cerebellar nuclei and transmits impulses to the region of cerebellum which controls movement.

The evolution of spatial arrangement of neurons is an essential process for the development and functioning of the cerebellum. Positioning of young neurons is under glial guidance [17, 18]. Importantly, the granule cell precursors (neuroblasts) move forward through adhesion on the long axonal processes of the Bergmann glia [19, 20]. The neural-glial reciprocal interaction between glial cells and neuroblasts [17, 21] is held up by adhesion protein called astrotactin that assists in adhesion of neurons to the glial cells [22, 23].

5. Cerebral structure

The three-zone positioning pattern cerebellum first-ependymal, second-mantle, and third-marginal layers of the neural tube is modified to vertical and horizontal positioning in the cerebrum.

Vertical positioning shows different vertical layers which interact with one another. As in cerebellum, in cerebrum, some of the neuroblasts move outwards from GNE and form the mantle zone and travel under glial guidance along the white matter to produce an additional layer of neurons at the outer layer of the cerebral cortex. This additional layer of grey matter (mantle) is called the neocortex. Neocortex is 2–5 mm thick, present on the surface of brain time-dependently differentiates into six layers (molecular layer, external granular layer, external pyramidal layer, internal granular layer, ganglionic layer and multiform layer) of neuronal cell bodies. Although layers are premature in nature and the maturity is not completed until the middle of childhood. Each vertical layer of the neocortex is unique and holds a specific function based on the types of neurons, and their connections with other neurons. For example, the inputs sent by thalamus are received by the neurons of layer 4, while output back to the thalamus is sent by the neurons of layer 6.

Horizontal positioning of the layers in cerebrum is more complex and they approximately form almost 40 regions that are regulated physiologically and have specific functions. For example, neurons in vertical cortical layer 6 horizontally possess both "visual cortex" and "auditory cortex". Auditory cortex is more anterior in position than the visual cortex. Visual cortex projects axons to the lateral geniculate nucleus of the thalamus (for vision), while auditory cortex projects axons to the medial geniculate nucleus of the thalamus (for hearing).

The vertical and horizontal arrangement in cerebrum depends on numerous multilineage neuroblasts derived from GNE. Further, on terminal mitotic division most of the neuroblasts of ventricular (ependymal) progress under glial guidance and lead to the formation of cortical plates located at the outer surface of the cortex of cerebrum.

To conclude, the neuroblasts with the early origin derived from GNE form the layer adjacent to the ventricle while neurons of later origin migrate through GNE and set apart to form the more exterior layers of the cortex. This positioning of cells forms an "inside-out" descent of expansion [24]. The neuroblast of the ventricular (ependymal) zone divides into neurons and glial cells in any of the cortical layers [25]. However, the fates of neuroblasts depend on the terminal division. The neuroblasts early in development are in their mid-S phase i.e., are in the way of division i.e., final division is not complete, hence likely become any neuron (for instance neurons of layers 2 or 6), at later stage of development of neuroblasts final mitosis is complete that give rise only to upper-level (layer 2) neurons [26]. The migration of the majority of these young neurons occurs in a radial manner on glial processes [27]. The migration initiates from the ventricular zone to the cortical plate. After neurogenesis, the generated young neurons (~12%) migrate laterally from one region of the cerebral cortex into another [28]. Further, the positioning of young neurons in different cortical areas are designated to unique functional domains. Once the neuronal cells make an appearance at their final designated cortical area, they may produce specific adhesion molecules that sort them together as brain nuclei [29].

6. Role of adult neural stem cells (NSCs) in neurogenesis

The cortical regions are composed of abundant neurons and glial cells produced from the differentiation of GNE-derived neuronal precursor cells/neuroblasts, which are self-sufficient to renew themselves as well as differentiate into multilineage neurons in the brain [30]. The above process of producing neurons and glial cells are termed neurogenesis and gliogenesis, respectively [31]. The largest NSCs/neuronal precursor cells/neuroblasts niches all through the life are essentially located in the adult ventricular-subventricular zone (V-SVZ) adjacent to the walls of the lateral ventricles [32] and the subgranular zone (SGZ) in the dentate gyrus of the hippocampus where new dentate granule cells are produced.

6.1 NSC model in the adult subventricular zone under basal conditions

V-SVZ produces large number of neuroblasts which travel a long distance through the rostral migratory stream (RMS) to the olfactory bulb (OB) in form of a chain, where they finally differentiate into granule cell type local interneurons [33]. Further, once reaching the core of the OB, immature neurons separate from the RMS through radial migration and then migrate towards glomeruli and differentiate into various subtypes of periglomerular (PG) interneurons. PG interneurons interconnect with the apical dendrites (often lack axons) of mitral and tufted cells inside the glomeruli [34]. The majority of interneurons are GABAergic granule cell neurons, which lack axons and form dendro-dendritic synapses with lateral dendrites of mitral and tufted cells in the external plexiform layer. In addition, few number of GABAergic PG interneurons and small percentage of interneurons are dopaminergic in nature. One report also suggested that very low percent of new interneurons are glutamatergic juxtaglomerular neurons in nature [35]. Transcript based markers have been identified for the five developmental stages of adult SVZ neurogenesis of the lateral ventricle and OB [1] activation of radial glia-like cells (GFAP, Vimentin and nestin positive) in the SVZ zone in the lateral ventricle (LV); [2] proliferation of transient amplifying cells/progenitor cells (Mash1 and low amount of nestin); [3] produce neuroblasts (Dlx2 positive) that migrate to OB; [4] subsequent chain migration of neuroblasts (Dlx2 positive) within the RMS and radial migration of immature neurons (Dlx2 and DCX positive) in the OB; [5] Synaptic Interaction through Interneurons (NeuN positive) and maturation of GC and PG neurons in the OB (reviewed by [33]) .

6.2 NSC model in the adult hippocampus under basal conditions

Adult SGZ in the dentate gyrus of the hippocampus possess proliferating radial and non-radial neuronal precursor cells that generate intermediate progenitors/transit amplifying cells, which in succession generate neuroblasts.

The multi-lineage radial precursors i.e., radial glia-like cells (RGLs or Type-1 cells) in dentate gyrus of adult hippocampus are identified through expression of transcripts like nestin, GFAP and Sox2. Besides transcript markers a distinguishing feature RGL possesses is radial branch which extends through the granule cell layer. Single RGL undergoes several rounds of self-renewal and differentiation to produce both neurons and astrocytes for a long period, displaying characteristic stem cell properties by each RGLs as evidenced through in vivo clonal assays [36].

Quiescent RGLs once triggered from quiescence stage i.e. G0 phase, RGLs moves towards formation of specific cell types like RGLs, non-radial precursors, proliferative intermediate progenitors (IPCs, or Type-2 cells) and astroglia, excluding the oligodendrocyte lineage. Later on the fate of RGLs may be decided whether they remain in a proliferative state, return to quiescence, or differentiate into an astrocyte.

Non-radial precursors generate new neurons in the adult SGZ and act as primary precursors [37]. They lack any radial process and few cells present as parallel extensions to the dentate granule cell layer. Unlike RGL, non-radial precursors express Sox2, but not GFAP [38] and more proliferative i.e., mostly present in cell cycle [37, 38]. They may or may not show involvement of IPCs and may generate new RGLs or astroglia, while maintaining the precursor state [36].

IPCs of the SGZ region of dentate gyrus rapidly proliferate and possess small tangential processes expressing Tbr2 as transcript marker [39]. They are derived from both radial and non-radial precursors [36, 38]. Afterwards they convert into secondary transient amplifying precursors and start expressing DCX and Prox1, markers of committed immature neurons [39]. IPCs re-enter cell cycle for self-renewal or produce astroglia or maintain as precursors over a long duration remains unclear.

In adult dentate non-neurogenic areas and SGZ region enrichment of another, progenitor population of NG2 cells have been identified [40] Major features of NG2 cells are long wispy processes, expression of specific proteogylcan NG2 as well as PDGF, Sox10 and Olig2 [41] has been observed. Presence of NG2 cells and oligodendrocytes in non-neurogenic areas differentiate them from RGLs in the adult SGZ [36] suggesting that they may have derived from different precursor populations with different embryonic origins. The consensus remains that NG2 cells may produce astroglia during development, and oligodendrocyte generation in the adult nervous system [41].

Astroglia, non-neuronal quiescent precursor cell type as proposed by absence of nestin expression, are a prospective third precursor population in the adult SGZ. Major characteristic features are horizontal or bushy morphology and expression of GFAP, S100β and Aldh1l1 markers [42]. The new astroglia generate from RGLs in the adult SGZ; afterwards they migrate to the hilus or molecular layer [36]. Hence, neuroblasts from NSCs in SGZ migrate short distances into the granule cell layer and mature into neurons, then integrate into functional circuits [43].

7. The effect of lncRNA on NSCs/NPCs pluripotency

Cell type- and tissue-specific long non-coding RNAs (lncRNAs) incorporate varying classes of transcripts that can control various fundamental molecular and cellular processes in organ development, disease and cancer. Here we will discuss the differential expression and unique function of lncRNAs in human brain development.

LncRNAs are present amply and specifically in different lineages of neurogenic cell-types which plays an important role in neuronal development [8]. For instance, Liu et al. [44] identified cell type-specific lncRNA and mRNA transcript pairs in developing neocortex; (a) radial glia-specific lncRNA *LOC646329*-mRNA *PAX6*, (b) maturing neuron-specific lncRNA *LINC00599-mRNA RTN1*, (c) interneuron-specific lncRNA *DLX6-AS1*-progenitor and differentiated cell-expressed mRNA *NNAT.* Maturing neurons of the cortical plate (CP) were enriched with *LINC00599*. The subpial granular layer interneuron showed predominance of unique *DLX6-AS1* [45, 46].

8. The function of lncRNAs in neurogenesis/neural differentiation

LncRNAs play a pivotal role in regulating epigenetic elements in NPCs or NSCs differentiation and neural development [47, 48]. Spatial and temporal expression of lncRNAs plays a very crucial role in neuronal development in the developing CNS [49]. However, the abundance and specificity of lncRNAs in different neurogenic cell-types or the specific functions show their involvement in development and cellular identity in the nervous system [1, 8].

Recently, a gene expression atlas of embryonic neurogenesis in Drosophila revealed complex spatiotemporal regulation of lncRNAs. This involved a significant set of 13 lncRNAs, on illustration they represented [1] time dependent appearance at subcellular and cellular levels, [2] moderate to excess expression in cytoplasmic or nuclear regions [3] were involved in precise RNA processing (for example splicing and nuclear-cytoplasmic commutation), during critical events in neurogenesis in Drosphila **Table 3** [50].

Interestingly, lncRNAs have undergone specific adaptive functions like selective loss during the evolution of neurogenesis [51]. LncRNA was a key determinant in NSCs or NPCs during cell-fate determination. Additionally, specific lncRNA types are involved in the different stages of NPCs or NSCs differentiation. The neuronal and astrocytic differentiation have been well explained based on a plethora of differentially expressed epigenetically modified lncRNA. It has also been suggested that different lncRNAs have biasness for neuronal differentiation compared to astrocytic differentiation. Although astrocytic differentiation is related more to the sense lncRNAs (lncRNA transcribed from the sense strand of exons possessing coding genes) [52]. Besides, the above functions lncRNAs also participate in synchronizing the fate of NSC differentiation into glia and neurons under physiological and pathological conditions [53, 54]. An overview of lncRNA involved in neurogenesis/neuronal differentiation, gliogenesis or synaptogenesis has been well described in **Table 4**.

CR30009	CR30009 is spliced and primarily exported to the cytoplasm	Increased expression in the early IC and in NBs (4–6 h and 6–8 h) constitutes the earliest neuroblast marker of the glial lineage However, was most highly enriched in glial cells stage 9/10 and stage 13/14	Specific expression in NBs and shows increased expression in glial cells
CR43283 (also known as cherub)	Specifically localized to the cytoplasm throughout embryogenesis and is clearly spliced, but harbors no coding potential and showed dynamic temporal regulation	Expression of cherub was strongly enriched in the earliest neuroblasts at 4–6 h, but enrichment quickly decreased in later neuroblasts (6–8 h); however, over time cherub became specifically expressed being strongly enriched in differentiated neurons and glia by the end of neurogenesis at 18–22 h	Specific expression in NBs and shows increased expression in differentiated neurons and glia
CR32730	Moderately enriched in the nuclear fraction in early and late embryos	CR32730 first detected in 4-6 h neuroblasts and was moderately enriched at 8–10 h in the neuronal, but not in the glial, population	Specific expression in NBs and shows increased expression in early neurons
CR46003	CR46003 was one of the most abundant and did not exhibit clear subcellular enrichment in either early or late embryos	First detected in the ventral column and was most highly enriched in early neuroblasts, but expression persisted in neuroblasts and early neurons	Specific expression in NBs and shows increased expression in early neurons
CR44024	Not predicted to exhibit distinct subcellular localization in early (6-8 h) embryos, but was moderately enriched in the cytoplasm at the end of embryogenesis (18–22 h)	Was first enriched in early neuroblasts and persisted through neuronal differentiation, and is predicted to be excluded from the intermediate and ventral columns and glia	Specific expression in NBs and persistent expression in neurons

Biological materials studied over the time course of neurogenesis: intermediate column (IC); ventral column (VC); neuroblasts (NBs); neurons; glia. Markers specifically used for RNA-FISH was NBs, Pros; neurons, Elav; glia, Repo (4–6 and 6–8 h (IC, VC, NBs); 6–8, 8–10 and 18–22 h (neurons and glia)) [50].

Table 3.
A list of high-confidence set of lncRNAs classified time dependently; distinct subcellular localization patterns and cell-specifically; moderate to overabundance in cytoplasmic or nuclear regions; and involved in highly specific RNA processing in neurogenesis in Drosphila.

9. The function of lncRNAs in neuronal differentiation

LncRNAs are cardinal for neuronal differentiation and for neurogenesis. They are specific to the brain region, especially SVZ, DG or Olfactory Bulb (OB). They exert their functions via interacting with transcription factors or binding to the promoter or enhancer regions of neighbouring/target genes, also act as competing endogenous RNA (ceRNA) against synergistic binding sequences of miRNA or are crucial signaling pathway modulators which regulate chromatin modification, transcription, and post-transcription.

LncRNA name	Mechanism	Biological function	References
Sox2ot	CpG island of Sox2, interacts with transcription factor YY1 and suppresses the expression of Sox2	Prohibit NSCs proliferation and advance neuronal differentiation	[55]
RMST	Target Sox2 promoter region	Promote neurogenesis	[56]
Kdm2b (also known as *Kancr*)	Bind with hnRNPAB and activate Kdm2b gene expression	Causes early neuronal differentiation of cortical projection neurons, hence promotes neurogenesis	[57]
Paupar	Bind with local epi-regulatorygenes-Pax6 and KAP1 through H3K9me3 deposition	Promote neurogenesis in neuroblastoma cells	[58, 59]
Gm21284	Interact with miR-30e-3p, miR-431 and miR-147	Inhibit NSCs proliferation while promote NSCs differentiation	[60]
1604	miR-200c/ZEB1/2 axis	Promote neural differentiation	[61]
Rik-201	Activated by C/EBPβ, miR-96/Sox6	Enhance neural differentiation	[62]
Rik-203	miR-467a-3p/Sox6, miR-101-3a/GSK-3β	Enhance neural differentiation	[62, 63]
MEG3	Act as a negative regulator of miR-128-3p while induced by the cAMP/ response element-binding protein (CREB) pathway	Promotes neuron differentiation	[64]
Malat1	Activate ERK/MAPK, inhibit PPAR/p53	Promote neural differentiation in neuroblastoma-derived Neuro-2a (N2a) cell	[65]
Pnky	Interact with RNA-binding protein (RBP)-PTBP1	Inhibit neural differentiation and neurogenesis	[30, 66]
lncR492	Interact with HuR and activate Wnt signalling	Inhibit neural differentiation of mouse embryonic stem cells	[67]
BDNF-AS	Targeting activating potassium uptake system protein (TrkB) signaling pathway	Inhibit eNSCs-derived neurite outgrowth and neural apoptosis	[68]
UCA1	miR-1 and its target Hes1	Promote NSCs differentiation to astrocyte not to neuron	[54]
lnOPC	lnOPC binds to upstream sequences of OLIG2	Promotes OPCs differentiation and oligodendrogenesis	[69]
lncOL1	Form a complex with Suz12, an oligodendrocyte maturation promoter	Promote oligodendrogenesis by promoting early maturation/differentiation of oligodendrocytes in neural development	[70]

LncRNA name	Mechanism	Biological function	References
lnc158	Promote regulatory transcription factor-nuclear factor-IB NFIB expressio	Promote oligodendrogenesis through enhanced oligodendrocyte-related genes expressions like and enhanced induction of oligodendrocyte lineage differentiation	[71]
Pcdh17it (immature lncRNa)		Oligodendrogenesis marker identified in new-born immature OLs	[72]
OLMALIN/-AS	OLMALINCAS, maps to the first exon of the dominant isoform of OLMALINC	Regulate oligodendrocyte maturation related genes	[73]
Synage (includes three isoforms of Gm2694)	Synage as a sponge for the sponge to microRNA miR-325-3p, act as scaffold for organizing the assembly of the LRP1-HSP90AA1-PSD-95 complex	Regulating synaptic stability in cerebella as distributed in the cytoplasm and synapses of cerebellar cells	[74]
GM12371	Nuclear-enriched	Prolific transcriptional regulator critical for synapse function in hippocampal neurons	[75]
Gm2694 (alias AK082312)	Enriched expression in the mouse cerebellar cortex		[76]
Gm2694 lncRNA (alias linc1582)		Associated with neuroectoderm differentiation	[77]
Gm2694 (alias Trincr1) was documented to	Regulate FGF/ERK signaling	Self-renewal of NSCs	[78]

Table 4.
The roles of lncRNAs on NSCs differentiation/neurogenesis, oligodendrogenesis and synapse stability.

10. Effect on lncRNA target genes expression

LncRNAs regulate neural development by binding to the proximal regions of the protein-coding genes expressions. Most importantly, evolutionarily conserved, nuclearly localized lncRNA Sox1 overlapping transcript (Sox1ot) and Sox2 overlapping transcript (Sox2ot) were identified in the developing brain. Overlapping transcripts Sox1ot and Sox2ot imbricate with Sox1 and Sox2 protein coding transcripts, respectively [79, 80]. Protein coding Sox1 and Sox2 transcripts function as pluripotent transcription factors to maintain the stemness of NPCs and NSCs [81]. Sox1ot and Sox2ot are highly expressed during neural development and are directly proportional to the Sox1 and Sox2 transcription factors abundance respectively [55, 82]. Mechanistically, overlapping transcript Sox2ot interacts with the transcriptional regulator YY1 and binds to CpG island which is present in the proximity of Sox2 locus and subsequently suppresses the Sox2 expression to restrain stemness of NSCs and NPCs [55]. LncRNA rhabdomyosarcoma 2-associated transcript (RMST) binds with promoter regions of Sox2 and regulates the downstream target genes and is critical for neurogenesis [56]. Another, lncRNA Kdm2b is uniquely transcribed from the bidirectional promoter along with Kdm2b. Epigenetically, lncRNA Kdm2b binds in cis manner with hnRNPAB and manages Kdm2b's transcription. Although lncRNA Kdm2b expression is transient and occurs only during early neuronal differentiation of cortical projection neurons [57]. LncRNA *Paupar*, regulates the function of transcriptional/epigenetic regulatory factors and modulates neuroblastoma cell growth. Most importantly, it directly binds to KAP1, which induces H3K9me3 methylation and modulates the expression of downstream target genes important for neuronal proliferation and differentiation. LncRNA *Paupar* epigenetically modulates (by binding H3K9me3 in cis manner) and controls Pax6 mediated neural differentiation and olfactory bulb neurogenesis [58, 59].

11. lncRNA as competing endogenous RNA (ceRNA) against miRNA

LncRNAs participate in neural development via acting as ceRNA of miRNA and indirectly regulate transcript expression in the cytoplasm [61, 83].

LncRNA Gm21284 promotes differentiation of NSCs to hippocampal cholinergic neurons by binding to miR-30e-3p, miR-431 and miR-147 and on silencing miRNAs impedes NSCs proliferation and enhances NSCs differentiation [60]. LncRNA1604 act as sponge to miR-200c and regulates important transcription factor zinc finger E-box binding homeobox1/2 (ZEB1/2) axis which promotes neural differentiation and on silencing miR-200c repress neural differentiation [61]. LncRNA isoforms also play an important role in neurogenesis. For instance, lncRNA RiK has two variants, Rik-201 and Rik-203. Both these variants get activated by CCAAT/enhancer-binding protein β (C/EBPβ) which are induced during neurogenesis. Mechanistically, Rik-201 triggers C/EBPβ, miR-96/Sox6 axis and [62] and lncRNA Rik-203 induces miR-467a-3p/Sox6, miR-101-3a/Glycogen Synthase Kinase-3β (GSK-3β) [62, 63] to promote neural differentiation. LncRNA MEG3 is also engaged in the process of neuron differentiation. Although it acts as a negative regulator of miR-128-3p it induces the cAMP/response element-binding protein (CREB) pathway [64].

12. LncRNAs as key signalling pathway modulators

LncRNAs moreover can contribute to neural differentiation through NSCs and may function as a key member of the signaling pathway. Neurite outgrowth is an essential act in the early neuronal-differentiation and self-renewal. The lncRNA Metastasis-associated lung adenocarcinoma transcript1 (Malat1) is a requisite for neurite growth in in vitro differentiation of neuroblastoma-derived Neuro-2a (N2a) cell as a model. Knockdown of Malat1 impeded neurite outgrowth and enhanced cell death in N2a cells. This owes to suppression of Mitogen-Activated Protein Kinase (MAPK) and activation of Peroxisome proliferator-activated receptor (PPAR) and p53 signalling pathways [65].

13. LncRNAs mediated repression of neuronal differentiation

As described above, most of the highly expressed lncRNAs promote neuronal differentiation, however, some other neuronal lncRNAs were revealed which blocks neuronal differentiation and plays an important role in brain development.

Nuclear localized lncRNA Pnky, was determined to be involved in neuronal development via inhibiting neuronal differentiation. Specifically, Pnky is expressed selectively in neural tissues that are enriched in SVZ-NSCs which are suppressed into mature neurons. Pnky binds to the pre-mRNA splicing regulator RNA-binding protein (RBP) polypyrimidine tract-binding protein (PTBP1). On silencing either Pnky or PTBP1 alters splicing signature of expressed mRNAs in the cell and subsequently induces neurogenesis in SVZ-NSCs. Hence, inverse correlation has been observed between expression of Pnky-PTBP1 complex and neurogenesis [30, 66]. Another lncRNA lncR492 acts as inhibitor of neuroectodermal differentiation via interacting with mRNA binding protein HuR and activating the Wnt signaling pathway [67]. Zhang et al. reported dose-dependent over expression of lncRNA brain derived neurotrophic factor antisense (BDNF-AS), inhibits neural growth in ketamine-treated mouse embryonic NSC-derived neurons. SiRNA mediated silencing of BDNF transcript expression improved neural apoptosis; inhibited neurite growth in NSC-derived neurons through stimulating potassium uptake system protein (TrkB) signaling pathway [68].

14. Role of lncRNAs in regulation of gliogenesis

Recent reports suggest that radial glial (RG) cells are considered for glial lineage along with a subpopulation of astrocytes. RG as matter of fact act as the NSCs that serve as progenitors for many differentiated neurons and glial cells during development and in the postnatal brain give rise to adult SVZ-NSCs that continue to produce neurons throughout adult life [84]. Importantly, at the inception of cortical development, NSCs or NPCs consecutively give rise to deep layer neurons trailed by surficial layer neurons; at later phase of cortical development, NSCs annihilate neurogenesis and move towards gliogenesis to attain gliogenic capability [85, 86]. Temporal NSCs transition from neurogenesis to gliogenesis is a prerequisite for proper cortical development [86, 87].

Several lncRNAs are considered as key regulators during neuronal-glial fate specification and oligodendrocyte lineage maturation. Time dependent overexpression of human urothelial carcinoma associated 1 (UCA1) was able to decide the direction of NSCs differentiation. Knockdown of UCA1 suggested suppression of NSCs proliferation and differentiation with decreased expression of nestin and the enhanced formation of the neurosphere. Further the silencing of UCA1 repressed NSCs differentiation into astrocytes rather NSCs were directed to differentiate as neurons due to the overexpression of miR-1 expression and decreased expression of its target gene-Hes1. Hence, UCA1 regulated the NSCs proliferation and differentiation through regulating Hes1 expression [54].

Dong et al. screened 5000 lncRNAs and identified lncRNAs that are modulated during oligodendrocyte precursor cell (OPC) differentiation from NSCs and play an essential role in oligodendrogenesis. Lnc-OPC was overexpressed in OPCs and is found to be highly conserved among placental mammals and predicts its role in brain development. Mechanistically, lnc-OPC binds to upstream regulatory elements of

OLIG2 and is directly proportional to the OLIG2 expression. Hence, overexpression of lnc-OPC enhances OPCs differentiation and oligodendrogenesis [69].

LncRNA has also emerged as an important regulator in oligodendrocyte mediated myelination and plays a crucial role in development and function of CNS [88, 89]. This was supported by dynamic co-expression signature of lncRNAs with protein coding genes at different stages of oligodendrocyte growth and myelination. Most importantly, highly conserved chromatin-associated lncRNA-lncOL1 has been identified during oligodendrocyte growth and myelination. Genetic knockdown of lncOL1 causes aberrations in myelination and remyelination processes after injury, while gain of function induces early oligodendrocyte differentiation i.e., maturation in neural development. Mechanically, lncOL1 forms a complex with a by binding to the promoter region of a member of polycomb repressive complex 2 (Suz12), involved in oligodendrocyte maturation [44]. Another lnc158 upregulates in NSCs and stimulates downstream various oligodendrocyte-related genes expressions including DNA binding transcription factor-nuclear factor-IB (NFIB) that regulates oligodendrocyte lineage differentiation [71]. Additionally, immature OL-specific lncRNA-Pcdh17 is a specific marker for newly born immature OLs and has been identified both in developing and adult forebrain of mice [72]. Interestingly, lncRNA oligodendrocyte maturation-associated long intervening non-coding RNA (OLMALINC) and its antisense counterpart, OLMALINCAS, both are equivalently and abundantly expressed in the white matter of human frontal cortex as opposed to grey matter and peripheral tissues and basically take part in modulation of human oligodendrocyte maturation related genes. OLMALINCAS, maps to the first exon of the major isoform of OLMALINC [73].

15. The role of lncRNAs in synaptogenesis

Synaptic stability in the developing and adult nervous system results due to the late phase long-term potentiation i.e., a continuous strengthening of synapses for long lasting increase in signal transmission between two neurons. The role of lncRNAs in modulating synaptic stability is ambiguous. Wang et al. [74], reported that cerebellum of the brain shows increased expression of lncRNA, Synage, to regulate synaptic stability. The lncRNA mediated synaptic stability is either lncRNA acting as a sponge or as a scaffold. As a sponge lncRNA Synage binds to miR-325-3p and alters the expression of downstream cerebellar synapse organizer identified in mouse, rhesus macaque, and human. Additionally, lncRNA Synage serves as a scaffold for rearranging the positioning of the LRP1-HSP90AA1-PSD-95 complex in Parallel fibre (PF)-Purkinje cell (PC) synapses. Knockdown of synage collapses cerebellar phenotype and leads to cerebellar degeneration, death of neurons, decline in synapse density which relates to synaptic pruning, decreased synaptic growth and synaptic plasticity during cerebellar development. Hence, the lncRNA Synage plays a major role in regulating synaptic stability and plays a crucial role during cerebellar development. GM12371 (nuclear enriched [75]) and Gm2694 (cerebellar cortex enriched [76]) (alias AK082312) also acts as a transcriptional regulator of synapse function.

16. Conclusion

Neural development related to NSCs/NPCs which constructs embryonic tissue architecture of CNS as well as exist as remnant in subventricular zone (SVZ) nearby the lateral wall of the lateral ventricles and the subgranular zone (SGZ) of hippocampus dentate gyrus (DG) of the brain is considered as a complex phenomenon. Advanced large-scale genome-wide RNA sequencing has been performed in various neuronal cells over the course of neural development to understand NSC self-renewal, neurogenesis, gliogenesis and synaptogenesis. This review has described in detail the functional roles of lncRNAs as ceRNA, by regulating proximal protein-coding genes expressions, and epigenetic modulations in regulation of NSCs/NPCs self-renewal, proliferation and differentiation into neuron or glial cells and synaptogenesis. This suggests that lncRNAs might be employed as potential selection biomarkers for identifying or screening suitable NPCs/NPCs. Importantly, a spatiotemporal expression of lncRNA as atlas of embryonic neurogenesis in Drosophila revealed a high- confidence set of 13 lncRNAs will open a new era of lncRNA based NSCs mediated neurogenesis and may help us to better understand the neuronal physiology. However, most of their function remains to be explored, more novel lncRNAs and their molecular mechanisms remain to be found and probed in-depth yet.

Acknowledgements

A special thanks to my Dr. Sanjay Kumar Singh for inspiring me to write this article and for financial support.

Abbreviations

Aldh1l1	aldehyde dehydrogenase 1 family member L1
AR	androgen receptor
BDNF	brain-derived neurotrophic factor
C/EBPβ	CCAAT/enhancer-binding protein β
ceRNA	ZEB1/2zinc finger E-box binding homeobox1/2
CNS	central nervous system
CO	cerebral cortex organoid
CP	cortical plate
CR	Cajal-Retzius
CREB	cAMP/response element-binding protein
CTIP2	COUP-TF-interacting protein 2
DCX	doublecortin
DG	dentate gyrus
Dlx2	Distal-Less Homeobox 2
EGL	external granule layer
ERK	extracellular signal regulated kinase
ESCs	embryonic stem cells
GSK-3β	glycogen synthase kinase-3β
IGL	internal granule layer
IPCs	intermediate progenitors
IZ	intermediate zone
Kdm2b	lysine demethylase 2B
LncRNAs	long non-coding RNAs
LV	lateral ventricle
GFAP	glial fibrillar protein

Malat1	metastasis-associated lung adenocarcinoma transcript1
MAPK	mitogen-activated protein kinase
MEG3	maternally expressed gene 3
MSNP1AS	Moesin pseudogene 1 antisense
N2a	Neuro-2a
NE	neuroepithelium
NEAT1	nuclear paraspeckle assembly transcript 11
NeuN	neuronal nuclei
NFIB	nuclear factor-IB
NG2	polydendrocytes
Notch	Notch receptor
NPCs	neural precursor/progenitor cells
NSCs	neural stem cells
OB	olfactory bulb
OCT3/4	POU class 5 homeobox 1
Olig2	oligodendrocyte transcription factor
OPC	oligodendrocyte precursor cells
OLMALINC	oligodendrocyte maturation-associated long intervening non-coding RNA
Paupar	PAX6 Upstream Antisense RNA
PAX6	Paired Box 6
PC	Purkinje cell
PDGF	platelet-derived growth factor
Pnky	long intergenic non-protein coding RNA PNKY
PF	parallel fiber
PPAR	peroxisome proliferator-activated receptor
Prox1	Prospero Homeobox 1
PSC	pluripotent stem cell
PTBP1	RNA-binding protein (RBP)-polypyrimidine tract-binding protein
RGLs	radial glia-like cells
RBP	RNA-binding protein
RG	radial glial
RMS	rostral migratory stream
RMST	rhabdomyosarcoma 2-associated transcript
RPS10P2-AS1	ribosomal protein S10 pseudogene 2 anti-sense 1
S100β	S100 calcium-binding protein B
SGZ	sub-granular zone
SHH	sonic hedgehog
Sox10	SRY-related HMG-box 10
Sox1ot	Sox1 overlapping transcript
Sox2ot	Sox2 overlapping transcript
Suz12	polycomb repressive complex 2
SVZ	subventricular zone
TALNEC2	tumor associated lncRNA expressed in chromosome 2
TBR1	T-box brain transcription factor 1
TBR2	T-box brain transcription factor 2
TGF-β	transforming growth factor-β
TREX	transiently expression of lncRNAs
Trincr1	TRIM71 interacting long noncoding RNA 1
TUNA	Tcl1 upstream neuron-associated lincRNA

UCA1	urothelial carcinoma associated 1
Wdr5	WD repeat domain 5
ZEB1/2	Zincfinger E-box binding homeobox ½

Author details

Neetu Singh
Molecular Biology Unit, Center for Advance Research, King George's Medical University, Lucknow, Uttar Pradesh

*Address all correspondence to: neetusingh@kgmcindia.edu

References

[1] Briggs JA, Wolvetang EJ, Mattick JS, Rinn JL, Barry G. Mechanisms of long non-coding RNAs in mammalian nervous system development, plasticity, disease, and evolution. Neuron. 2015;**88**(5):861-877. DOI: 10.1016/j.neuron.2015.09.045

[2] Knauss JL, Sun T. Regulatory mechanisms of long noncoding RNAs in vertebrate central nervous system development and function. Neuroscience. 2013;**235**:200-214. DOI: 10.1016/j.neuroscience.2013.01.022. Epub 2013 Jan 18

[3] Quan Z, Zheng D, Qing H. Regulatory roles of long non-coding RNAs in the central nervous system and associated neurodegenerative diseases. Frontiers in Cellular Neuroscience. 2017;**11**:175. DOI: 10.3389/fncel.2017.00175

[4] Salvatori B, Biscarini S, Morlando M. Non-coding RNAs in nervous system development and disease. Frontiers in Cell and Development Biology. 2020;**8**:273. DOI: 10.3389/fcell.2020.00273

[5] Field AR, Jacobs FMJ, Fiddes IT, Phillips APR, Reyes-Ortiz AM, LaMontagne E, et al. Structurally conserved primate LncRNAs are transiently expressed during human cortical differentiation and influence cell-type-specific genes. Stem Cell Reports. 2019;**12**(2):245-257. DOI: 10.1016/j.stemcr.2018.12.006. Epub 2019 Jan 10

[6] Lachmann A, Torre D, Keenan AB, Jagodnik KM, Lee HJ, Wang L, et al. Massive mining of publicly available RNA-seq data from human and mouse. Nature Communications. 2018;**9**(1):1366. DOI: 10.1038/s41467-018-03751-6

[7] Su AI, Wiltshire T, Batalov S, Lapp H, Ching KA, Block D, et al. A gene atlas of the mouse and human protein-encoding transcriptomes. Proceedings of the National Academy of Sciences of the United States of America. 2004;**101**(16):6062-6067. DOI: 10.1073/pnas.0400782101. Epub 2004 Apr 9

[8] Liu SJ, Nowakowski TJ, Pollen AA, Lui JH, Horlbeck MA, Attenello FJ, et al. Single-cell analysis of long non-coding RNAs in the developing human neocortex. Genome Biology. 2016;**17**:67

[9] Singh N. Role of mammalian long non-coding RNAs in normal and neuro oncological disorders. Genomics. 2021;**113**(5):3250-3273. DOI: 10.1016/j.ygeno.2021.07.015. Epub 2021 Jul 21

[10] Sauer FC. Mitosis in the neural tube. The Journal of Comparative Neurology. 1935;**62**:377-405

[11] Fujita S. Application of light and electron microscopy to the study of the cytogenesis of the forebrain. In: Hassler R, Stephen H, editors. Evolution of the Forebrain. New York: Plenum; 1966. pp. 180-196

[12] Jacobson M. Cessation of DNA synthesis in retinal ganglion cells correlated with the time of specification of their central connections. Developmental Biology. 1968;**17**:219-232

[13] Chenn A, McConnell SK. Cleavage orientation and the asymmetric inheritance of Notch1 immunoreactivity in mammalian neurogenesis. Cell. 1995;**82**:631-641

[14] Letourneau PC. Regulation of neuronal morphogenesis by cell-substratum adhesion. Soc. Neurosci. Symp. 1977;**2**:67-81

[15] Jacobson M. Developmental Neurobiology. 2nd ed. New York: Plenum; 1991

[16] Wallace VA. Purkinje cell-derived Sonic hedgehog regulates granule neuron precursor cell proliferation in the developing mouse cerebellum. Current Biology. 1999;**9**:445-448

[17] Hatten ME. Riding the glial monorail: A common mechanism for glial-guided neuronal migration in different regions of the mammalian brain. Trends in Neurosciences. 1990;**13**:179-184

[18] Rakic P. Mode of cell migration to superficial layers of fetal monkey neocortex. The Journal of Comparative Neurology. 1972;**145**:61-84

[19] Rakic P, Sidman RL. Organization of cerebellar cortex secondary to deficit of granule cells in weaver mutant mice. The Journal of Comparative Neurology. 1973;**152**:133-162

[20] Rakic P. Cell migration and neuronal ectopias in the brain. In: Bergsma D, editor. Morphogenesis and Malformations of Face and Brain, Birth Defects Original Article Series. Vol. 11(7). New York: Alan R. Liss; 1975. pp. 95-129

[21] Komuro H, Rakic P. Selective role of N-type calcium channels in neuronal migration. Science. 1992;**157**:806-809

[22] Edmondson JC, Liem RKH, Kuster JC, Hatten ME. Astrotactin: A novel neuronal cell surface antigen that mediates neuronal-astroglial interactions in cerebellar microcultures. The Journal of Cell Biology. 1988;**106**:505-517

[23] Fishell G, Hatten ME. Astrotactin provides a receptor system for glia-guided neuronal migration. Development. 1991;**113**:755-765

[24] Rakic P. Neurons in rhesus visual cortex: Systematic relation between time of origin and eventual disposition. Science. 1974;**183**:425-427

[25] Walsh C, Cepko CL. Clonally related cortical cells show several migration patterns. Science. 1988;**241**:1342-1345

[26] Frantz GD, McConnell SK. Restriction of late cerebral cortical progenitors to an upper-layer fate. Neuron. 1996;**17**:55-61

[27] O'Rourke NA, Dailey ME, Smith SJ, McConnell SK. Diverse migratory pathways in the developing cerebral cortex. Science. 1992;**258**:299-302

[28] Walsh C, Cepko CL. Widespread dispersion of neuronal clones across functional regions of the cerebral cortex. Science. 1992;**255**:434-440

[29] Matsunami H, Takeichi M. Fetal brain subdivisions defined by T- and E- cadherins expressions: Evidence for the role of cadherin activity in region-specific, cell-cell adhesion. Developmental Biology. 1995;**172**:466-478

[30] Ramos AD, Andersen RE, Liu SJ, Nowakowski TJ, Hong SJ, Gertz C, et al. The long noncoding RNA Pnky regulates neuronal differentiation of embryonic and postnatal neural stem cells. Cell Stem Cell. 2015;**16**:439-447

[31] Fawal MA, Davy A. Impact of metabolic pathways and epigenetics on neural stem cells. Epigenet Insights. 2018;**11**:2516865718820946

[32] Morizur L, Chicheportiche A, Gauthier LR, Daynac M, Boussin FD, Mouthon MA. Distinct molecular signatures of quiescent and activated adult neural stem cells reveal specific interactions with their

microenvironment. Stem Cell Reports. 2018;**11**:565-577

[33] Ming GL, Song H. Adult neurogenesis in the mammalian brain: Significant answers and significant questions. Neuron. 2011;**70**:687-702

[34] Lledo PM, Alonso M, Grubb MS. Adult neurogenesis and functional plasticity in neuronal circuits. Nature Reviews. Neuroscience. 2006;**7**:179-193

[35] Brill MS, Ninkovic J, Winpenny E, Hodge RD, Ozen I, Yang R, et al. Adult generation of glutamatergic olfactory bulb interneurons. Nature Neuroscience. 2009;**12**:1524-1533

[36] Bonaguidi MA, Wheeler MA, Shapiro JS, Stadel RP, Sun GJ, Ming GL, et al. In vivo clonal analysis reveals self-renewing and multipotent adult neural stem cell characteristics. Cell. 2011;**145**:1142-1155

[37] Suh H, Consiglio A, Ray J, Sawai T, D'Amour KA, Gage FH. In vivo fate analysis reveals the multipotent and self-renewal capacities of Sox2+ neural stem cells in the adult hippocampus. Cell Stem Cell. 2007;**1**:515-528

[38] Lugert S, Basak O, Knuckles P, Haussler U, Fabel K, Gotz M, et al. Quiescent and active hippocampal neural stem cells with distinct morphologies respond selectively to physiological and pathological stimuli and aging. Cell Stem Cell. 2010;**6**:445-456

[39] Hodge RD, Kowalczyk TD, Wolf SA, Encinas JM, Rippey C, Enikolopov G, et al. Intermediate progenitors in adult hippocampal neurogenesis: Tbr2 expression and coordinate regulation of neuronal output. The Journal of Neuroscience. 2008;**28**:3707-3717

[40] Encinas JM, Michurina TV, Peunova N, Park JH, Tordo J, Peterson DA, et al. Division-coupled astrocytic differentiation and age-related depletion of neural stem cells in the adult hippocampus. Cell Stem Cell. 2011;**8**:566-579

[41] Zhu X, Hill RA, Dietrich D, Komitova M, Suzuki R, Nishiyama A. Age-dependent fate and lineage restriction of single NG2 cells. Development. 2011;**138**:745-753

[42] Seri B, Garcia-Verdugo JM, Collado-Morente L, McEwen BS, Alvarez-Buylla A. Cell types, lineage, and architecture of the germinal zone in the adult dentate gyrus. The Journal of Comparative Neurology. 2004;**478**:359-378

[43] Bonaguidi MA, Song J, Ming GL, Song H. A unifying hypothesis on mammalian neural stem cell properties in the adult hippocampus. Current Opinion in Neurobiology. 2012;**22**:754-761

[44] Liu SJ, Horlbeck MA, Cho SW, Birk HS, Malatesta M, He D, et al. CRISPRi-based genome-scale identification of functional long noncoding RNA loci in human cells. Science. 2017;**355**(6320):aah7111. DOI: 10.1126/science.aah7111. Epub 2016 Dec 15

[45] Hansen DV, Lui JH, Flandin P, Yoshikawa K, Rubenstein JL, Alvarez-Buylla A, et al. Non-epithelial stem cells and cortical interneuron production in the human ganglionic eminences. Nature Neuroscience. 2013;**16**:1576-1587

[46] Rakic S, Zecevic N. Emerging complexity of layer I in human cerebral cortex. Cerebral Cortex. 2003;**13**:1072-1083

[47] Ayana R, Singh S, Pati S. Decoding crucial LncRNAs implicated in neurogenesis and neurological

disorders. Stem Cells and Development. 2017;**26**:541-553

[48] Yao B, Jin P. Unlocking epigenetic codes in neurogenesis. Genes & Development. 2014;**28**:1253-1271

[49] Goff LA, Groff AF, Sauvageau M, Trayes-Gibson Z, Sanchez-Gomez DB, Morse M, et al. Spatiotemporal expression and transcriptional perturbations by long noncoding RNAs in the mouse brain. Proceedings of the National Academy of Sciences of the United States of America. 2015;**112**:6855-6862

[50] McCorkindale AL, Wahle P, Werner S, Jungreis I, Menzel P, Shukla CJ, et al. A gene expression atlas of embryonic neurogenesis in Drosophila reveals complex spatiotemporal regulation of lncRNAs. Development. 2019;**146**:dev175265

[51] Lewitus E, Huttner WB. Neurodevelopmental LincRNA microsyteny conservation and mammalian brain size evolution. PLoS One. 2015;**10**:e0131818

[52] Prajapati B, Fatma M, Maddhesiya P, Sodhi MK, Fatima M, Dargar T, et al. Identification and epigenetic analysis of divergent long non-coding RNAs in multilineage differentiation of human neural progenitor cells. RNA Biology. 2019;**16**:13-24

[53] Wang L, Deng Y, Duan D, Sun S, Ge L, Zhuo Y, et al. Hyperthermia influences fate determination of neural stem cells with lncRNAs alterations in the early differentiation. PLoS One. 2017;**12**:e0171359

[54] Zheng J, Yi D, Liu Y, Wang M, Zhu Y, Shi H. Long nonding RNA UCA1 regulates neural stem cell differentiation by controlling miR-1/Hes1 expression. American Journal of Translational Research. 2017;**9**:3696-3704

[55] Knauss JL, Miao N, Kim SN, Nie Y, Shi Y, Wu T, et al. Long noncoding RNA Sox2ot and transcription factor YY1 co-regulate the differentiation of cortical neural progenitors by repressing Sox2. Cell Death & Disease. 2018;**9**:799

[56] Ng SY, Bogu GK, Soh BS, Stanton LW. The long noncoding RNA RMST interacts with SOX2 to regulate neurogenesis. Molecular Cell. 2013;**51**:349-359

[57] Li W, Shen W, Zhang B, Tian K, Li Y, Mu L, et al. Long noncoding RNA LncKdm2b regulates cortical neuronal differentiation by cis-activating Kdm2b. Protein & Cell. 2020;**11**(3):161-186

[58] Pavlaki I, Alammari F, Sun B, Clark N, Sirey T, Lee S, et al. The long non-coding RNA Paupar promotes KAP1-dependent chromatin changes and regulates olfactory bulb neurogenesis. The EMBO Journal. 2018;**37**(10):e98219

[59] Vance KW, Sansom SN, Lee S, Chalei V, Kong L, Cooper SE, et al. The long non-coding RNA Paupar regulates the expression of both local and distal genes. The EMBO Journal. 2014;**33**:296-311

[60] Cheng X, Li H, Zhao H, Li W, Qin J, Jin G. Function and mechanism of long non-coding RNA Gm21284 in the development of hippocampal cholinergic neurons. Cell & Bioscience. 2019;**9**:72

[61] Weng R, Lu C, Liu X, Li G, Lan Y, Qiao J, et al. Long noncoding RNA-1604 orchestrates neural differentiation through the miR-200c/ZEB axis. Stem Cells. 2018;**36**:325-336

[62] Zhang L, Xue Z, Yan J, Wang J, Liu Q, Jiang H. LncRNA Riken-201 and Riken-203 modulates neural development by regulating the Sox6 through sequestering miRNAs. Cell Proliferation. 2019a;**52**:e12573

[63] Zhang L, Yan J, Liu Q, Xie Z, Jiang H. LncRNA Rik-203 contributes to anesthesia neurotoxicity via microRNA-101a-3p and GSK-3beta-mediated neural differentiation. Scientific Reports. 2019;**9**:6822

[64] Gao Y, Zhang R, Wei G, Dai S, Zhang X, Yang W, et al. Long noncoding RNA maternally expressed 3 increases the expression of neuronspecific genes by targeting miR-128-3p in all-trans retinoic acid-induced neurogenic differentiation from amniotic epithelial cells. Frontiers in Cell and Development Biology. 2019;**7**:342

[65] Chen L, Feng P, Zhu X, He S, Duan J, Zhou D. Long non-coding RNA Malat1 promotes neurite outgrowth through activation of ERK/MAPK signalling pathway in N2a cells. Journal of Cellular and Molecular Medicine. 2016;**20**:2102-2110

[66] Grammatikakis I, Gorospe M. Identification of neural stem cell differentiation repressor complex Pnky-PTBP1. Stem Cell Investigation. 2016;**3**:10

[67] Winzi M, Casas Vila N, Paszkowski-Rogacz M, Ding L, Noack S, Theis M, et al. The long noncoding RNA lncR492 inhibits neural differentiation of murine embryonic stem cells. PLoS One. 2018;**13**:e0191682

[68] Zheng X, Lin C, Li Y, Ye J, Zhou J, Guo P. Long noncoding RNA BDNF-AS regulates ketamine-induced neurotoxicity in neural stem cell derived neurons. Biomedicine & Pharmacotherapy. 2016;**82**:722-728

[69] Dong X, Chen K, Cuevas-Diaz Duran R, You Y, Sloan SA, Zhang Y, et al. Comprehensive identification of long non-coding RNAs in purified cell types from the brain reveals functional LncRNA in OPC fate determination. PLoS Genetics. 2015;**11**:e1005669

[70] He D, Wang J, Lu Y, Deng Y, Zhao C, Xu L, et al. lncRNA functional networks in oligodendrocytes reveal stage-specific myelination control by an lncOL1/Suz12 complex in the CNS. Neuron. 2017;**93**:362-378

[71] Li Y, Guo B, Yang R, Xiao Z, Gao X, Yu J, et al. A novel long noncoding RNA lnc158 promotes the differentiation of mouse neural precursor cells into oligodendrocytes by targeting nuclear factor-IB. Neuroreport. 2018;**29**:1121-1128

[72] Kasuga Y, Fudge AD, Zhang Y, Li H. Characterization of a long noncoding RNA Pcdh17it as a novel marker for immature premyelinating oligodendrocytes. Glia. 2019;**67**:2166-2177

[73] Mills JD, Kavanagh T, Kim WS, Chen BJ, Waters PD, Halliday GM, et al. High expression of long intervening non-coding RNA OLMALINC in the human cortical white matter is associated with regulation of oligodendrocyte maturation. Molecular Brain. 2015;**8**:2

[74] Wang F, Wang Q, Liu B, Mei L, Ma S, Wang S, et al. The long noncoding RNA Synage regulates synapse stability and neuronal function in the cerebellum. Cell Death and Differentiation. 2021;**28**(9):2634-2650. DOI: 10.1038/s41418-021-00774-3. Epub 2021 Mar 24

[75] Raveendra BL, Swarnkar S, Avchalumov Y, Liu X-A, Grinman E, Badal K, et al. Long noncoding RNA GM12371 acts as a transcriptional regulator of synapse function. Proceedings of the National Academy of Sciences. 2018;**115**:E10197

[76] Mercer TR, Dinger ME, Sunkin SM, Mehler MF, Mattick JS. Specific expression

of long noncoding RNAs in the mouse brain. Proceedings of the National Academy of Sciences of the United States of America. 2008;**105**:716-721

[77] Guttman M, Donaghey J, Carey BW, Garber M, Grenier JK, Munson G, et al. lincRNAs act in the circuitry controlling pluripotency and differentiation. Nature. 2011;**477**:295-300

[78] Li YP, Duan FF, Zhao YT, Gu KL, Liao LQ, Su HB, et al. A TRIM71 binding long noncoding RNA Trincr1 represses FGF/ERK signaling in embryonic stem cells. Nature Communications. 2019;**10**:1368

[79] Askarian-Amiri ME, Seyfoddin V, Smart CE, Wang J, Kim JE, Hansji H, et al. Emerging role of long non-coding RNA SOX2OT in SOX2 regulation in breast cancer. PLoS One. 2014;**9**:e102140

[80] Kan L, Israsena N, Zhang Z, Hu M, Zhao LR, Jalali A, et al. Sox1 acts through multiple independent pathways to promote neurogenesis. Developmental Biology. 2004;**269**(2):580-594. DOI: 10.1016/j.ydbio.2004.02.005

[81] Zhang S, Cui W. Sox2, a key factor in the regulation of pluripotency and neural differentiation. World Journal of Stem Cells. 2014;**6**:305-311

[82] Ahmad A, Strohbuecker S, Tufarelli C, Sottile V. Expression of a SOX1 overlapping transcript in neural differentiation and cancer models. Cellular and Molecular Life Sciences. 2017;**74**:4245-4258

[83] Tay Y, Rinn J, Pandolfi PP. The multilayered complexity of ceRNA crosstalk and competition. Nature. 2014;**505**:344-352

[84] Kriegstein A, Alvarez-Buylla A. The glial nature of embryonic and adult neural stem cells. Annual Review of Neuroscience. 2009;**32**:149-184. DOI: 10.1146/annurev.neuro.051508.135600

[85] Benito-Muñoz M, Matute C, Cavaliere F. Adenosine A1 receptor inhibits postnatal neurogenesis and sustains astrogliogenesis from the subventricular zone. Glia. 2016;**64**(9):1465-1478. DOI: 10.1002/glia.23010. Epub 2016 Jun 15

[86] Ohtsuka T, Shimojo H, Matsunaga M, Watanabe N, Kometani K, Minato N, et al. Gene expression profiling of neural stem cells and identification of regulators of neural differentiation during cortical development. Stem Cells. 2011;**29**(11):1817-1828. DOI: 10.1002/stem.731

[87] Lein ES, Belgard TG, Hawrylycz M, Molnár Z. Transcriptomic perspectives on neocortical structure, development, evolution, and disease. Annual Review of Neuroscience. 2017;**40**:629-652. DOI: 10.1146/annurev-neuro-070815-013858. Epub 2017 Jun 29

[88] Emery B, Lu QR. Transcriptional and epigenetic regulation of oligodendrocyte development and myelination in the central nervous system. Cold Spring Harbor Perspectives in Biology. 2015;7:a020461

[89] Zuchero JB, Barres BA. Intrinsic and extrinsic control of oligodendrocyte development. Current Opinion in Neurobiology. 2013;**23**:914-920

Chapter 8

Interactions of lncRNAs and miRNAs in Digestive System Tumors

Hussein Al-Dahmoshi, Noor Al-Khafaji, Moaed E. Al-Gazally, Maha F. Smaism, Zena Abdul Ameer Mahdi and Suhad Y. Abed

Abstract

Noncoding RNA (ncRNA) includes short (miRNA) and long (lncRNA) that have important regulatory role in different biological processes. One of the important issue in which ncRNA involved is tumor induction and suppression. miRNA and lncRNA were vital players in many tumors including digestive system tumors. This study includes studying the role of 140 hsa-miR including miR-1 to miR-140 and their sponger lncRNA in esophageal and stomach cancers by 249 studies. The review revealed that each miR may play as oncogene only or tumor suppressor via upregulation and downregulation regulatory proteins in cell cycles and activation of physiological cascades. Some of miR have dual role in same type of tumor as oncogene and suppressive miR. Same thing is for lncRNA tacting as oncogenic via sponging some of miR when overexpressed to upregulate oncogenic protein or acting as suppression lncRNA when overexpressed to downregulate some oncogenic proteins activated by miR. The current review concludes the vital role of ncRNA (both miRNA and lncRNA) in some digestive system tumors as oncogene-promoting cancer viability, invasiveness, proliferation, and metastasis or as tumor suppressor inhibiting tumorigenicity or inducing apoptosis.

Keywords: miRNA, lncRNA, sponge, oncogene, tumor suppressor, esophageal tumors, gastric cancers

1. Introduction

Ribonucleic acids (RNAs) are important nucleic acids for cell life and are classified as coding and non-coding RNA (ncRNAs). MicroRNAs (miRNAs) are a class of short noncoding RNAs (ncRNAs) (22 nts) that play important roles in posttranscriptional gene regulation. The majority of miRNAs are transcribed from DNA sequences into primary miRNAs and processed into precursor miRNAs, and finally mature miRNAs [1]. Long noncoding RNAs (lncRNAs) (more than 200 nts) may regulate cell proliferation, apoptosis, migration, invasion, and maintenance of stemness during cancer development [2, 3]. miRNA has a role in many tumors and upregulation/downregulation status of them may influence tumorigenesis, proliferation, metastasis, and chemoresistance [4, 5]. miRNAs implicated as oncogene of repressors for sets of cancers of liver: focal nodular hyperplasia (FNH) [6], hepatocellular adenoma (HCA) [7], hepatocellular carcinoma (HCC) [8], and cholangiocarcinomas (CCA) [9]. miRNAs were also implicated in pancreatic cancers: pancreatic endocrine tumors (PET) [10], pancreatic ductal adenocarcinoma (PDAC), and pancreatic acinar cell carcinoma (PACC) [11]. Esophageal squamous-cell carcinoma (ESCC) [12], and esophageal adenocarcinoma (EAC) [13], stomach adenocarcinoma (STAD) [14], colon adenocarcinoma (COAD) [15] were also influenced by miRNAs. The current review focused on 140 types of miR (miR-1 to miR-140) as oncogenic or tumor suppressor miR in different digestive system tumors.

1.1 Esophageal cancers

Esophageal cancer is a disease in which malignant (cancer) cells form in the tissues of the esophagus. It is characterized by its high mortality rate and poor prognosis. This disease is the sixth cause of cancer-related deaths and the eighth most common cancer worldwide with a 5-year survival rate of less than 25% [15]. Esophageal cancer occurs as either squamous cell carcinomas (ESCC) or adenocarcinoma (EAC). ncRNA including miRNA and lncRNA has a vital role in esophageal cancers either as oncogenic or as tumor suppressor [16, 17].

1.1.1 lncRNA/miR interaction in esophageal squamous cell carcinoma (ESCC)

Esophageal squamous cell carcinoma (ESCC) is a cancer that forms in the thin, flat cells lining the inside of the esophagus. It accounts for about 90% of esophageal cancers. miRNA can play a vital role in cancer regulation and may be an oncogene or tumor suppressor gene when overexpressed. In esophageal squamous cell carcinoma (ESCC), miR-1, −22, −26, −27, −29, −30, −33, −34, −98, −99, −100, −101, −107, −122, −124, −125, −127, −128, −129, −133, −134, −136, −137, −138, −139, and − 140 were downregulated in ESCC tissues compared with normal one acting as tumor suppressor and targeting different genes [18–43]. In contrast, the expression of miR-7, −9, −10, −16, −17, −18, −19, −20, −21, −23, −24, −25, −28, −31, −32, −92, −93, −96, −103, −105, −106, −126, −130-, and miR-135 was upregulated in ESCC acting as oncogene [44–66], as shown in **Table 1**.

Actually, lncRNA may have oncogenic activity acting as molecular sponge to inhibit activity of tumor suppressor miR. lncRNA opposite in action with tumor suppressor miR will act as oncogenic lncRNA, as shown in **Table 2**. HOX transcript antisense RNA (HOTAIR) expression increased in ESCC and inhibit the activity of miR-1. HOTAIR can be used as diagnostic marker of ESCC. miR-1 exert its suppressive action on ESCC via gene suppression of hepatocyte-growth factor (CCND1, CDK4, and MET). HOTAIR-mediated sponging of miR-1 leads to upregulation of those growth factors leading to ESCC proliferation and propagation [67]. Zinc finger E-box binding homeobox 1 (ZEB1) is transcriptional factor responsible for metastasis in ESCC, which is dysregulated by miR-33 to improve the outcome of ESCC. Differentiation antagonizing nonprotein coding RNA (DANCR) is lncRNA, which downregulates miR-33 and upregulates ZEB1 and so participates in worseness of ESCC [68]. Another lncRNA called MIR31HG acts on miR-34 leading to upregulation of c-Met promoting ESCC [69]. SNHG16 is also lncRNA of miR-98 that directly binds to enhancer of zeste homolog 2 (EZH2) and promotes ESCC propagation [70]. ANRIL is lncRNA of miR-99, which also promotes ESCC proliferation *via* downregulation of

miRNA	Expression in ESCC	Role in ESCC	Target gene	Ref.
miR-1	Downregulated	Tumor-suppressor	NOTCH2, LASP1	[18]
miR-22	Downregulated	Tumor-suppressor	PTEN, C-MYC	[19]
miR-26	Downregulated	Tumor-suppressor	MYCBP	[20]
miR-27	Downregulated	Tumor-suppressor	FBXW7	[21]
miR-29	Downregulated	Tumor-suppressor	FBXO31	[22]
miR-30	Downregulated	Tumor-suppressor	ITGA5, PDGFRB	[23]
miR-33	Downregulated	Tumor-suppressor	ZEB1	[24]
miR-34	Downregulated	Tumor-suppressor	c-MET, FOXM1	[25]
miR-98	Downregulated	Tumor-suppressor	EZH2	[26]
miR-99	Downregulated	Tumor-suppressor	CCND1, CCNA2	[27]
miR-100	Downregulated	Tumor-suppressor	CXCR7	[28]
miR-101	Downregulated	Tumor-suppressor	COX-2	[29]
miR-107	Downregulated	Tumor-suppressor	CDC42	[30]
miR-122	Downregulated	Tumor-suppressor	KIF22	[31]
miR-124	Downregulated	Tumor-suppressor	BCAT1	[32]
miR-125	Downregulated	Tumor-suppressor	p38-MAPK	[33]
miR-127	Downregulated	Tumor-suppressor	FMNL3	[34]
miR-128	Downregulated	Tumor-suppressor	ZEB1	[35]
miR-129	Downregulated	Tumor-suppressor	CTBP2	[36]
miR-133	Downregulated	Tumor-suppressor	COL1A1	[37]
miR-134	Downregulated	Tumor-suppressor	FOXM1	[38]
miR-136	Downregulated	Tumor-suppressor	MUC1	[39]
miR-137	Downregulated	Tumor-suppressor	EZH2, PXN	[40]
miR-138	Downregulated	Tumor-suppressor	NF-κB	[41]
miR-139	Downregulated	Tumor-suppressor	NR5A2	[42]
miR-140	Downregulated	Tumor-suppressor	ZEB1	[43]
miR-7	Downregulated	Tumor-suppressor	HOXB13	[44]
miR-9	Overexpressed	Oncogene	E-cadherin, FOXO1	[45]
miR-10	Overexpressed	Oncogene	FOXO3, KLF4	[46]
miR-16	Overexpressed	Oncogene	RECK, SOX6	[47]
miR-17	Overexpressed	Oncogene	RBL2	[48]
miR-18	Overexpressed	Oncogene	KRAS	[49]
miR-19	Overexpressed	Oncogene	CDC42, RAC1	[50]
miR-20	Overexpressed	Oncogene	RB1, TP53INP1	[51]
miR-21	Overexpressed	Oncogene	TPM1, PTEN	[52]
miR-23	Overexpressed	Oncogene	EBF3	[53]
miR-24	Overexpressed	Oncogene	FBXW7	[54]
miR-25	Overexpressed	Oncogene	PTEN, ZNF512B	[55]
miR-28	Overexpressed	Oncogene	ARF6	[56]
miR-31	Overexpressed	Oncogene	LATS2	[57]
miR-32	Overexpressed	Oncogene	CXXC5	[58]

miRNA	Expression in ESCC	Role in ESCC	Target gene	Ref.
miR-92	Overexpressed	Oncogene	PTEN	[59]
miR-93	Overexpressed	Oncogene	TGFβR2	[60]
miR-96	Overexpressed	Oncogene		[61]
miR-103	Overexpressed	Oncogene	CDH11, NR3C1	[62]
miR-105	Overexpressed	Oncogene	SPARCL1, FAK	[63]
miR-106	Overexpressed	Oncogene	PTEN	[64]
miR-126	Overexpressed	Oncogene	STAT3	[65]
miR-135	Overexpressed	Oncogene	RERG	[66]

Table 1.
Oncogenic/tumor-suppressor miR among ESCC.

lncRNA	Expression of lncRNA in ESCC	Target miR	Target gene	Ref.
HOTAIR	Overexpressed	miR-1	CCND1, CDK4, and MET	[67]
DANCR	Overexpressed	miR-33	ZEB1	[68]
MIR31HG	Overexpressed	miR-34	c-Met	[69]
SNHG16	Overexpressed	miR-98	EZH2	[70]
ANRIL	Overexpressed	miR-99	—	[71]
MALAT1	Overexpressed	miR-101	—	[72]
FAM201A	Overexpressed	miR-101	mTOR	[73]
LINC00152	Overexpressed	miR-107	Rab10	[74]
LINC01296	Overexpressed	miR-122	mTOR	[75]
ZFAS1	Overexpressed	miR-124	STAT3	[76]
HOTAIR	Overexpressed	miR-125	HK2	[77]
NEAT1	Overexpressed	miR-129	CTBP2	[36]
H19	Overexpressed	miR-138	EZH2	[78]
BCAR4	Overexpressed	miR-139	ELAVL1	[79]
SNHG16	Overexpressed	miR-140	ZEB1	[43]
LincIN	Overexpressed	miR-7	HOXB13	[80]
MEG3	Downregulated	miR-9	E-cadherin, FOXO1	[81]
FAM83H-AS1	Overexpressed	miR-10	—	[82]
PART1	Downregulated	miR-18	SOX6	[83]
GAS5	Downregulated	miR-21	RECK	[84]
AC012073.1	Downregulated	miR-93	—	[85]

Table 2.
Oncogenic/tumor suppressor lncRNA among ESCC.

miR-99 [71]. MALAT1 lncRNA may decrease the expression of miR-101 and promote ESCC proliferation and metastasis via upregulation of [72]. Additionally, FAM201A lncRNA acts as a sponge for miR-101 and upregulates mTOR [73]. miR-107 targeting Ras-related protein Rab-10 (Rab10) and decreasing their expression and preventing ESCC propagation. LINC00152 is sponge lncRNA of miR-107, which promotes ESCC *via* overexpression of Rab10 upon miR-107 sponging [74]. Additionally LINC01296 sponge miR-122 and increasing mTOR expression [75]. ZFAS1 lncRNA was found to promote the proliferation, migration, and invasion of ESCC by upregulating STAT3 and downregulating miR-124 [76]. HOTAIR could increase the expression of hexokinase 2 (HK2) in ESCC through sponging of miR-125 [77]. Nuclear paraspeckle assembly transcript 1 (NEAT1) is lncRNA that sponge miR-129 and upregulates their target, CTBP2, promoting ESCC viability and invasion [36]. H19 lncRNA inhibits the effect of miR-138 and promotes EZH2 thereby promoting ESCC [78]. Breast cancer antiestrogen resistance 4 (BCAR4) lncRNA act to sponged miR-139-3p, leading to upregulation of ELAVL1 and promoting tumorigenesis of ESCC [79]. SNHG16 lncRNA squeegee miR-140 and upregulates their target, ZEB1, thereby promoting ESCC [43]. lncRNA LincIN has been reported to be overexpressed and to be involved in the metastasis of breast cancer. LincIN has the potential role in ESCC invasion and metastasis *via* upregulation of HOXB13 and downregulation of miR-7 + enhancement of binding between NF90 on primary miR-7. It seem that no sponge lncRNA were documented for miR-22, −26, −27, −29, −30, −100, −127, −128, −133, −134, −136, and miR-137 in ESCC yet.

lncRNA can act as tumor suppressor counteracting the effect of oncogenic miR. Maternally expressed gene 3 (MEG3) is tumor suppressor lncRNA of miR-9. MEG3 decreased expression was seen in ESCC. Expression level of MEG3 was significantly increased in cancer cells after being treated with the DNA methyltransferase inhibitor 5-Aza-dC, leading to decreased miR-9 and increased E-cadherin and FOXO1 expression [81]. miR-10 can be sponged by lncRNA FAM83H-AS1 in ESCC [82]. Prostate androgen-regulated transcript 1 (PART1) lncRNA was downregulated in ESCC and, when overexpressed, will sponge oncogenic miR-18 leading to upregulation of SOX6 thereby inhibiting ESCC proliferation and metastasis [83]. Growth arrest-specific 5 (GAS5) lncRNA is seen to be elevated in radiation-sensitive ESCC tissues, leading to dysregulation of miR-21 and increasing the level of its target, RECK [84]. lncRNA called AC012073.1 is seen to bind competitively to miR-93 in ESCC [85] as shown in **Table 2**.

1.1.2 lncRNA/miR interaction in esophageal adenocarcinoma (EAC)

Esophageal adenocarcinoma (EAC) is a malignancy classically seen in the distal esophagus. The incidence of EAC is seven times more common in men than in women [86]. lncRNA and miRNA can either be oncogenic promoting tumor proliferation, invasion, and metastasis or acting as a tumor suppressor via targeting specific protein and signaling pathways. It seems few studies were conducted on miR role in tumorigenesis or anti-tumor in EAC, but many studies highlighted the pivotal role of lncRNA. lncRNA called miR205HG was found to have tumor suppressory effect on EAC when overexpressed *via* downregulation of the Hedgehog (Hh) signaling pathway [87]. lncRNA HOTAIR expression was upregulated in EAC tumor acting as oncogene via regulating NTRK2, NP1, CHRDL1, NTRK2, HOXC8, and IL11. Inversely lncRNA CYP1B1-AS1 was downregulated in EAC acting as tumor supressor [88]. Two lncRNA called AFAP1-AS1 and HNF1A-AS1 were shown to be

lncRNA	Expression of lncRNA in EAC	Target miR	Target gene	Ref.
miR205HG	Downregulated	NA	Hedgehog	[87]
HOTAIR	Overexpressed	NA	NTRK2, NP1, CHRDL1, NTRK2, HOXC8 and IL11	[88]
CYP1B1-AS1	Downregulated	NA	NA	[88]
AFAP1-AS1	Overexpressed	NA	NA	[89]
HNF1A-AS1	Overexpressed	NA	H19	[90]
PVT1	Overexpressed	NA	LATS1, YAP1	[91]
MIR22HG	Overexpressed	NA	STAT3	[92]
BDNF-AS	Downregulated	miR-214	JAG1	[92]
ADAMTS9- AS2	Downregulated	NA	CDH3	[93]
LINC00662	Overexpressed	NA	Wnt/β-catenin	[94]

Table 3.
Oncogenic/tumor suppressor lncRNA among EAC.

overexpressed in EAC acting as oncogene [89, 90]. PVT1 lncRNA was also documented as oncogene via upregulation of YAP1 in EAC tissues [91]. Also, MIR22HG lncRNA has same effect on PVT1 (oncogenic) via activation of STAT3/c-Myc/p-FAK pathway. Tumor suppressor lncRNA like BDNF-AS and ADAMTS9- AS2 can exert their suppressive activity via sponging miR-214 and CDH3, respectively [92, 93]. Another oncogenic lncRNA, LINC00662, utilizes its effect *via* activating Wnt/β-catenin signaling (**Table 3**) [94].

1.2 Stomach cancers

Gastric or stomach cancers were also regulated by miR/lncRNA interactions. miR-1 directly targets the MET gene and downregulates its expression acting as tumor suppressor [95]. MET is an oncogene and its activation results from the binding of hepatocyte growth factor (HGF), leading to tumor growth, metastasis, migration, and drug resistance [96]. Targeting MET by miR-1 will deactivate it, and MET can restore its activity by oncogenic lncRNA called LINC00242 when sponging the miR-1 [97]. miR-7 also acting as a tumor suppressor in gastric cancer may be *via* degradation of EGFR mRNA, and thus, the oncogenic lncRNA UCA1 can sponge miR-7, leading to enhancing the expression of EGFR and promoting cell metastasis and migration [98]. miR-9 is implicated as oncogenic *via* downregulation of CDX2 and promotes gastric cancer cell proliferation [99] and may act as tumor suppressor that can be sponged by HULC lncRNA via upregulation of MYH9 [100]. miR-17, −18, −19, and − 20 were documented as oncogenic ncRNA among gastric cancer patients. Oncogenic miR-17 targeting PTEN and EGR2 to enhance proliferation and metastasis of stomach cancer, and this effect can be sponged by lncRNA HOTAIRM1 or LINC01939, which suppressed proliferation and migration of GC cell acting as tumor suppressor lncRNA [101, 102]. Inversely, lncRNA NEAT1 was overexpressed in gastric cancers and positively related with miR-17 *via* activation of GSK3β [103]. By targeting IRF2, miR-18 enhances proliferation and metastasis of gastric cancer [104]. Sponging of miR-19 by lncRNA CASC2 can increase the sensitivity to cisplatin and so it acts as tumor suppressor [105, 106].

<>Oncogenic miR-21 can promote gastric cancer cell viability and progression via downregulation of some tumor suppressor genes like PTEN, RECK, and PDCD4 [107]. Inhibiting miR-21 expression by lncRNA MEG3 can inhibit gastric cancer growth and metastasis [108]. miR-22 acts to suppress gastric cancer via upregulating MMP14, NET1, and Snail while lncRNA CTC-497E21.4 can squeegee miR-22 and promote proliferation and invasion [109]. miR-24 and miR-25 were upregulated in gastric cancer tissues and may promote the occurrence, development, infiltration, and metastasis of gastric cancer. As oncogenic miR-24 inhibits the CDKN1B and CHEK1 and miR-25 targeting FOXO3 [110, 111]. Tumor suppressor lncRNA GATA6-AS acts to inhibit gastric cancer progression by sponging miR-25 [112]. Targeting PTEN, miR-26 acts as oncogenic and upregulated in gastric cancer tissues promoting proliferation and invasion. Additionally, miR-26 can target EZH2 and can be suppressed by tumor suppressor lncRNA TET1–3 [113, 114]. miR-27 is additional oncogenic miR acting on HOXA10 [115]. By inhibiting the phosphorylation of AKT protein in gastric cancer cells, miR-28 acts as inhibiting progression and metastasis and can be sponged by LOC400043 [116, 117]. Low expression was seen in gastric cancer tissues for miR-29 highlighting their role as tumor suppressor targeting CCND2 and MMP2, and can be sponged by lncRNA MEG3 [118, 119]. As tumor suppressor, miR-30 is responsible for inhibiting gastric cancer and increasing sensitivity to anticancer drugs when upregulated [120], and lncRNA PVT1, HNF1A-AS1, and DLEU2 can sponge miR-30 and upregulating Snail protein, PI3K/AKT signaling pathway and ETS2, respectively, promoting gastric cancer cell proliferation and metastasis [121–123].

Conversely, it can be acting as oncogenic miR through P53/ROS-mediated regulation of the mitochondrial apoptotic pathway [124]. miR-31 acts as a vital tumor suppressor ncRNA by inhibiting E2F2s and RhoA expression, also upregulation of miR-31 targeting ITGA5 may suppress tumor cell invasion and metastasis by indirectly regulating PI3K/AKT signaling pathway in human SGC7901 GC cells [125, 126]. lncRNA MIR31HG can encourage gastric cancer cell proliferation and invasion via sponging miR-31 [127]. Another oncogenic miR is miR-32, which augments tumorigenesis of gastric cell cancer by targeting KLF4 and KLF2, and at the same time can be sponged by SNHG5 lncRNA [128]. Gastric cancer suppresivity of miR-33 and miR-34 by targeting CDK6, CCND1, and PIM1 via miR-33 and Bcl-2, Notch, and HMGA2 via miR-34 [129, 130].

Overexpression of miR-43 was seen in gastric cancer tissues that promotes proliferation and metastasis by targeting VEZT [131]. miR-92 suppresses proliferation of gastric cancer and induces apoptosis by targeting EP4, Notch1 [132], and by targeting SOX4 while sponging of miR-92 by lncRNA PITPNA-AS1 and MT1JP can promote gastric cancer migration via upregulation of SOX4 and FBXW7 respectively [133, 134]. Oncogenic miR-93 can promote tumorigenesis by downregulation of IFNAR1 or PTEN [135, 136], and gastric cancer suppressor lncRNA PTENP1, GPC5-AS1, and CA3-AS1 can achieve gastric cancer inhibition by sponging miR93 and upregulating PTEN, GPC5, and PTG3 respectively [136–138]. Dual effect of miR-95 targeting EMP1 as oncogene or tumor suppressor by targeting Slug [139, 140]. Oncogenic miR-96 can target *ZDHHC5*, KIF26A, and FOXO3 promoting gastric cancer cell viability [141, 142]. Downregulation of BCAT1 Treg and CCND2 by miR-98 as a tumor suppressor for gastric cancer [143, 144] and TTTY15 lncRNA can sponge miR-98 and upregulate CCND2 [145]. Tumor suppressor miR-100 can inhibit cell proliferation and induce apoptosis in human gastric cancer via downregulating many proteins, such as BMPR2 [146], ZBTB7A [147], and CXCR7 [148], or acting as oncogene via their antiapoptotic role by inhibiting ubiquitination-mediated p53 degradation [149] and upregulation of HS3ST2 [150]. Contrariwise, oncogenic lncRNA such as HAGLROS [151] and MIR100HG [152] were sponging miR-100 and promote tumorigenesis via activation of the mTORC1 signaling pathway [151], PI3K/AKT/mTOR pathway [153, 154].

Tumor suppressor miR-101 targeting: ANXA2 [155], ZEB1 [156], SOCS2 [157], PI3K/AKT/mTOR [158], EZH2 [159], and AMPK [160] and sponged by LINC01303 and lncRNA XIST by upregulating EZH2 [159, 161], lncRNA SPRY4-IT1 by upregulating AMPK [160], lncRNA SNHG6 by upregulating ZEB1 [162] and lncRNA LINC00943 [163]. Dual oncogenic and tumor suppressive effects of miR-103 were elucidated in gastric cancer. It was found that overexpressed caveolin-1 and RAB10 were targets for suppressive miR-103 [164, 165] while miR-103 acting as oncogenic by downregulation of KLF4 [166]. lncRNA LINC00152 acting as oncogenic by sponging miR-103 and upregulation of RAB10 [165]. miR-105 inhibits gastric cancer cell metastasis, by targeting SOX9 and YY1 [167–169]. miR-106 play an oncogenic role in gastric cancer [170]. lncRNA GPC5-AS1 acting as tumor suppressor for gastric cancer via sponging miR-106 and upregulation of GPC5 [137]. Like miR-103, miR-107 has onogenic and tumor suppressive effects in gastric cancers, oncogenic by downregulation of PTEN [171], NF1 [172], and HIF-1α [173] suppressive by targeting BDNF [174]. lncRNA ZFR and PCAT18 counteracting oncogenic effect of miR-107 by upregulation of PTEN [171, 175]. Suppresivity of miR-122 may be linked to their target downregulation including DUSP4 [176], LYN [177], MYC [178], MMP-9 [179], GIT-1 [180], and VEGFD [181] while their effect can be sponged by lncRNA LINC01296, CRART16, and promoting metastasis by upregulation of MMP-9 and VEGFD respectively [179, 181]. Same thing for miR-124, they inhibit gastric cancer by downregulating many oncogenes like SPHK1 [182], ROCK1 [183], RAC1 and SP1 [184], EZH2 [185, 186], DNMT3B [187], and ITGB3 [188]. lncRNA MALAT1, LINC00511, LINC00240, and HOXA11-AS were overexpressed in gastric cancer as oncogene promoting cancer cell viability, proliferation, and metastasis via sponging miR-124 and upregulating EZH2, DNMT3B and ITGB3 respectively [185–188]. Tumor suppresivity of miR-125 on gastric cancers was attributed to downregulation of many proteins inhibiting proliferation and metastasis: MCL1, BRMS1, VEGF-A, and HER2 [189–192], while lncRNA PVT1 was the only oncogenic ncRNA sponging miR-125 in gastric cancer [193]. Tumor suppressor miR-126 can inhibit proliferation and metastasis of gastric cancers by downregulation of CRKL, VEGF-A, CXCR4, ADAM9, BRCC3, and PIK3R2 [194–199] while TMPO-AS1 and HOTAIR were two oncogenic lncRNA promoting invasion and metastasis by upregulation of BRCC3 and PIK3R2, and sponging miR-126 [198, 199]. As tumor suppressor acting to downregulate MAPK4, WNT7a, SORT1, and MTDH by miR-127 and inhibiting gastric cancer invasion [200–203]. SORT1 and MTDH can be upregulated by sponging miR-127 by lncRNA circ_0110389 and circALPL respectively [202, 203]. Four lncRNA were found to be oncogenic and sponging the tumor suppressor miR-128 and upregulating their targets leading to promoting gastric cancer proliferation and metastasis: lncRNA CCL2 with PARP2, lncRNA HCP5 with HMGA2, lncRNA PCAT1 with ZEB1, and lncRNA LINC01091 with ELF4 [204–207]. Additional 4 oncogenic lncRNA were upregulated in gastric cancer tissues and downregulated miR-129: GACAT2, GACAT3, AC130710, and PCGEM1, which upregulate P4HA2 [208–210]. Oncogenic miR-130 promotes gastric cancer invasion and metastasis by downregulation of TGFβR2, C-MYB, and GCNT4 [211–213] while lncRNA MRPL39 acts to suppress the metastasis by sponging miR-130 [214]. Tumor suppressor miR-132 inhibits gastric tumor invasiveness and metastasis via downregulation of MUC13, CD44 and fibronectin1 (FN1), KIF21B, and PXN [215–218], while lncRNA XIST can sponge miR-132 and upregulate PXN [218]. miR-134 and their lncRNA can have dual effects as tumor suppressor or oncogene and vice versa. By targeting and downregulation of GOLPH3, YY1 and YWHAZ [219–221] miR-134 acting as gastric cancer suppressor while acting as oncogene to deactivate PTEN while lncRNA circPTK2 can sponge miR-134 to activate PTEN inhibiting proliferation and metastasis [222]. Inversely lncRNA LUCAT1 can act as oncogene sponging suppressor miR-134 and upregulation of YWHAZ [221]. Oncogenic miR-135 can downregulate E2F1 and DAPK2 [223] and upregulate WNT [224] while miR-135 can act as gastric cancer suppressor down-regulating SMAD2 [225]. Gastric cancer metastasis and invasion can be promoted by sponging of miR-136 by lncRNA circ_0110389 and circ_100876 leading to upregulation of SORT1 and MIEN1 respectively [202, 226]. Sponging of miR-137 by lncRNA like DSCR8, NCK1-AS1, and circHECTD1 can promote invasion and proliferation of gastric cancer by upregulation of CDC42, NUP43, and PBX3 respectively [227–229]. miR-138 inhibits gastric cancer vitality and progression by downregulation of ITGA2, PLAU, FOXC1, and SIRT2, which can be upregulated after sponging miR-138 by lncRNA UBE2CP3, TRPM2-AS, MCM3AP-AS1, and LINC00152 respectively

miRNA	Expression in ESCC	Role in ESCC	Target gene	Ref.
miR-1	Downregulated	Tumor-suppressor	MET	[95]
miR-7	Downregulated	Tumor-suppressor	EGFR	[243]
miR-9	Overexpressed	Oncogenic	CDX2	[99]
miR-9	Downregulated	Tumor-suppressor	MYH9	[100]
miR-17	Overexpressed	Oncogenic	PTEN, EGR2	[101, 102]
miR-18	Overexpressed	Oncogenic	IRF2	[104]
miR-19	Overexpressed	Oncogenic	NA	[106]
miR-20	Overexpressed	Oncogenic	NA	[106]
miR-21	Overexpressed	Oncogenic	PTEN, RECK, and PDCD4	[107]
miR-22	Downregulated	Tumor-suppressor	MMP14, NET1, and Snail	[109]
miR-24	Overexpressed	Oncogenic	CDKN1B and CHEK1	[110]
miR-25	Overexpressed	Oncogenic	FOXO3	[111]
miR-26	Overexpressed	Oncogenic	PTEN, EZH2	[113]
miR-27	Overexpressed	Oncogenic	HOXA10	[115]
miR-28	Downregulated	Tumor-suppressor	AKT	[116]
miR-29	Downregulated	Tumor-suppressor	CCND2, MMP2	[118]
miR-30	Downregulated	Tumor-suppressor	beclin-1, Snail, and ETS2	[120, 121, 123]
miR-30	Overexpressed	Oncogenic	P53	[124]

miRNA	Expression in ESCC	Role in ESCC	Target gene	Ref.
miR-31	Downregulated	Tumor-suppressor	E2F2s, RhoA, and ITGA5	[125–127]
miR-32	Overexpressed	Oncogenic	KLF4, KLF2	[128, 244]
miR-33	Downregulated	Tumor-suppressor	CDK6, CCND1, and PIM1	[129]
miR-34	Downregulated	Tumor-suppressor	Bcl-2, Notch, and HMGA2	[130]
miR-43	Overexpressed	Oncogenic	VEZT	[131]
miR-92	Downregulated	Tumor-suppressor	EP4, Notch1, SOX4, and FBXW7	[132–134]
miR-93	Overexpressed	Oncogenic	IFNAR1, PTEN GPC5, and PTG3	[135–138]
miR-95	Overexpressed	Oncogenic	EMP1	[139]
miR-95	Downregulated	Tumor-suppressor	Slug	[140]
miR-96	Overexpressed	Oncogenic	ZDHHC5, KIF26A, and FOXO3	[141, 142]
miR-98	Downregulated	Tumor-suppressor	BCAT1, Treg, and CCND2	[143–145]
miR-100	Downregulated	Tumor-suppressor	BMPR2, ZBTB7A	[146–148]
miR-100	Overexpressed	Oncogenic	p53, HS3ST2	[149, 150]
miR-101	Downregulated	Tumor-suppressor	ANXA2, ZEB1, SOCS2, PI3K/AKT/mTOR, EZH2, and AMPK	[155–159]
miR-103	Downregulated	Tumor-suppressor	Caveolin-1, RAB10	[164, 165]
miR-103	Overexpressed	Oncogenic	KLF4	[166]
miR-105	Downregulated	Tumor-suppressor	SOX9, YY1	[167–169]
miR-106	Overexpressed	Oncogenic	NA	[170, 245]
miR-107	Overexpressed	Oncogenic	PTEN, NF1, and HIF1α	[171–173]
miR-107	Downregulated	Tumor-suppressor	BDNF	[174]
miR-122	Downregulated	Tumor-suppressor	DUSP4, LYN, MYC, MMP-9, and GIT-1	[176–180]
miR-124	Downregulated	Tumor-suppressor	SPHK1, ROCK1, RAC1, and SP1	[182–184]
miR-125	Downregulated	Tumor-suppressor	MCL1, BRMS1, VEGF-A, and HER2	[189–192]
miR-126	Downregulated	Tumor-suppressor	CRKL, VEGF-A, CXCR4, ADAM9, BRCC3, and PIK3R2	[194–199]
miR-127	Downregulated	Tumor-suppressor	MAPK4, WNT7a, SORT1, and MTDH	[200–203]

miRNA	Expression in ESCC	Role in ESCC	Target gene	Ref.
miR-128	Downregulated	Tumor-suppressor	PARP2, HMGA2, ZEB1, and ELF4	[204–207]
miR-129	Downregulated	Tumor-suppressor	P4HA2	[210]
miR-130	Overexpressed	Oncogenic	TGFβR2, C-MYB, and GCNT4	[211–213]
miR-132	Downregulated	Tumor-suppressor	MUC13, CD44, fibronectin1 (FN1), KIF21B, and PXN	[215–218]
miR-134	Downregulated	Tumor-suppressor	GOLPH3, YY1, and YWHAZ	[219–221]
miR-134	Overexpressed	Oncogenic	PTEN	[222]
miR-136	Downregulated	Tumor-suppressor	SORT1, MIEN1	[202, 226]
miR-137	Downregulated	Tumor-suppressor	CDC42, NUP43, and PBX3	[227–229]
miR-138	Downregulated	Tumor-suppressor	ITGA2, PLAU, FOXC1, and SIRT2	[230–233]
miR-139	Downregulated	Tumor-suppressor	MYB, MMP11, PRKAA1, ELK1, and SOX4	[234–238]
miR-140	Downregulated	Tumor-suppressor	ATG5, SOX4, ADAM10, and NDRG3	[239–242]

Table 4.
Oncogenic/tumor suppressor miR among stomach cancer.

lncRNA	Expression of lncRNA in Stomach cancer	Target miR	Target gene	Ref.
LINC00242	Overexpressed	miR-1	MET	[97]
UCA1	Overexpressed	miR-7	EGFR	[98]
HULC	Overexpressed	miR-9	MYH9	[100]
HOTAIRM1	Downregulated	miR-17	PTEN	[101]
LINC01939	Downregulated	miR-17	EGR2	[102]
NEAT1	Overexpressed	miR-17	GSK3β	[103]
CASC2	Downregulated	miR-19	NA	[105]
MEG3	Downregulated	miR-21	PTEN	[108]
CTC-497E21.4	Overexpressed	miR-22	NET1	[109]
GATA6-AS	Downregulated	miR-22	FOXO3	[112]
TET1–3	Downregulated	miR-26	EZH2	[114]
LOC400043	Overexpressed	miR-28	AKT	[117]
MEG3	Overexpressed	miR-29	CCND2, MMP2	[119]
PVT1	Overexpressed	miR-30	Snail	[121]

lncRNA	Expression of lncRNA in Stomach cancer	Target miR	Target gene	Ref.
HNF1A-AS1	Overexpressed	miR-30	PI3K/AKT	[122]
DLEU2	Overexpressed	miR-30	ETS2	[123]
MIR31HG	Overexpressed	miR-31	E2F2s, RhoA, and ITGA5	[127]
SNHG5	Downregulated	miR-32	KLF4	[128]
PITPNA-AS1	Overexpressed	miR-92	SOX4	[133]
MT1JP	Overexpressed	miR-92	FBXW7	[134]
PTENP1	Downregulated	miR-93	PTEN, GPC5, and PTG3	[136–138]
TTTY15	Overexpressed	miR-98	CCND2	[145]
HAGLROS	Overexpressed	miR-100	mTORC1 signaling pathway	[151]
MIR100HG	Overexpressed	miR-100	PI3K/AKT/mTOR pathway	[152–154]
LINC01303	Overexpressed	miR-100	EZH2	[159]
SPRY4-IT1	Overexpressed	miR-100	AMPK	[160]
XIST	Overexpressed	miR-100	EZH2	[161]
SNHG6	Overexpressed	miR-100	ZEB1	[162]
LINC00943	Overexpressed	miR-100	NA	[163]
LINC00152	Overexpressed	miR-103	RAB10	[165]
GPC5-AS1	Downregulated	miR-106	GPC5	[137]
ZFR	Downregulated	miR-107	PTEN	[171]
PCAT18	Downregulated	miR-107	PTEN	[175]
LINC01296	Overexpressed	miR-122	MMP-9	[179]
CRART16	Overexpressed	miR-122	VEGFD	[180]
MALAT1	Overexpressed	miR-124	EZH2	[185]
LINC00511	Overexpressed	miR-124	EZH2	[186]
LINC00240	Overexpressed	miR-124	DNMT3B	[187]
HOXA11-AS	Overexpressed	miR-124	ITGB3	[188]
PVT1	Overexpressed	miR-125	NA	[193]
BRCC3	Overexpressed	miR-126	BRCC3	[198]
PIK3R2	Overexpressed	miR-126	PIK3R2	[199]
circ_0110389	Overexpressed	miR-127	SORT1	[202]
circALPL	Overexpressed	miR-127	MTDH	[203]
CCL2	Overexpressed	miR-128	PARP2	[204]
HCP5	Overexpressed	miR-128	HMGA2	[205]
PCAT1	Overexpressed	miR-128	ZEB1	[206]

lncRNA	Expression of lncRNA in Stomach cancer	Target miR	Target gene	Ref.
LINC01091	Overexpressed	miR-128	ELF4	[207]
GACAT2,	Overexpressed	miR-129	NA	[208]
GACAT3	Overexpressed	miR-129	NA	[208]
AC130710	Overexpressed	miR-129	NA	[209]
PCGEM1	Overexpressed	miR-129	NA	[210]
MRPL39	Downregulated	miR-130	NA	[214]
XIST	Overexpressed	miR-132	PXN	[218]
circPTK2	Downregulated	miR-134	PTEN	[222]
LUCAT1	Overexpressed	miR-134	YWHAZ	[221]
circ_0110389	Overexpressed	miR-136	SORT1	[202]
circ_100876	Overexpressed	miR-136	MIEN1	[226]
DSCR8	Overexpressed	miR-137	CDC42	[227]
NCK1-AS1	Overexpressed	miR-137	NUP43	[228]
circHECTD1	Overexpressed	miR-137	PBX3	[229]
UBE2CP3	Overexpressed	miR-138	ITGA2	[230]
TRPM2-AS	Overexpressed	miR-138	PLAU	[231]
MCM3AP-AS1	Overexpressed	miR-138	FOXC1	[232]
LINC00152	Overexpressed	miR-138	SIRT2	[233]
SNHG3	Overexpressed	miR-139	MYB	[234]
CTBP1-AS2	Overexpressed	miR-139	MMP11	[235]
LINC00152	Overexpressed	miR-139	PRKAA1	[236]
Circ-PTPDC1	Overexpressed	miR-139	ELK1	[237]
circ_0000218	Overexpressed	miR-139	SOX4	[238]
CCAT1	Overexpressed	miR-140	ATG5	[239]
TMPO-AS1	Overexpressed	miR-140	SOX4	[240]
SNHG1	Overexpressed	miR-140	ADAM10	[241]
SNHG20	Overexpressed	miR-140	NDRG3	[242]

Table 5.
Oncogenic/tumor suppressor lncRNA among stomach cancer.

[230–233]. Same miR-138, miR-139 is tumor suppressor ncRNA inhibiting of tumorgenicity and their effect can be sponged by lncRNA, which promote tumorigenicity via upregulation of MYB, MMP11, PRKAA1, ELK1, and SOX4 by lncRNA SNHG3, CTBP1-AS2, LINC00152, Circ-PTPDC1, and circ_0000218 respectively [234–238]. Tumor suppresivity of miR-140 in gastric cancer was achieved via decreasing the expression of ATG5, SOX4, ADAM10, and NDRG3. Inverse effect (oncogenic) on gastric cancer can be accomplished by lncRNA CCAT1, TMPO-AS1, SNHG1, and SNHG20, which upregulate previously mentioned proteins respectively [239–242] (**Tables 4** and **5**).

2. Conclusion

The current review concludes the vital role of ncRNA (both miRNA and lncRNA) in some digestive system tumors either as an oncogene-promoting cancer viability, invasiveness, proliferation, and metastasis or as a tumor suppressor inhibiting tumorigenicity or inducing apoptosis.

Conflict of interest

There is no "conflict of interest" for this work.

Author details

Hussein Al-Dahmoshi[1*], Noor Al-Khafaji[1], Moaed E. Al-Gazally[2], Maha F. Smaism[3], Zena Abdul Ameer Mahdi[4] and Suhad Y. Abed[5]

1 Biology Department, College of Science, University of Babylon, Hilla, Iraq

2 College of Medicine, University of Al-Ameed, Karbala-Iraq

3 College of Medicine, University of Babylon, Babylon, Hilla, Iraq

4 College of Pharmacy, Ahlabayt University, Karbala, Iraq

5 Department of Biology, College of Science, Mustansiriyah University, Baghdad, Iraq

*Address all correspondence to: dr.dahmoshi83@gmail.com

References

[1] O'Brien J, Hayder H, Zayed Y, Peng C. Overview of microRNA biogenesis, mechanisms of actions, and circulation. Frontiers in Endocrinology. 2018;**9**:402. DOI: 10.3389/fendo.2018.00402

[2] Batista PJ, Chang HY. Long noncoding RNAs: Cellular address codes in development and disease. Cell. 2013;**152**(6):1298-1307. DOI: 10.1016/j.cell/2013/02/012

[3] Yuan JH, Yang F, Wang F, Ma JZ, Guo YJ, Tao QF, et al. A long noncoding RNA activated by TGF-β promotes the invasion-metastasis cascade in hepatocellular carcinoma. Cancer Cell. 2014;**25**(5):666-681. DOI: 10.1016/j.ccr.2014.03.010

[4] Forterre A, Komuro H, Aminova S, Harada M. A comprehensive review of cancer microRNA therapeutic delivery strategies. Cancers. 2020;**12**(7):1852. DOI: 10.3390/cancers12071852

[5] Tan W, Liu B, Qu S, Liang G, Luo W, Gong C. MicroRNAs and cancer: Key paradigms in molecular therapy. Oncology Letters. 2018;**15**(3):2735-2742. DOI: 10.3892/ol.2017.7638

[6] Lendvai G, Szekerczés T, Gyöngyösi B, Schlachter K, Kontsek E, Pesti A, et al. MicroRNA expression in focal nodular hyperplasia in comparison with cirrhosis and hepatocellular carcinoma. Pathology Oncology Research. 2019;**25**(3):1103-1109. DOI: 10.1007/s12253-018-0528-z

[7] Wang H, Yang G, Yu Y, Peibing Gu PG. MicroRNA-490-3p suppresses the proliferation and invasion of hepatocellular carcinoma cells via targeting TMOD3. Oncology Letters. 2020;**20**(4):1. DOI: 10.3892/ol.2020.11956

[8] Han TS, Hur K, Cho HS, Ban HS. Epigenetic associations between lncRNA/circRNA and miRNA in hepatocellular carcinoma. Cancers. 2020;**12**(9):2622. DOI: 10.3390/cancers12092622

[9] Guan C, Zhao Y, Wang W, Hu Z, Liu L, Li W, et al. Knockdown of lncRNA SNHG20 suppressed the proliferation of cholangiocarcinoma by sponging miR-520f-3p. Cancer Biotherapy & Radiopharmaceuticals. 2020;**12**(1):1-13. DOI: 10.1089/cbr.2020.4042

[10] Li K, Han H, Gu W, Cao C, Zheng P. Long non-coding RNA LINC01963 inhibits progression of pancreatic carcinoma by targeting miR-641/TMEFF2. Biomedicine & Pharmacotherapy. 2020;**129**:110346. DOI: 10.1016/j.biopha.2020.110346

[11] Miao H, Lu J, Guo Y, Qiu H, Zhang Y, Yao X, et al. LncRNA TP73-AS1 enhances the malignant properties of pancreatic ductal adenocarcinoma by increasing MMP14 expression through miRNA-200a sponging. Journal of Cellular and Molecular Medicine. 2021;**25**(7):3654-3664. DOI: 10.1111/jcmm.16425

[12] Ye Z, Fang J, Wang Z, Wang L, Li B, Liu T, et al. Bioinformatics-based analysis of the lncRNA–miRNA–mRNA and TF regulatory networks reveals functional genes in esophageal squamous cell carcinoma. Bioscience Reports. 2020;**40**(8):1-15. DOI: 10.1042/BSR20201727

[13] Ghafouri-Fard S, Shoorei H, Dashti S, Branicki W, Taheri M. Expression profile of lncRNAs and miRNAs in esophageal cancer: Implications in diagnosis, prognosis, and therapeutic response. Journal of Cellular Physiology. 2020;**235**(12):9269-9290. DOI: 10.1002/jcp.29825

[14] Jin Y, Cao J, Hu X, Cheng H. Long noncoding RNA TUG1 upregulates VEGFA to enhance malignant behaviors in stomach adenocarcinoma by sponging miR-29c-3p. Journal of Clinical Laboratory Analysis. 2021;**35**(12):e24106. DOI: 10.1002/jcla.24106

[15] Arnal MJ, Arenas ÁF, Arbeloa ÁL. Esophageal cancer: Risk factors, screening and endoscopic treatment in Western and eastern countries. World Journal of Gastroenterology WJG. 2015;**21**(26):7933-7943

[16] Yang M, Wei L, Sun J, Zhang N, Shen Y, Wang T, et al. Novel implications of microRNAs, long noncoding RNAs and circular RNAs in drug resistance of esophageal cancer. Frontiers in Cell and Development Biology. 2021;**9**:1-14. DOI: 10.3389/fcell.2021.764313

[17] Chan JJ, Tay Y. Noncoding RNA: RNA regulatory networks in cancer. International Journal of Molecular Sciences. 2018;**19**(5):1310. DOI: 10.3390/ijms19051310

[18] Liu W, Li M, Chen X, Zhu S, Shi H, Zhang D, et al. MicroRNA-1 suppresses proliferation, migration and invasion by targeting Notch2 in esophageal squamous cell carcinoma. Scientific Reports. 2018;**8**(1):5183. DOI: 10.1038/s41598-018-23421-3

[19] Yang C, Ning S, Li Z, Qin X, Xu W. miR-22 is down-regulated in esophageal squamous cell carcinoma and inhibits cell migration and invasion. Cancer Cell International. 2014;**14**(1):138. DOI: 10.1186/s12935-014-0138-0

[20] Li J, Liang Y, Lv H, Meng H, Xiong G, Guan X, et al. miR-26a and miR-26b inhibit esophageal squamous cancer cell proliferation through suppression of c-MYC pathway. Gene. 2017;**625**:1-9. DOI: 10.1016/j.gene.2017.05.001

[21] Wu XZ, Wang KP, Song HJ, Xia JH, Jiang Y, Wang YL. MiR-27a-3p promotes esophageal cancer cell proliferation via F-box and WD repeat domain-containing 7 (FBXW7) suppression. International Journal of Clinical and Experimental Medicine. 2015;**8**(9):15556-15562

[22] Visone R, Petrocca F, Croce CM. Micro-RNAs in gastrointestinal and liver disease. Gastroenterology. 2008;**135**(6):1866-1869. DOI: 10.1053/j.gastro.2008.10.074

[23] Xu J, Lv H, Zhang B, Xu F, Zhu H, Chen B, et al. miR-30b-5p acts as a tumor suppressor microRNA in esophageal squamous cell carcinoma. Journal of Thoracic Disease. 2019;**11**(7):3015-3029. DOI: 10.21037/jtd.2019.07.50

[24] Gao C, Wei J, Tang T, Huang Z. Role of microRNA-33a in malignant cells. Oncology Letters. 2020;**20**(3):2537-2556. DOI: 10.3892/ol.2020.11835

[25] Zhou H, Yang L, Xu X, Lu M, Guo R, Li D, et al. miR-34a inhibits esophageal squamous cell carcinoma progression via regulation of FOXM1. Oncology Letters. 2019;**17**(1):706-712. DOI: 10.3892/ol.2018.9593

[26] Huang SD, Yuan Y, Zhuang CW, Li BL, Gong DJ, Wang SG, et al. MicroRNA-98 and microRNA-214 post-transcriptionally regulate enhancer of zeste homolog 2 and inhibit migration and invasion in human esophageal squamous cell carcinoma. Molecular Cancer. 2012;**11**(1):51. DOI: 10.1186/1476-4598-11-51

[27] Mei LL, Qiu YT, Huang MB, Wang WJ, Bai J, Shi ZZ. MiR-99a suppresses proliferation, migration and invasion of esophageal squamous cell carcinoma cells through inhibiting the IGF1R signaling pathway. Cancer Biomarkers. 2017;**20**(4):527-537. DOI: 10.3233/CBM-170345

[28] Zhou SM, Zhang F, Chen XB, Jun CM, Jing X, Wei DX, et al. miR-100 suppresses the proliferation and tumor growth of esophageal squamous cancer cells via targeting CXCR7. Oncology Reports. 2016;**35**(6):3453-3459. DOI: 10.3892/or.2016.4701

[29] Shao Y, Li P, Zhu ST, Yue JP, Ji XJ, He Z, et al. Cyclooxygenase-2, a potential therapeutic target, is regulated by miR-101 in esophageal squamous cell carcinoma. PLoS One. 2015;**10**(11):e0140642. DOI: 10.1371/journal.pone.0140642

[30] Sharma P, Saini N, Sharma R. miR-107 functions as a tumor suppressor in human esophageal squamous cell carcinoma and targets Cdc42. Oncology Reports. 2017;**37**(5):3116-3127. DOI: 10.3892/or.2017.5546

[31] Wang J, Yu PY, Yu JP, Luo JD, Sun ZQ, Sun F, et al. KIF22 promotes progress of esophageal squamous cell carcinoma cells and is negatively regulated by miR-122. American Journal of Translational Research. 2021;**13**(5):4152-4166

[32] Zeng B, Zhang X, Zhao J, Wei Z, Zhu H, Fu M, et al. The role of DNMT1/hsa-miR-124-3p/BCAT1 pathway in regulating growth and invasion of esophageal squamous cell carcinoma. BMC Cancer. 2019;**19**(1):609. DOI: 10.1186/s12885-019-5815-x

[33] Cheng C, Mao Q, Shi M, Lu H, Shen B, Xiao T, et al. miR-125b prevent the progression of esophageal squamous cell carcinoma through the p38-MAPK signaling pathway. Journal of Gastrointestinal Oncology. 2020;**11**(6):1113-1122. DOI: 10.21037/jgo-20-546

[34] Gao X, Wang X, Cai K, Wang W, Ju Q, Yang X, et al. MicroRNA-127 is a tumor suppressor in human esophageal squamous cell carcinoma through the regulation of oncogene FMNL3. European Journal of Pharmacology. 2016;**791**:603-610. DOI: 10.1016/j.ejphar.2016.09.025

[35] Zhao L, Li R, Xu S, Li Y, Zhao P, Dong W, et al. Tumor suppressor miR-128-3p inhibits metastasis and epithelial–mesenchymal transition by targeting ZEB1 in esophageal squamous-cell cancer. Acta biochim biophys Sin (Shanghai). 2018;**50**(2):171-180. DOI: 10.1093/abbs/gmx132

[36] Li Y, Chen D, Gao X, Li X, Shi G. LncRNA NEAT1 regulates cell viability and invasion in esophageal squamous cell carcinoma through the miR-129/CTBP2 axis. Disease Markers. 2017;**2017**:5314649. DOI: 10.1155/2017/5314649

[37] Yin Y, Du L, Li X, Zhang X, Gao Y. miR-133a-3p suppresses cell proliferation, migration, and invasion and promotes apoptosis in esophageal squamous cell carcinoma. Journal of Cellular Physiology. 2019;**234**(8):12757-12770. DOI: 10.1002/jcp.27896

[38] Yuan Y, Wang Q, Cao F, Han B, Xu L. MiRNA-134 suppresses esophageal squamous cell carcinoma progression by targeting FOXM1. International Journal of Clinical and Experimental Pathology. 2019;**12**(6):2130-2138

[39] Huang HZ, Yin YF, Wan WJ, Xia D, Wang R, Shen XM. Up-regulation of microRNA-136 induces apoptosis and radiosensitivity of esophageal squamous cell carcinoma cells by inhibiting the expression of MUC1. Experimental and Molecular Pathology. 2019;**110**:104278. DOI: 10.1016/j.yexmp.2019.104278

[40] Xu S, Li X, Li L, Wang Y, Geng C, Guo F, et al. CTCF-silenced miR-137

contributes to EMT and radioresistance in esophageal squamous cell carcinoma. Cancer Cell International. 2021;**21**(1):155. DOI: 10.1186/s12935-020-01740-8

[41] Gong H, Song L, Lin C, Liu A, Lin X, Wu J, et al. Downregulation of miR-138 sustains NF-κB activation and promotes lipid raft formation in esophageal squamous cell carcinoma. Clinical Cancer Research. 2013;**19**(5):1083-1093. DOI: 10.1158/1078-0432.CCR-12-3169

[42] Liu R, Yang M, Meng Y, Liao J, Sheng J, Pu Y, et al. Tumor-suppressive function of miR-139-5p in esophageal squamous cell carcinoma. PLoS One. 2013;**8**(10):e77068. DOI: 10.1371/journal.pone.0077068

[43] Zhang K, Chen J, Song H, Chen LB. SNHG16/miR-140-5p axis promotes esophagus cancer cell proliferation, migration and EMT formation through regulating ZEB1. Oncotarget. 2018;**9**(1):1028-1040. DOI: 10.18632/oncotarget.23178

[44] Su C, Han Y, Zhang H, Li Y, Yi L, Wang X, et al. RS-7 targeting miR-7 modulates the progression of non-small cell lung cancer in a manner dependent on NF-κB signalling. Journal of Cellular and Molecular Medicine. 2018;**22**(6):3097-3107

[45] Song Y, Li J, Zhu Y, Dai Y, Zeng T, Liu L, et al. MicroRNA-9 promotes tumor metastasis via repressing E-cadherin in esophageal squamous cell carcinoma. Oncotarget. 2014;**5**(22):11669-11680. DOI: 10.18632/oncotarget.2581

[46] Lu YF, Yu JR, Yang Z, Zhu GX, Gao P, Wang H, et al. Promoter hypomethylation mediated upregulation of MicroRNA-10b-3p targets FOXO3 to promote the progression of esophageal squamous cell carcinoma (ESCC). Journal of Experimental & Clinical Cancer Research. 2018;**37**(1):301. DOI: 10.1186/s13046-018-0966-1

[47] Li BX, Yu Q, Shi ZL, Li P, Fu S. Circulating microRNAs in esophageal squamous cell carcinoma: Association with locoregional staging and survival. International Journal of Clinical and Experimental Medicine. 2015;**8**(5):7241-7250

[48] Xu H, Meng XR, Zhou Y, Wang F. Expression of microRNA-17-5p in esophageal squamous cell carcinoma and its effects on cell proliferation and invasion. Zhonghua Zhong liu za zhi [Zhonghua Zhong Liu Za Zhi]. 2020;**42**(2):105-113. DOI: 10.3760/cma.j.issn.0253-3766.2020.02.004

[49] Hirajima S, Komatsu S, Ichikawa D, Takeshita H, Konishi H, Shiozaki A, et al. Clinical impact of circulating miR-18a in plasma of patients with oesophageal squamous cell carcinoma. British Journal of Cancer. 2013;**108**(9):1822-1829. DOI: 10.1038/bjc.2013.148

[50] Zhong H, Xu Y, Wang J, Cao Q, Hu L, Sun D. Overexpression of microRNA-19a-3p promotes lymph node metastasis of esophageal squamous cell carcinoma via the RAC1/CDC42-PAK1 pathway. Translational Cancer Research. 2021;**10**(6):2694-2706. DOI: 10.21037/tcr-21-254

[51] Yu J, Chen S, Niu Y, Liu M, Zhang J, Yang Z, et al. Functional significance and therapeutic potential of miRNA-20b-5p in esophageal squamous cell carcinoma. Molecular Therapy-Nucleic Acids. 2020;**21**:315-331. DOI: 10.1016/j.omtn.2020.05.015

[52] Komatsu S, Ichikawa D, Kawaguchi T, Takeshita H, Miyamae M, Ohashi T, et al. Plasma microRNA profiles: Identification of miR-23a as a novel biomarker for chemoresistance in esophageal

squamous cell carcinoma. Oncotarget. 2016;**7**(38):62034-62048. DOI: 10.18632/oncotarget.11500

[53] Maghsudlu M, Farashahi Yazd E, Amiriani T. Increased expression of MiR-27a and MiR-24-2 in esophageal squamous cell carcinoma. Journal of Gastrointestinal Cancer. 2020;**51**(1):227-233. DOI: 10.1007/s12029-019-00232-x

[54] Wu C, Li M, Hu C, Duan H. Clinical significance of serum miR-223, miR-25 and miR-375 in patients with esophageal squamous cell carcinoma. Molecular Biology Reports. 2014;**41**(3):1257-1266. DOI: 10.1007/s11033-013-2970-z

[55] Zhang J, Yao Y, Li H, Ye S. miR-28-3p inhibits prostate cancer cell proliferation, migration and invasion, and promotes apoptosis by targeting ARF6. Experimental and Therapeutic Medicine. 2021;**22**(5):1205. DOI: 10.3892/etm.2021.10639

[56] Gao Y, Yi J, Zhang K, Bai F, Feng B, Wang R, et al. Downregulation of MiR-31 stimulates expression of LATS2 via the hippo pathway and promotes epithelial-mesenchymal transition in esophageal squamous cell carcinoma. Journal of Experimental & Clinical Cancer Research. 2017;**36**(1):161. DOI: 10.1186/s13046-017-0622-1

[57] Liu YT, Zong D, Jiang XS, Yin L, Wang LJ, Wang TT, et al. miR-32 promotes esophageal squamous cell carcinoma metastasis by targeting CXXC5. Journal of Cellular Biochemistry. 2019;**120**(4):6250-6263. DOI: 10.1002/jcb.27912

[58] Li X, Guo S, Min L, Guo Q, Zhang S. miR-92a-3p promotes the proliferation, migration and invasion of esophageal squamous cell cancer by regulating PTEN. International Journal of Molecular Medicine. 2019;**44**(3):973-981. DOI: 10.3892/ijmm.2019.4258

[59] Cai Y, Ruan W, Ding J, Wei N, Wang J, Zhang H, et al. miR-93-5p regulates the occurrence and development of esophageal carcinoma epithelial cells by targeting TGFβR2. International Journal of Molecular Medicine. 2021;**47**(3):1. DOI: 10.3892/ijmm.2020.4836

[60] Yao L, Zhang Y, Zhu Q, Li X, Zhu S, Gong L, et al. Downregulation of microRNA-1 in esophageal squamous cell carcinoma correlates with an advanced clinical stage and its overexpression inhibits cell migration and invasion. International Journal of Molecular Medicine. 2015;**35**(4):1033-1041. DOI: 10.3892/ijmm.2015.2094

[61] Gao DC, Hou B, Zhou D, Liu QX, Zhang K, Lu X, et al. Tumor-derived exosomal miR-103a-2-5p facilitates esophageal squamous cell carcinoma cell proliferation and migration. European Review for Medical and Pharmacological Sciences. 2020;**24**(11):6097-6110. DOI: 10.26355/eurrev_202006_21505

[62] He B, Zhang K, Han X, Su C, Zhao J, Wang G, et al. Extracellular vesicle-derived miR-105-5p promotes malignant phenotypes of esophageal squamous cell carcinoma by targeting SPARCL1 via FAK/AKT signaling pathway. Frontiers in Genetics. 2022;**13**:1-14. DOI: 10.3389/fgene.2022.819699

[63] Zhang J, Chen D, Liang S, Wang J, Liu C, Nie C, et al. miR-106b promotes cell invasion and metastasis via PTEN mediated EMT in ESCC. Oncology Letters. 2018;**15**(4):4619-4626. DOI: 10.3892/ol.2018.7861

[64] Li M, Meng X, Li M. MiR-126 promotes esophageal squamous cell carcinoma via inhibition of apoptosis and autophagy. Aging (Albany NY). 2020;**12**(12):12107-12118. DOI: 10.18632/aging.103379

[65] Yu T, Cao R, Li S, Fu M, Ren L, Chen W, et al. MiR-130b plays an oncogenic role by repressing PTEN expression in esophageal squamous cell carcinoma cells. BMC Cancer. 2015;**15**(1):29. DOI: 10.1186/s12885-015-1031-5

[66] Zhang Y, Ren S, Yuan F, Zhang K, Fan Y, Zheng S, et al. miR-135 promotes proliferation and stemness of oesophageal squamous cell carcinoma by targeting RERG. Artificial Cells Nanomedicine Biotechnology. 2018;**46**(suppl. 2):1210-1219. DOI: 10.1080/21691401.2018.1483379

[67] Jiang S, Zhao C, Yang X, Li X, Pan Q, Huang H, et al. miR-1 suppresses the growth of esophageal squamous cell carcinoma in vivo and in vitro through the downregulation of MET, cyclin D1 and CDK4 expression. International Journal of Molecular Medicine. 2016;**38**(1):113-122. DOI: 10.3892/ijmm.2016.2619

[68] Zhang C, Wang L, Yang J, Fu Y, Li H, Xie L, et al. MicroRNA-33a-5p suppresses esophageal squamous cell carcinoma progression via regulation of lncRNA DANCR and ZEB1. European Journal of Pharmacology. 2019;**861**:172590. DOI: 10.1016/j.ejphar.2019.172590

[69] Chu J, Jia J, Yang L, Qu Y, Yin H, Wan J, et al. LncRNA MIR31HG functions as a ceRNA to regulate c-met function by sponging miR-34a in esophageal squamous cell carcinoma. Biomedicine & Pharmacotherapy. 2020;**128**:110313. DOI: 10.1016/j.biopha.2020.110313

[70] Cao X, Xu J, Yue D. LncRNA-SNHG16 predicts poor prognosis and promotes tumor proliferation through epigenetically silencing p21 in bladder cancer. Cancer Gene Therapy. 2018;**25**(1-2):10-17. DOI: 10.1038/s41417-017-0006-x

[71] Zhang EB, Kong R, Yin DD, You LH, Sun M, Han L, et al. Long noncoding RNA ANRIL indicates a poor prognosis of gastric cancer and promotes tumor growth by epigenetically silencing of miR-99a/miR-449a. Oncotarget. 2014;**5**(8):2276-2292. DOI: 10.18632/oncotarget.1902

[72] Wang X, Li M, Wang Z, Han S, Tang X, Ge Y, et al. Silencing of long noncoding RNA MALAT1 by miR-101 and miR-217 inhibits proliferation, migration, and invasion of esophageal squamous cell carcinoma cells. The Journal of Biological Chemistry. 2015;**290**(7):3925-3935. DOI: 10.1074/jbc.M114.596866

[73] Chen M, Liu P, Chen Y, Chen Z, Shen M, Liu X, et al. Long noncoding RNA FAM201A mediates the radiosensitivity of esophageal squamous cell cancer by regulating ATM and mTOR expression via miR-101. Frontiers in Genetics. 2018;**9**:611. DOI: 10.3389/fgene.2018.00611

[74] Zhou Z, Huang F. Long non-coding RNA LINC00152 regulates cell proliferation, migration and invasion in esophageal squamous cell carcinoma via miR-107/Rab10 axis. Oncotargets and Therapy. 2019;**12**:8553-8567. DOI: 10.2147/OTT.S221515

[75] Wang B, Liang T, Li J. Long noncoding RNA LINC01296 is associated with poor prognosis in ESCC and promotes ESCC cell proliferation, migration and invasion. European Review for Medical and Pharmacological Sciences. 2018;**22**(14):4524-4531. DOI: 10.26355/eurrev_201807_15507

[76] Li Z, Qin X, Bian W, Li Y, Shan B, Yao Z, et al. Exosomal lncRNA ZFAS1 regulates esophageal squamous cell carcinoma cell proliferation, invasion, migration and apoptosis via

microRNA-124/STAT3 axis. Journal of Experimental & Clinical Cancer Research. 2019;**38**(1):477. DOI: 10.1186/s13046-019-1473-8

[77] Ma J, Fan Y, Feng T, Chen F, Xu Z, Li S, et al. HOTAIR regulates HK2 expression by binding endogenous miR-125 and miR-143 in oesophageal squamous cell carcinoma progression. Oncotarget. 2017;**8**(49):86410-86422. DOI: 10.18632/oncotarget.21195

[78] Hong Y, He H, Sui W, Zhang J, Zhang S, Yang D. Long non-coding RNA H1 promotes cell proliferation and invasion by acting as a ceRNA of miR-138 and releasing EZH2 in oral squamous cell carcinoma. International Journal of Oncology. 2018;**52**(3):901-912. DOI: 10.3892/ijo.2018.4247

[79] Yan S, Xu J, Liu B, Ma L, Feng H, Tan H, et al. Long non-coding RNA BCAR4 aggravated proliferation and migration in esophageal squamous cell carcinoma by negatively regulating p53/p21 signaling pathway. Bioengineered. 2021;**12**(1):682-696. DOI: 10.1080/21655979.2021.1887645

[80] Tan Z, Zhou P, Zhu Z, Wang Y, Guo Z, Shen M, et al. Upregulated long non-coding RNA LincIN promotes tumor progression via the regulation of nuclear factor 90/microRNA-7/HOXB13 in esophageal squamous cell carcinoma. International Journal of Molecular Medicine. 2021;**47**(5):1-2. DOI: 10.3892/ijmm.2021.4911

[81] Dong Z, Zhang A, Liu S, Lu F, Guo Y, Zhang G, et al. Aberrant methylation-mediated silencing of lncRNA MEG3 functions as a ceRNA in esophageal cancer. Molecular Cancer Research. 2017;**15**(7):800-810. DOI: 10.1158/1541-7786.MCR-16-0385

[82] Feng B, Wang G, Liang X, Wu Z, Wang X, Dong Z, et al. 83H-AS1 promotes oesophageal squamous cell carcinoma progression via miR-10a-5p/Girdin axis. Journal of Cellular and Molecular Medicine. 2020;**24**(16):8962-8976

[83] Zhao Y, Zhang Q, Liu H, Wang N, Zhang X, Yang S. lncRNA part 1. Oncology Reports. 2021;**45**(3):1118-1132. DOI: 10.3892/or.2021.7931

[84] Lin J, Liu Z, Liao S, Li E, Wu X, Zeng W. Elevation of long non-coding RNA GAS5 and knockdown of microRNA-21 up-regulate RECK expression to enhance esophageal squamous cell carcinoma cell radio-sensitivity after radiotherapy. Genomics. 2020;**112**(3):2173-2185. DOI: 10.1016/j.ygeno.2019.12.013

[85] Zhang J, Xiao F, Qiang G, Zhang Z, Ma Q, Hao Y, et al. Novel lncRNA panel as for prognosis in esophageal squamous cell carcinoma based on ceRNA network mechanism. Computational and Mathematical Methods in Medicine. 2021;**2021**:8020879. DOI: 10.1155/2021/8020879

[86] Jain S, Dhingra S. Pathology of esophageal cancer and Barrett's esophagus. Annals of Cardiothoracic Surgery. 2017;**6**(2):99-109. DOI: 10.21037/acs.2017.03.06

[87] Song JH, Tieu AH, Cheng Y, Ma K, Akshintala VS, Simsek C, et al. Novel long noncoding rna mir205hg functions as an esophageal tumor-suppressive hedgehog inhibitor. Cancers. 2021;**13**(7):1707. DOI: 10.3390/cancers13071707

[88] Yu Y, Chen X, Cang S. Cancer-related long noncoding RNAs show aberrant expression profiles and competing endogenous RNA potential in esophageal adenocarcinoma. Oncology Letters. 2019;**18**(5):4798-4808. DOI: 10.3892/ol.2019.10808

[89] Wu W, Bhagat TD, Yang X, Song JH, Cheng Y, Agarwal R, et al. Hypomethylation of noncoding DNA regions and overexpression of the long noncoding RNA, AFAP1-AS1. Barrett's esophagus and esophageal adenocarcinoma. Gastroenterology. 2013;**144**(5):956-966.e4. DOI: 10.1053/j.gastro.2013.01.019

[90] Yang X, Song JH, Cheng Y, Wu W, Bhagat T, Yu Y, et al. Long non-coding RNA HNF1A-AS1 regulates proliferation and migration in oesophageal adenocarcinoma cells. Gut. 2014;**63**(6):881-890. DOI: 10.1136/gutjnl-2013-305266

[91] Xu Y, Li Y, Jin J, Han G, Sun C, Pizzi MP, et al. LncRNA PVT1 up-regulation is a poor prognosticator and serves as a therapeutic target in esophageal adenocarcinoma. Molecular Cancer. 2019;**18**(1):141. DOI: 10.1186/s12943-019-1064-5

[92] Su W, Guo C, Wang L, Wang Z, Yang X, Niu F, et al. LncRNA MIR22HG abrogation inhibits proliferation and induces apoptosis in esophageal adenocarcinoma cells via activation of the STAT3/c-Myc/FAK signaling. Aging (Albany, NY). 2019;**11**(13):4587-4596. DOI: 10.18632/aging.102071

[93] Liu D, Wu K, Yang Y, Zhu D, Zhang C, Zhao S. Long noncoding RNA ADAMTS9-AS2 suppresses the progression of esophageal cancer by mediating CDH3 promoter methylation. Molecular Carcinogenesis. 2020;**59**(1):32-44. DOI: 10.1002/mc.23126

[94] Pang J, Pan H, Yang C, Meng P, Xie W, Li J, et al. Prognostic value of immune-related multi-IncRNA signatures associated with tumor microenvironment in esophageal cancer. Frontiers in Genetics. 2021;**12**:722601. DOI: 10.3389/fgene.2021.722601

[95] Han C, Zhou Y, An Q, Li F, Li D, Zhang X, et al. MicroRNA-1 (miR-1) inhibits gastric cancer cell proliferation and migration by targeting MET. Tumour Biology. 2015;**36**(9):6715-6723. DOI: 10.1007/s13277-015-3358-6

[96] Siemens H, Neumann J, Jackstadt R, Mansmann U, Horst D, Kirchner T, et al. Detection of miR-34a promoter methylation in combination with elevated expression of c-met and beta-catenin predicts distant metastasis of colon cancer. Clinical Cancer Research. 2013;**19**(3):710-720. DOI: 10.1158/1078-0432.CCR-12-1703

[97] Deng P, Li K, Gu F, Zhang T, Zhao W, Sun M, et al. LINC00242/miR-1-3p/G6PD axis regulates Warburg effect and affects gastric cancer proliferation and apoptosis. Molecular Medicine. 2021;**27**(1):9. DOI: 10.1186/s10020-020-00259-y

[98] Yang Z, Shi X, Li C, Wang X, Hou K, Li Z, et al. Long non-coding RNA UCA1 upregulation promotes the migration of hypoxia-resistant gastric cancer cells through the miR-7-5p/EGFR axis. Experimental Cell Research. 2018;**368**(2):194-201. DOI: 10.1016/j.yexcr.2018.04.030

[99] Rotkrua P, Akiyama Y, Hashimoto Y, Otsubo T, Yuasa Y. MiR-9 downregulates CDX2 expression in gastric cancer cells. International Journal of Cancer. 2011;**129**(11):2611-2620. DOI: 10.1002/ijc.25923

[100] Liu T, Liu Y, Wei C, Yang Z, Chang W, Zhang X. LncRNA HULC promotes the progression of gastric cancer by regulating miR-9-5p/MYH9 axis. Biomedicine & Pharmacotherapy.

2020;**121**:109607. DOI: 10.1016/j.biopha.2019.109607

[101] Lu R, Zhao G, Yang Y, Jiang Z, Cai J, Zhang Z, et al. Long noncoding RNA HOTAIRM1 inhibits cell progression by regulating miR-17-5p/PTEN axis in gastric cancer. Journal of Cellular Biochemistry. 2019;**120**(4):4952-4965. DOI: 10.1002/jcb.27770

[102] Chen M, Fan L, Zhang SM, Li Y, Chen P, Peng X, et al. LINC01939 inhibits the metastasis of gastric cancer by acting as a molecular sponge of miR-17-5p to regulate EGR2 expression. Cell Death & Disease. 2019;**10**(2):70. DOI: 10.1038/s41419-019-1344-4

[103] Wang CL, Wang D, Yan BZ, Fu JW, Qin L. Long non-coding RNA NEAT1 promotes viability and migration of gastric cancer cell lines through up-regulation of microRNA-17. European Review for Medical and Pharmacological Sciences. 2018;**22**(13):4128-4137. DOI: 10.26355/eurrev_201807_15405

[104] Chen YJ, Wu H, Zhu JM, Li XD, Luo SW, Dong L, et al. MicroRNA-18a modulates P53 expression by targeting IRF2 in gastric cancer patients. Journal of Gastroenterology and Hepatology. 2016;**31**(1):155-163. DOI: 10.1111/jgh.13041

[105] Li Y, Lv S, Ning H, Li K, Zhou X, Xv H, et al. Down-regulation of CASC2 contributes to cisplatin resistance in gastric cancer by sponging miR-19a. Biomedicine & Pharmacotherapy. Dec 2018;**1**(108):1775-1782

[106] Fan B, Shen C, Wu M, Zhao J, Guo Q, Luo Y. miR-17-92 cluster is connected with disease progression and oxaliplatin/capecitabine chemotherapy efficacy in advanced gastric cancer patients: A preliminary study. Medicine. 2018;**97**(35):e12007. DOI: 10.1097/MD.0000000000012007

[107] Kim SY, Jeon TY, Choi CI, Kim DH, Kim DH, Kim GH, et al. Validation of circulating miRNA biomarkers for predicting lymph node metastasis in gastric cancer. The Journal of Molecular Diagnostics. 2013;**15**(5):661-669. DOI: 10.1016/j.jmoldx.2013.04.004

[108] Dan J, Wang J, Wang Y, Zhu M, Yang X, Peng Z, et al. LncRNA-MEG3 inhibits proliferation and metastasis by regulating miRNA-21 in gastric cancer. Biomedicine & Pharmacotherapy. 2018;**99**:931-938. DOI: 10.1016/j.biopha.2018.01.164

[109] Zong W, Feng W, Jiang Y, Cao Y, Ke Y, Shi X, et al. LncRNA CTC-497E21.4 promotes the progression of gastric cancer via modulating miR-22/NET1 axis through RhoA signaling pathway. Gastric Cancer. 2020;**23**(2):228-240

[110] Dong X, Liu Y. Expression and significance of miR-24 and miR-101 in patients with advanced gastric cancer. Oncology Letters. 2018;**16**(5):5769-5774. DOI: 10.3892/ol.2018.9324

[111] Nho RS, Hergert P. FoxO3a and disease progression. World Journal of Biological Chemistry. 2014;**5**(3):346-354. DOI: 10.4331/wjbc.v5.i3.346

[112] Li D, Wang T, Lai J, Zhang T, Zhu X, Zeng D, et al. Long non-coding RNA GATA6-AS inhibits gastric cancer cell proliferation by downregulating microRNA-25-3p. Oncology Letters. 2019;**18**(5):4639-4644. DOI: 10.3892/ol.2019.10803

[113] Ding K, Wu Z, Wang N, Wang X, Wang Y, Qian P, et al. MiR-26a performs converse roles in proliferation and metastasis of different gastric cancer

cells via regulating of PTEN expression. Pathology, Research and Practice. 2017;**213**(5):467-475. DOI: 10.1016/j.prp.2017.01.026

[114] Deng M, Zhang R, He Z, Qiu Q, Lu X, Yin J, et al. TET-mediated sequestration of miR-26 drives EZH2 expression and gastric carcinogenesis. Cancer Research. 2017;**77**(22):6069-6082. DOI: 10.1158/0008-5472.CAN-16-2964

[115] Song B, Yan G, Hao H, Yang B. rs11671784 G/a and rs895819 a/G polymorphisms inversely affect gastric cancer susceptibility and miR-27a expression in a Chinese population. Medical Science Monitor. 2014;**20**:2318-2326. DOI: 10.12659/MSM.892499

[116] Xiao F, Cheng Z, Wang P, Gong B, Huang H, Xing Y, et al. MicroRNA-28-5p inhibits the migration and invasion of gastric cancer cells by suppressing AKT phosphorylation. Oncology Letters. 2018;**15**(6):9777-9785. DOI: 10.3892/ol.2018.8603

[117] Militello G, Weirick T, John D, Döring C, Dimmeler S, Uchida S. Screening and validation of lncRNAs and circRNAs as miRNA sponges. Briefings in Bioinformatics. 2017;**18**(5):780-788. DOI: 10.1093/bib/bbw053

[118] Gong J, Li J, Wang Y, Liu C, Jia H, Jiang C, et al. Characterization of microRNA-29 family expression and investigation of their mechanistic roles in gastric cancer. Carcinogenesis. 2014;**35**(2):497-506. DOI: 10.1093/carcin/bgt337

[119] Wei GH, Wang X. lncRNA MEG3 inhibit proliferation and metastasis of gastric cancer via p53 signaling pathway. European Review for Medical and Pharmacological Sciences. 2017;**21**(17):3850-3856

[120] Du X, Liu B, Luan X, Cui Q, Li L. miR-30 decreases multidrug resistance in human gastric cancer cells by modulating cell autophagy. Experimental and Therapeutic Medicine. 2018;**15**(1):599-605. DOI: 10.3892/etm.2017.5354

[121] Wang L, Xiao B, Yu T, Gong L, Wang Y, Zhang X, et al. lncRNA PVT1 promotes the migration of gastric cancer by functioning as ceRNA of miR-30a and regulating snail. Journal of Cellular Physiology. 2021;**236**(1):536-548. DOI: 10.1002/jcp.29881

[122] Liu HT, Ma RR, Lv BB, Zhang H, Shi DB, Guo XY, et al. LncRNA-HNF1A-AS1 functions as a competing endogenous RNA to activate PI3K/AKT signalling pathway by sponging miR-30b-3p in gastric cancer. British Journal of Cancer. 2020;**122**(12):1825-1836. DOI: 10.1038/s41416-020-0836-4

[123] Han S, Qi Y, Xu Y, Wang M, Wang J, Wang J, et al. lncRNA DLEU2 promotes gastric cancer progression through ETS2 via targeting miR-30a-5p. Cancer Cell International. 2021;**21**(1):376. DOI: 10.1186/s12935-021-02074-9

[124] Wang J, Jiao Y, Cui L, Jiang L. miR-30 functions as an oncomir in gastric cancer cells through regulation of P53-mediated mitochondrial apoptotic pathway. Bioscience, Biotechnology, and Biochemistry. 2017;**81**(1):119-126. DOI: 10.1080/09168451.2016.1238294

[125] Wang H, Zhang X, Liu Y, Ni Z, Lin Y, Duan Z, et al. Downregulated miR-31 level associates with poor prognosis of gastric cancer and its restoration suppresses tumor cell malignant phenotypes by inhibiting E2F2. Oncotarget. 2016;**7**(24):36577

[126] Korourian A, Roudi R, Shariftabrizi A, Madjd Z. MicroRNA-31

inhibits RhoA-mediated tumor invasion and chemotherapy resistance in MKN-45 gastric adenocarcinoma cells. Experimental Biology and Medicine. 2017;**242**(18):1842-1847

[127] Zhang XB, Song L, Wen HJ, Bai XX, Li ZJ, Ma LJ. Upregulation of microRNA-31 targeting integrin α5 suppresses tumor cell invasion and metastasis by indirectly regulating PI3K/AKT pathway in human gastric cancer SGC7901 cells. Tumor Biology. 2016;**37**(6):8317-8325

[128] Zhao L, Han T, Li Y, Sun J, Zhang S, Liu Y, et al. The lncRNA SNHG5/miR-32 axis regulates gastric cancer cell proliferation and migration by targeting KLF4. The FASEB Journal. 2017;**31**(3):893-903. DOI: 10.1096/fj.201600994R

[129] Wang Y, Zhou X, Shan B, Han J, Wang F, Fan X, et al. Downregulation of microRNA-33a promotes cyclin-dependent kinase 6, cyclin D1 and PIM1 expression and gastric cancer cell proliferation. Molecular Medicine Reports. 2015;**12**(5):6491-6500. DOI: 10.3892/mmr.2015.4296

[130] Ji Q, Hao X, Meng Y, Zhang M, DeSano J, Fan D, et al. Restoration of tumor suppressor miR-34 inhibits human p53-mutant gastric cancer tumorspheres. BMC Cancer. 2008;**8**(1):266. DOI: 10.1186/1471-2407-8-266

[131] Guo X, Jing C, Li L, Zhang L, Shi Y, Wang J, et al. Down-regulation of VEZT gene expression in human gastric cancer involves promoter methylation and miR-43c. Biochemical and Biophysical Research Communications. 2011;**404**(2):622-627. DOI: 10.1016/j.bbrc.2010.12.026

[132] Shin VY, Siu MT, Liu X, Ng EKO, Kwong A, Chu KM. MiR-92 suppresses proliferation and induces apoptosis by targeting EP4/Notch1 axis in gastric cancer. Oncotarget. 2018;**9**(36):24209-24220. DOI: 10.18632/oncotarget.24819

[133] Liu L, Dai A, Zhang Z, Ning M, Han D, Li L, et al. LncRNA PITPNA-AS1 promotes gastric cancer by increasing SOX4 expression via inhibition of miR-92a-3p. Aging (Albany, NY). 2021;**13**(17):21191-21201. DOI: 10.18632/aging.203403

[134] Zhang Y, Guo L, Li Y, Feng G, Teng F, Li W, et al. MicroRNA-494 promotes cancer progression and targets adenomatous polyposis coli in colorectal cancer. Molecular Cancer. 2018;**17**(1):1-11. DOI: 10.1186/s12943-017-0753-1

[135] Ma DH, Li BS, Liu JJ, Xiao YF, Yong X, Wang SM, et al. miR-93-5p/IFNAR1 axis promotes gastric cancer metastasis through activating the STAT3 signaling pathway. Cancer Letters. 2017;**408**:23-32. DOI: 10.1016/j.canlet.2017.08.017

[136] Zhang R, Guo Y, Ma Z, Ma G, Xue Q, Li F, et al. Long non-coding RNA PTENP1 functions as a ceRNA to modulate PTEN level by decoying miR-106b and miR-93 in gastric cancer. Oncotarget. 2017;**8**(16):26079-26089. DOI: 10.18632/oncotarget.15317

[137] Bo G, Liu Y, Li W, Wang L, Zhao L, Tong D, et al. The novel lncRNA GPC5-AS1 stabilizes GPC5 mRNA by competitively binding with miR-93/106a to suppress gastric cancer cell proliferation. Aging (Albany, NY). 2022;**14**(4):1767-1781. DOI: 10.18632/aging.203901

[138] Zhang XY, Zhuang HW, Wang J, Shen Y, Bu YZ, Guan BG, et al. Long noncoding RNA CA3-AS1 suppresses gastric cancer migration and invasion by sponging miR-93-5p and targeting

BTG3. Gene Therapy. 2020;**29**(9):1-9. DOI: 10.1038/s41434-020-00201-1

[139] Ni Q, Zhang Y, Tao R, Li X, Zhu J. MicroRNA-95-3p serves as a contributor to cisplatin resistance in human gastric cancer cells by targeting EMP1/PI3K/AKT signaling. Aging (Albany, NY). 2021;**13**(6):8665-8687. DOI: 10.18632/aging.202679

[140] Zhang W, Sun J, Chen J, Xu C, Zhang L. Downregulation of miR-95 in gastric cancer promotes EMT via regulation of slug, thereby promoting migration and invasion. Oncology Reports. 2019;**41**(2):1395-1403. DOI: 10.3892/or.2018.6911

[141] Zhou HY, Wu CQ, Bi EX. MiR-96-5p inhibition induces cell apoptosis in gastric adenocarcinoma. World Journal of Gastroenterology. 2019;**25**(47):6823-6834. DOI: 10.3748/wjg.v25.i47.6823

[142] Ma RR, Zhang H, Chen HF, Zhang GH, Tian YR, Gao P. MiR-19a/miR-96-mediated low expression of KIF26A suppresses metastasis by regulating FAK pathway in gastric cancer. Oncogene. 2021;**40**(14):2524-2538. DOI: 10.1038/s41388-020-01610-7

[143] Zhan P, Shu X, Chen M, Sun L, Yu L, Liu J, et al. miR-98-5p inhibits gastric cancer cell stemness and chemoresistance by targeting branched-chain aminotransferases 1. Life Sciences. 2021;**276**:119405. DOI: 10.1016/j.lfs.2021.119405

[144] Xu QF, Peng HP, Lu XR, Hu Y, Xu ZH, Xu JK. Oleanolic acid regulates the Treg/Th17 imbalance in gastric cancer by targeting IL-6 with miR-98-5p. Cytokine. 2021;**148**:155656. DOI: 10.1016/j.cyto.2021.155656

[145] Wen X, Han W, Liu C. Long non-coding RNA TTTY15 silencing inhibits gastric cancer progression by sponging microRNA-98-5p to down-regulate cyclin D2 expression. Bioengineered. 2022;**13**(3):7380-7391. DOI: 10.1080/21655979.2022.2047398

[146] Peng CW, Yue LX, Zhou YQ, Tang S, Kan C, Xia LM, et al. miR-100-3p inhibits cell proliferation and induces apoptosis in human gastric cancer through targeting to BMPR2. Cancer Cell International. 2019;**19**(1):354. DOI: 10.1186/s12935-019-1060-2

[147] Shi DB, Wang YW, Xing AY, Gao JW, Zhang H, Guo XY, et al. C/EBPα-induced miR-100 expression suppresses tumor metastasis and growth by targeting ZBTB7A in gastric cancer. Cancer Letters. 2015;**369**(2):376-385. DOI: 10.1016/j.canlet.2015.08.029

[148] Cao Y, Song J, Ge J, Song Z, Chen J, Wu C. MicroRNA-100 suppresses human gastric cancer cell proliferation by targeting CXCR7. Oncology Letters. 2018;**15**(1):453-458. DOI: 10.3892/ol.2017.7305

[149] Gong Y, Yang G, Wang Q, Wang Y, Zhang X. NME2 is a master suppressor of apoptosis in gastric cancer cells via transcriptional regulation of miR-100 and other survival factors. Molecular Cancer Research. 2020;**18**(2):287-299. DOI: 10.1158/1541-7786.MCR-19-0612

[150] Yang G, Gong Y, Wang Q, Wang Y, Zhang X. The role of miR-100-mediated notch pathway in apoptosis of gastric tumor cells. Cellular Signalling. 2015;**27**(6):1087-1101. DOI: 10.1016/j.cellsig.2015.02.013

[151] Chen JF, Wu P, Xia R, Yang J, Huo XY, Gu DY, et al. STAT3-induced lncRNA HAGLROS overexpression contributes to the malignant progression of gastric cancer cells via mTOR signal-mediated inhibition of autophagy.

Molecular Cancer. 2018;**17**(1):6. DOI: 10.1186/s12943-017-0756-y

[152] Li J, Xu Q, Wang W, Sun S. MIR100HG: A credible prognostic biomarker and an oncogenic lncRNA in gastric cancer. Bioscience Reports. 2019;**39**(4):1-8. DOI: 10.1042/BSR20190171

[153] Zheng Y, Tan K, Huang H. Retracted: Long noncoding RNA HAGLROS regulates apoptosis and autophagy in colorectal cancer cells via sponging miR-100 to target ATG5 expression. Journal of Cellular Biochemistry. 2019;**120**(3):3922-3933. DOI: 10.1002/jcb.27676

[154] Zhang W, Zhang Y, Xi S. Upregulation of lncRNA HAGLROS enhances the development of nasopharyngeal carcinoma via modulating miR-100/ATG14 axis-mediated PI3K/AKT/mTOR signals. Artificial Cells Nanomedicine Biotechnology. 2019;**47**(1):3043-3052. DOI: 10.1080/21691401.2019.1640233

[155] Bao J, Xu Y, Wang Q, Zhang J, Li Z, Li D, et al. miR-101 alleviates chemoresistance of gastric cancer cells by targeting ANXA2. Biomedicine & Pharmacotherapy. 2017;**92**:1030-1037. DOI: 10.1016/j.biopha.2017.06.011

[156] Imamura T, Komatsu S, Ichikawa D, Miyamae M, Okajima W, Ohashi T, et al. Low plasma levels of miR-101 are associated with tumor progression in gastric cancer. Oncotarget. 2017;**8**(63):106538-106550. DOI: 10.18632/oncotarget.20860

[157] Zhou X, Xia Y, Li L, Zhang G. MiR-101 inhibits cell growth and tumorigenesis of helicobacter pylori related gastric cancer by repression of SOCS2. Cancer Biology & Therapy. 2015;**16**(1):160-169. DOI: 10.4161/15384047.2014.987523

[158] Riquelme I, Tapia O, Leal P, Sandoval A, Varga MG, Letelier P, et al. miR-101-2, miR-125b-2 and miR-451a act as potential tumor suppressors in gastric cancer through regulation of the PI3K/AKT/mTOR pathway. Cellular Oncology (Dordrecht). 2016;**39**(1):23-33. DOI: 10.1007/s13402-015-0247-3

[159] Cao C, Xu Y, Du K, Mi C, Yang C, Xiang L, et al. LINC01303 functions as a competing endogenous RNA to regulate EZH2 expression by sponging miR-101-3p in gastric cancer. Journal of Cellular and Molecular Medicine. 2019;**23**(11):7342-7348

[160] Cao S, Lin L, Xia X, Wu H. lncRNA SPRY4-IT1 regulates cell proliferation and migration by sponging miR-101-3p and regulating AMPK expression in gastric cancer. Molecular Therapy-Nucleic Acids. 2019;**17**:455-464. DOI: 10.1016/j.omtn.2019.04.030

[161] Chen DL, Ju HQ, Lu YX, Chen LZ, Zeng ZL, Zhang DS, et al. Long non-coding RNA XIST regulates gastric cancer progression by acting as a molecular sponge of miR-101 to modulate EZH2 expression. Journal of Experimental & Clinical Cancer Research. 2016;**35**(1):142. DOI: 10.1186/s13046-016-0420-1

[162] Yan K, Tian J, Shi W, Xia H, Zhu Y. LncRNA SNHG6 is associated with poor prognosis of gastric cancer and promotes cell proliferation and EMT through epigenetically silencing p27 and sponging miR-101-3p. Cellular Physiology and Biochemistry. 2017;**42**(3):999-1012. DOI: 10.1159/000478682

[163] Xu Y, Ji T, An N, Wang X, Zhang H, Xu F. LINC00943 is correlated with gastric cancer and regulates cancer cell proliferation and chemosensitivity via hsa-miR-101-3p. International Journal of Clinical Oncology. 2021;**26**(9):1650-1660. DOI: 10.1007/s10147-021-01945-5

[164] Zhang Y, Qu X, Li C, Fan Y, Che X, Wang X, et al. miR-103/107 modulates multidrug resistance in human gastric carcinoma by downregulating Cav-1. Tumour Biology. 2015;**36**(4):2277-2285. DOI: 10.1007/s13277-014-2835-7

[165] Wei F, Wang Y, Zhou Y, Li Y. Long noncoding RNA CYTOR triggers gastric cancer progression by targeting miR-103/RAB10. Acta Biochimica et Biophysica Sinica (Shanghai). 2021;**53**(8):1044-1054. DOI: 10.1093/abbs/gmab071

[166] Zheng J, Liu Y, Qiao Y, Zhang L, Lu S. miR-103 promotes proliferation and metastasis by targeting KLF4 in gastric cancer. International Journal of Molecular Sciences. 2017;**18**(5):910. DOI: 10.3390/ijms18050910

[167] Shang JC, Yu GZ, Ji ZW, Wang XQ, Xia L. MiR-105 inhibits gastric cancer cells metastasis, epithelial-mesenchymal transition by targeting SOX9. European Review for Medical and Pharmacological Sciences. 2019;**23**(14):6160-6169. DOI: 10.26355/eurrev_201907_18429

[168] Jin M, Zhang GW, Shan CL, Zhang H, Wang ZG, Liu SQ, et al. Up-regulation of miRNA-105 inhibits the progression of gastric carcinoma by directly targeting SOX9. European Review for Medical and Pharmacological Sciences. 2019;**23**(9):3779-3789. DOI: 10.26355/eurrev_201905_17804

[169] Zhou GQ, Han F, Shi ZL, Yu L, Li XF, Yu C, et al. DNMT3A-mediated down-regulation of microRNA-105 promotes gastric cancer cell proliferation. European Review for Medical and Pharmacological Sciences. 2017;**21**(15):3377-3383

[170] Hou X, Zhang M, Qiao H. Diagnostic significance of miR-106a in gastric cancer. International Journal of Clinical and Experimental Pathology. 2015;**8**(10):13096-13101

[171] Liu T, Liu S, Xu Y, Shu R, Wang F, Chen C, et al. Circular RNA-ZFR inhibited cell proliferation and promoted apoptosis in gastric cancer by sponging miR-130a/miR-107 and modulating PTEN. Cancer Research and Treatment. 2018;**50**(4):1396-1417. DOI: 10.4143/crt.2017.537

[172] Wang S, Ma G, Zhu H, Lv C, Chu H, Tong N, et al. miR-107 regulates tumor progression by targeting NF1 in gastric cancer. Scientific Reports. 2016;**6**(1):36531. DOI: 10.1038/srep36531

[173] Ayremlou N, Mozdarani H, Mowla SJ, Delavari A. Increased levels of serum and tissue miR-107 in human gastric cancer: Correlation with tumor hypoxia. Cancer Biomarkers. 2015;**15**(6):851-860. DOI: 10.3233/CBM-150529

[174] Wei J, Xu H, Wei W, Wang Z, Zhang Q, De W, et al. circHIPK3 promotes cell proliferation and migration of gastric cancer by sponging miR-107 and regulating BDNF expression. Oncotargets and Therapy. 2020;**13**:1613-1624. DOI: 10.2147/OTT.S226300

[175] Chen P, Zhao X, Wang H, Zheng M, Wang Q, Chang W. The down-regulation of lncRNA PCAT18 promotes the progression of gastric cancer via MiR-107/PTEN/PI3K/AKT signaling pathway. Oncotargets and Therapy. 2019;**12**:11017-11031. DOI: 10.2147/OTT.S225235

[176] Xu X, Gao F, Wang J, Tao L, Ye J, Ding L, et al. MiR-122-5p inhibits cell migration and invasion in gastric cancer by down-regulating DUSP4. Cancer Biology & Therapy. 2018;**19**(5):427-435. DOI: 10.1080/15384047.2018.1423925

[177] Meng L, Chen Z, Jiang Z, Huang T, Hu J, Luo P, et al. MiR-122-5p suppresses the proliferation, migration, and invasion of gastric cancer cells by targeting

LYN. Acta Biochimica et Biophysica Sinica (Shanghai). 2020;**52**(1):49-57. DOI: 10.1093/abbs/gmz141

[178] Pei ZJ, Zhang ZG, Hu AX, Yang F, Gai Y. miR-122-5p inhibits tumor cell proliferation and induces apoptosis by targeting MYC in gastric cancer cells. Die Pharmazie. 2017;**72**(6):344-347. DOI: 10.1691/ph.2017.6404

[179] Qin QH, Yin ZQ, Li Y, Wang BG, Zhang MF. Long intergenic noncoding RNA 01296 aggravates gastric cancer cells progress through miR-122/MMP-9. Biomedicine & Pharmacotherapy. 2018;**97**:450-457. DOI: 10.1016/j.biopha.2017.10.066

[180] Jiao Y, Zhang L, Li J, He Y, Zhang X, Li J. Exosomal miR-122-5p inhibits tumorigenicity of gastric cancer by downregulating GIT1. The International Journal of Biological Markers. 2021;**36**(1):36-46. DOI: 10.1177/1724600821990677

[181] Zhang J, Pang X, Lei L, Zhang J, Zhang X, Chen Z, et al. LncRNA CRART16/miR-122-5p/FOS axis promotes angiogenesis of gastric cancer by upregulating VEGFD expression. Aging (Albany, NY). 2022;**14**(9):4137-4157. DOI: 10.18632/aging.204078

[182] Xia J, Wu Z, Yu C, He W, Zheng H, He Y, et al. miR-124 inhibits cell proliferation in gastric cancer through down-regulation of SPHK1. The Journal of Pathology. 2012;**227**(4):470-480. DOI: 10.1002/path.4030

[183] Hu CB, Li QL, Hu JF, Zhang Q, Xie JP, Deng L. miR-124 inhibits growth and invasion of gastric cancer by targeting ROCK1. Asian Pacific Journal of Cancer Prevention. 2014;**15**(16):6543-6546. DOI: 10.7314/apjcp.2014.15.16.6543

[184] Liu F, Hu H, Zhao J, Zhang Z, Ai X, Tang L, et al. miR-124-3p acts as a potential marker and suppresses tumor growth in gastric cancer. Biomedicine Reports. 2018;**9**(2):147-155. DOI: 10.3892/br.2018.1113

[185] Zhu B, Cui H, Xu W. Hydrogen inhibits the proliferation and migration of gastric cancer cells by modulating lncRNA MALAT1/miR-124-3p/EZH2 axis. Cancer Cell International. 2021;**21**(1):70. DOI: 10.1186/s12935-020-01743-5

[186] Huang HG, Tang XL, Huang XS, Zhou L, Hao YG, Zheng YF. Long noncoding RNA LINC00511 promoted cell proliferation and invasion via regulating miR-124-3p/EZH2 pathway in gastric cancer. European Review for Medical and Pharmacological Sciences. 2020;**24**(8):4232-4245. DOI: 10.26355/eurrev_202004_21003

[187] Li Y, Yan J, Wang Y, Wang C, Zhang C, Li G. LINC00240 promotes gastric cancer cell proliferation, migration and EMT via the miR-124-3p/DNMT3B axis. Cell Biochemistry and Function. 2020;**38**(8):1079-1088. DOI: 10.1002/cbf.3551

[188] Cheng Y, Yang L, Shi G, Chen P, Li L, Fang H, et al. Ninjurin 2 rs118050317 gene polymorphism and endometrial cancer risk. Cancer Cell International. 2021;**21**(1):1. DOI: 10.1186/s12935-020-01646-5

[189] Wu S, Liu F, Xie L, Peng Y, Lv X, Zhu Y, et al. miR-125b suppresses proliferation and invasion by targeting MCL1 in gastric cancer. BioMed Research International. 2015;**2015**:365273. DOI: 10.1155/2015/365273

[190] Cao Y, Tan S, Tu Y, Zhang G, Liu Y, Li D, et al. MicroRNA-125a-5p inhibits invasion and metastasis of gastric cancer cells by targeting BRMS1 expression. Oncology Letters. 2018;**15**(4):5119-5130. DOI: 10.3892/ol.2018.7983

[191] Dai J, Wang J, Yang L, Xiao Y, Ruan Q. miR-125a regulates angiogenesis of gastric cancer by targeting vascular endothelial growth factor a. International Journal of Oncology. 2015;**47**(5):1801-1810. DOI: 10.3892/ijo.2015.3171

[192] Fassan M, Pizzi M, Realdon S, Balistreri M, Guzzardo V, Zagonel V, et al. The HER2-miR125a5p/miR125b loop in gastric and esophageal carcinogenesis. Human Pathology. 2013;**44**(9):1804-1810. DOI: 10.1016/j.humpath.2013.01.023

[193] Niu J, Song X, Zhang X. Regulation of lncRNA PVT1 on miR-125 in metastasis of gastric cancer cells. Oncology Letters. 2020;**19**(2):1261-1266. DOI: 10.3892/ol.2019.11195

[194] Wang J, Chen X, Li P, Su L, Yu B, Cai Q, et al. CRKL promotes cell proliferation in gastric cancer and is negatively regulated by miR-126. Chemico-Biological Interactions. 2013;**206**(2):230-238. DOI: 10.1016/j.cbi.2013.09.003

[195] Chen H, Li L, Wang S, Lei Y, Ge Q, Lv N, et al. Reduced miR-126 expression facilitates angiogenesis of gastric cancer through its regulation on VEGF-A. Oncotarget. 2014;**5**(23):11873-11885. DOI: 10.18632/oncotarget.2662

[196] Xiao J, Lai H, Wei SH, Ye ZS, Gong FS, Chen LC. Lnc RNA HOTAIR promotes gastric cancer proliferation and metastasis via targeting miR-126 to active CXCR 4 and RhoA signaling pathway. Cancer Medicine. 2019;**8**(15):6768-6779. DOI: 10.1002/cam4.1302

[197] Wang J, Zhou Y, Fei X, Chen X, Yan J, Liu B, et al. ADAM9 functions as a promoter of gastric cancer growth which is negatively and post-transcriptionally regulated by miR-126. Oncology Reports. 2017;**37**(4):2033-2040. DOI: 10.3892/or.2017.5460

[198] Hu Y, Zhang Y, Ding M, Xu R. Long noncoding RNA TMPO-AS1/miR-126-5p/BRCC3 axis accelerates gastric cancer progression and angiogenesis via activating PI3K/Akt/mTOR pathway. Journal of Gastroenterology and Hepatology. 2021;**36**(7):1877-1888

[199] Yan J, Dang Y, Liu S, Zhang Y, Zhang G. LncRNA HOTAIR promotes cisplatin resistance in gastric cancer by targeting miR-126 to activate the PI3K/AKT/MRP1 genes. Tumor Biology. 2016;**37**(12):16345-16355

[200] Guo LH, Li H, Wang F, Yu J, He JS. The tumor suppressor roles of miR-433 and miR-127 in gastric cancer. International Journal of Molecular Sciences. 2013;**14**(7):14171-14184. DOI: 10.3390/ijms140714171

[201] Wang L, Wang X, Jiang X. miR-127 suppresses gastric cancer cell migration and invasion via targeting Wnt7a. Oncology Letters. 2019;**17**(3):3219-3226. DOI: 10.3892/ol.2019.9955

[202] Liang M, Yao W, Shi B, Zhu X, Cai R, Yu Z, et al. Circular RNA hsa_circ_0110389 promotes gastric cancer progression through upregulating SORT1 via sponging miR-127-5p and miR-136-5p. Cell Death & Disease. 2021;**12**(7):639. DOI: 10.1038/s41419-021-03903-5

[203] Wu P, Ye D, Li J, Yan F, Jin X, Zhang Z, et al. circALPL sponges miR-127 to promote gastric cancer progression by enhancing MTDH expression. Journal of Cancer. 2021;**12**(16):4924-4932. DOI: 10.7150/jca.49942

[204] Ma L, Jiang Y, Wu N. Long non-coding RNA CCL2 promoted gastric cancer function via miR-128/PARP2 signal pathway. Bioengineered. 2022;**13**(1):1602-1611. DOI: 10.1080/21655979.2021.2020548

[205] Liang L, Kang H, Jia J. HCP5 contributes to cisplatin resistance in gastric cancer through miR-128/HMGA2 axis. Cell Cycle. 2021;**20**(11):1080-1090. DOI: 10.1080/15384101.2021.1924948

[206] Guo Y, Yue P, Wang Y, Chen G, Li Y. PCAT-1 contributes to cisplatin resistance in gastric cancer through miR-128/ZEB1 axis. Biomedicine & Pharmacotherapy. 2019;**118**:109255. DOI: 10.1016/j.biopha.2019.109255

[207] Wang Q, Zhang C, Cao S, Zhao H, Jiang R, Li Y. Tumor-derived exosomes orchestrate the microRNA-128-3p/ELF4/CDX2 axis to facilitate the growth and metastasis of gastric cancer via delivery of LINC01091. Cell Biology and Toxicology. 2022:1-8. DOI: 10.1007/s10565-022-09728-y

[208] Xu C, Shao Y, Xia T, Yang Y, Dai J, Luo L, et al. lncRNA-AC130710 targeting by miR-129-5p is upregulated in gastric cancer and associates with poor prognosis. Tumour Biology. 2014;**35**(10):9701-9706. DOI: 10.1007/s13277-014-2274-5

[209] Zhang T, Piao HY, Guo S, Zhao Y, Wang Y, Zheng ZC, et al. LncRNA PCGEM1 enhances metastasis and gastric cancer invasion through targeting of miR-129-5p to regulate P4HA2 expression. Experimental and Molecular Pathology. 2020;**116**:104487. DOI: 10.1016/j.yexmp.2020.104487

[210] Chen S, Li P, Xiao B, Guo J. Long noncoding RNA HMlincRNA717 and AC130710 have been officially named as gastric cancer associated transcript 2 (GACAT2) and GACAT3, respectively. Tumor Biology. 2014;**35**(9):8351-8352

[211] Duan J, Zhang H, Qu Y, Deng T, Huang D, Liu R, et al. Onco-miR-130 promotes cell proliferation and migration by targeting TGFβR2 in gastric cancer. Oncotarget. 2016;**7**(28):44522-44533. DOI: 10.18632/oncotarget.9936

[212] Yang H, Zhang H, Ge S, Ning T, Bai M, Li J, et al. Exosome-derived miR-130a activates angiogenesis in gastric cancer by targeting C-MYB in vascular endothelial cells. Molecular Therapy. 2018;**26**(10):2466-2475. DOI: 10.1016/j.ymthe.2018.07.023

[213] Hu W, Zheng X, Liu J, Zhang M, Liang Y, Song M. MicroRNA MiR-130a-3p promotes gastric cancer by targeting glucosaminyl N-acetyl transferase 4 (GCNT4) to regulate the TGF-β1/SMAD3 pathway. Bioengineered. 2021;**12**(2):11634-11647. DOI: 10.1080/21655979.2021.1995099

[214] Yu MJ, Zhao N, Shen H, Wang H. Long noncoding RNA MRPL39 inhibits gastric cancer proliferation and progression by directly targeting miR-130. Genetic Testing and Molecular Biomarkers. 2018;**22**(11):656-663. DOI: 10.1089/gtmb.2018.0151

[215] He L, Qu L, Wei L, Chen Y, Suo J. Reduction of miR-132-3p contributes to gastric cancer proliferation by targeting MUC13. Molecular Medicine Reports. 2017;**15**(5):3055-3061. DOI: 10.3892/mmr.2017.6347

[216] Liu F, Cheng Z, Li X, Li Y, Zhang H, Li J, et al. A novel Pak1/ATF2/miR-132 signaling axis is involved in the hematogenous metastasis of gastric cancer cells. Molecular Therapy-Nucleic Acids. 2017;**8**:370-382. DOI: 10.1016/j.omtn.2017.07.005

[217] Liu B, Qiang L, Guan B, Ji Z. Targeting kinesin family member 21B by miR-132-3p represses cell proliferation, migration and invasion in gastric cancer. Bioengineered. 2022;**13**(4):9006-9018. DOI: 10.1080/21655979.2022.2054755

[218] Li P, Wang L, Li P, Hu F, Cao Y, Tang D, et al. Silencing lncRNA XIST exhibits antiproliferative and proapoptotic effects on gastric cancer cells by up-regulating microRNA-132 and down-regulating PXN. Aging. 2021;**13**(10):14469-14481. DOI: 10.18632/aging.103635

[219] Liu Y, Sun Y, Zhao A. MicroRNA-134 suppresses cell proliferation in gastric cancer cells via targeting of GOLPH3. Oncology Reports. 2017;**37**(4):2441-2448. DOI: 10.3892/or.2017.5488

[220] Zhong BZ, Wang Q, Liu F, He JL, Xiong Y, Cao J. Effects of mir-384 and mir-134-5p acting on yy1 signaling transduction on biological function of gastric cancer cells. Oncotargets and Therapy. 2020;**13**:9631-9641. DOI: 10.2147/OTT.S259988

[221] Chi J, Liu T, Shi C, Luo H, Wu Z, Xiong B, et al. Long non-coding RNA LUCAT1 promotes proliferation and invasion in gastric cancer by regulating miR-134-5p/YWHAZ axis. Biomedicine & Pharmacotherapy. 2019;**118**:109201. DOI: 10.1016/j.biopha.2019.109201

[222] Fan HN, Zhao XY, Liang R, Chen XY, Zhang J, Chen NW, et al. CircPTK2 inhibits the tumorigenesis and metastasis of gastric cancer by sponging miR-134-5p and activating CELF2/PTEN signaling. Pathology-Research and Practice. 2021;**227**:153615

[223] Yan LH, Chen ZN, Li-Li CJ, Wei WE, Mo XW, et al. miR-135a promotes gastric cancer progression and resistance to oxaliplatin. Oncotarget. 2016;**7**(43):70699-70714. DOI: 10.18632/oncotarget.12208

[224] Wu Y, Hu G, Wu R, Gong N. High expression of miR-135b predicts malignant transformation and poor prognosis of gastric cancer. Life Sciences. 2020;**257**:118133. DOI: 10.1016/j.lfs.2020.118133

[225] He Y, Wu L, Dai Y, Li J, Liu S. MicroRNA-135 inhibits gastric cancer metastasis by targeting SMAD2. European Review for Medical and Pharmacological Sciences. 2019;**23**(21):9436-9444. DOI: 10.26355/eurrev_201911_19437

[226] Yu X, Xiao W, Song H, Jin Y, Xu J. Liu X CircRNA_100876 sponges miR-136 to promote proliferation and metastasis of gastric cancer by upregulating MIEN1 expression. Gene. 2020;**748**:144678. DOI: 10.1016/j.gene.2020.144678

[227] Chen Z, Xu C, Pan X, Cheng G, Liu M, Li J, et al. lncRNA DSCR8 mediates miR-137/Cdc42 to regulate gastric cancer cell proliferation, invasion, and cell cycle as a competitive endogenous RNA. Molecular Therapy-Oncolytics. 2021;**22**:468-482. DOI: 10.1016/j.omto.2021.05.010

[228] Li W, Duan J, Shi W, Lei L, Lv P. Long non-coding RNA NCK1-AS1 serves an oncogenic role in gastric cancer by regulating miR-137/NUP43 axis. Oncotargets and Therapy. 2020;**13**:9929-9939. DOI: 10.2147/OTT.S259336

[229] Lu Y, Li L, Li L, Wu G, Liu G. Circular RNA circHECTD1 prevents Diosbulbin-B-sensitivity via miR-137/PBX3 axis in gastric cancer. Cancer Cell International. 2021;**21**(1):264. DOI: 10.1186/s12935-021-01957-1

[230] Li D, She J, Hu X, Zhang M, Sun R, Qin S. The ELF3-regulated lncRNA UBE2CP3 is over-stabilized by RNA–RNA interactions and drives gastric cancer metastasis via miR-138-5p/ITGA2 axis. Oncogene. 2021;**40**(35):5403-5415. DOI: 10.1038/s41388-021-01948-6

[231] Sun J, Zhou F, Xue J, Ji C, Qu Y, Pan Y. Long non-coding RNA

TRPM2-AS regulates microRNA miR-138-5p and PLAU (plasminogen activator, urokinase) to promote the progression of gastric adenocarcinoma. Bioengineered. 2021;**12**(2):9753-9765. DOI: 10.1080/21655979.2021.1995101

[232] Sun H, Wu P, Zhang B, Wu X, Chen W. MCM3AP-AS1 promotes cisplatin resistance in gastric cancer cells via the miR-138/FOXC1 axis. Oncology Letters. 2021;**21**(3):1. DOI: 10.3892/ol.2021.12472

[233] Wang J, Wu J, Wang L, Min X, Chen Z. The LINC00152/miR-138 axis facilitates gastric cancer progression by mediating SIRT2. Journal of Oncology. 2021;**2021**:1173869. DOI: 10.1155/2021/1173869

[234] Xie Y, Rong L, He M, Jiang Y, Li H, Mai L, et al. LncRNA SNHG3 promotes gastric cancer cell proliferation and metastasis by regulating the miR-139-5p/MYB axis. Aging (Albany, NY). 2021;**13**(23):25138-25152. DOI: 10.18632/aging.203732

[235] Yang Y, Gao M, Li Y, Li M, Ma Q. LncRNA CTBP1-AS2 facilitates gastric cancer progression via regulating the miR-139-3p/MMP11 axis. Oncotargets and Therapy. 2020;**13**:11537-11547. DOI: 10.2147/OTT.S264394

[236] Sun K, Hu P, Xu F. LINC00152/miR-139-5p regulates gastric cancer cell aerobic glycolysis by targeting PRKA. Biomedicine & Pharmacotherapy. 2018;**97**:1296-1302. DOI: 10.1016/j.biopha.2017.11.015

[237] Li Z, Cheng Y, Fu K, Lin Q, Zhao T, Tang W, et al. Circ-PTPDC1 promotes the progression of gastric cancer through sponging Mir-139-3p by regulating ELK1 and functions as a prognostic biomarker. International Journal of Biological Sciences. 2021;**17**(15):4285-4304. DOI: 10.7150/ijbs.62732

[238] Xia G, Wang A, Li L. Hsa_circ_0000218/hsa-miR-139-3p/SOX4 regulatory feedback circuit influences the proliferation and apoptosis of gastric cancer cells. Cytotechnology. 2022;**74**(1):89-98. DOI: 10.1007/s10616-021-00509-9

[239] Yang F, Peng ZX, Ji WD, Yu JD, Qian C, Liu JD, et al. LncRNA CCAT1 upregulates ATG5 to enhance autophagy and promote gastric cancer development by absorbing miR-140-3p. Digestive Diseases and Sciences. 2021;**6**:1-7. DOI: 10.1007/s10620-021-07187-9

[240] Sun Y, Han C. Long non-coding RNA TMPO-AS1 promotes cell migration and invasion by sponging miR-140-5p and inducing SOX4-mediated EMT in gastric cancer. Cancer Management and Research. 2020;**12**:1261-1268. DOI: 10.2147/CMAR.S235898

[241] Guo W, Huang J, Lei P, Guo L, Li X. LncRNA SNHG1 promoted HGC-27 cell growth and migration via the miR-140/ADAM10 axis. International Journal of Biological Macromolecules. 2019;**122**:817-823. DOI: 10.1016/j.ijbiomac.2018.10.214

[242] Guo H, Yang S, Li S, Yan M, Li L, Zhang H. LncRNA SNHG20 promotes cell proliferation and invasion via miR-140-5p-ADAM10 axis in cervical cancer. Biomedicine & Pharmacotherapy. 2018;**102**:749-757. DOI: 10.1016/j.biopha.2018.03.024

[243] Kong D, Piao YS, Yamashita S, Oshima H, Oguma K, Fushida S, et al. Inflammation-induced repression of tumor suppressor miR-7 in gastric tumor cells. Oncogene. 2012;**31**(35):3949-3960. DOI: 10.1038/onc.2011.558

[244] Wang Q, He Y, Kan W, Li F, Ji X, Wu X, et al. microRNA-32-5p targets KLF2 to promote gastric cancer by

activating PI3K/AKT signaling pathway. American Journal of Translational Rcscarch. 2019;**11**(8):4895-4908

[245] Peng Q, Shen Y, Lin K, Zou L, Shen Y, Zhu Y. Comprehensive and integrative analysis identifies microRNA-106 as a novel non-invasive biomarker for detection of gastric cancer. Journal of Translational Medicine. 2018;**16**(1):127. DOI: 10.1186/s12967-018-1510-y

Chapter 9

MicroRNAs and Male Infertility

Mohsin Munawar, Irfana Liaqat and Shaukat Ali

Abstract

Spermatozoan production is tightly controlled by the multistep process of spermatogenesis and spermiogenesis. Physiological and molecular disruption in spermatogenesis can lead to various reproductive disorders including male infertility. Male infertility is associated with various etiologies, but mechanism is not determined yet. MicroRNAs (miRNAs) are almost 22 nucleotides long, non-protein coding RNA that play an essential role in posttranscriptional regulations in various biological processes including spermatogenesis. The current review is aimed to summarize the recent literature on the role of miRNAs in male infertility and spermatogenesis and their potential in diagnosis, prognosis, and therapy of the disease. miRNAs have shown tremendous potential to be used as diagnostic and prognostic marker and therapeutic target in diseases related to male infertility. Experimental evidence reveals that aberrant expression of miRNAs affects different cell types and different stages of spermatogenesis, which ultimately leads to male infertility. To exploit the full potential of miRNAs, characterization of unidentified miRNAs is required to understand the miRNA-mediated regulatory mechanism related to male infertility.

Keywords: miRNAs, male infertility, spermatogenesis, spermiogenesis, non-coding RNA, therapeutic agents

1. Introduction

Infertility is the inability to conceive spontaneously in 1 year by a sexually active, non-contracepting couple. Primary infertility, the complete inability to conceive, ranges from 2 to 5%, while secondary infertility, indicating cessation of further fertility, globally has a prevalence rate of 20%. Approximately 15% (48.5 million) of couples cannot conceive worldwide [1].

Among infertile men, the etiology of 30–40% of cases remains unknown, so considered idiopathic male infertility [2]. The possible causes of male infertility are physiological anomalies, immunological factors, some genetic abnormalities [3], and some environmental toxicants, which can disturb the reproductive health of male by disturbing steroidogenesis, spermatogenesis, and histopathological structures [4]. Among all these possible causes of male infertility, several types of small non-coding RNAs, including microRNAs (miRNAs), are expressed in the male germ line and impair the mammalian spermatogenesis [5, 6].

Protein coding genes represent only 1.5%of the genome, which can be increased by up to 2% if untranslated regions (UTRs) are also included. The remaining 98% genome, the non-protein-coding region, has been considered a “black box” until the characterization of non-coding RNAs (ncRNAs) was done using novel nucleotide sequencing technologies. ncRNAs are present in cellular compartments, participating in multiple biological functions, including the male reproductive system, whereas some are identified in extracellular fluids, correctly named as circulating ncRNAs, where they can be detected in exosomes, bound on lipoprotein and free circulating molecules [7].

Ambros and his colleagues 1993 discovered the miRNA and then revealed the ncRNAs as gene regulators in eukaryotes [8, 9]. *Lin-4* and *let-7* in *Caenorhabditis elegans* were first discovered ncRNAs, later classified as miRNAs. Thus far, almost 38579 entries have been recorded, and among these, up to 1982 miRNAs are only from the human genome [10]. miRNAs code is either located in the intergenic region or introns of genes of the whole genome. In contrast, nearly half of total miRNAs are arranged nearby (within 50kb of another miRNA code) to form clusters. These clusters range from 2 to 46 miRNAs; C19MC is the major known cluster of miRNAs located on chromosome 19 in primates [11]. It is predicted that over 30% of mammalian and 60% of human genes are regulated by miRNAs [12, 13].

miRNAs are small RNA molecules, derived from the genome-encoded-precursor loop, consisting of almost 19–23 nucleotides. They are conserved in species and so regulate the expression of the mRNAs by recognizing the targeted mRNA through base-pair binding to the 3′UTR [14, 15].

2. miRNA nomenclature

MicroRNAs (prefix; "miR" for mature sequence whereas precursor hairpins are labeled as "mir") are named by using the number in sequential order, such as miR-1, miR-2. Despite the discovery of identical miRNAs in different organisms, the same number is assigned. Lettered suffix such as miR-1a and miR-1b is assigned to the sequences whose mature miRNAs sequences differ at one of two positions. Numbered suffix (e.g., miR-1-1 and miR-1-2) is used to label the identical miRNAs that have originated from distinct hairpin loci. The -3p and -5p suffixes refer to the arm from which the mature miRNA sequence originates. Detailed guidelines for naming the miRNAs can be seen in [16, 17].

3. MicroRNAs: biogenesis

miRNAs have a vital role as epigenetic regulators. The enzyme (Dicer protein) used for the biosynthesis of miRNA plays a very crucial role for the developmental processes [18]. During miRNAs biogenesis, following steps will be followed sequentially as elaborated in **Figure 1**:

i. Primarily, a long imperfect ~80 nt hairpin-like structure primary microRNA (pri-miRNA) is transcribed by RNA polymerase (RNA pol) II from intergenic non-coding region or intragenic region intron (untranslated region of protein-coding genes).

ii. Secondarily, pri-miRNA undergoes two steps enzymes (Drosha and Dicer from RNase III superfamily) catalyzed reaction.

   a. Pri-miRNA (~80-nt hairpin structure) is excised to form an intermediate precursor (pre-) miRNA (~65–70 nt) processed by Nuclear *Drosha-DGCR8*

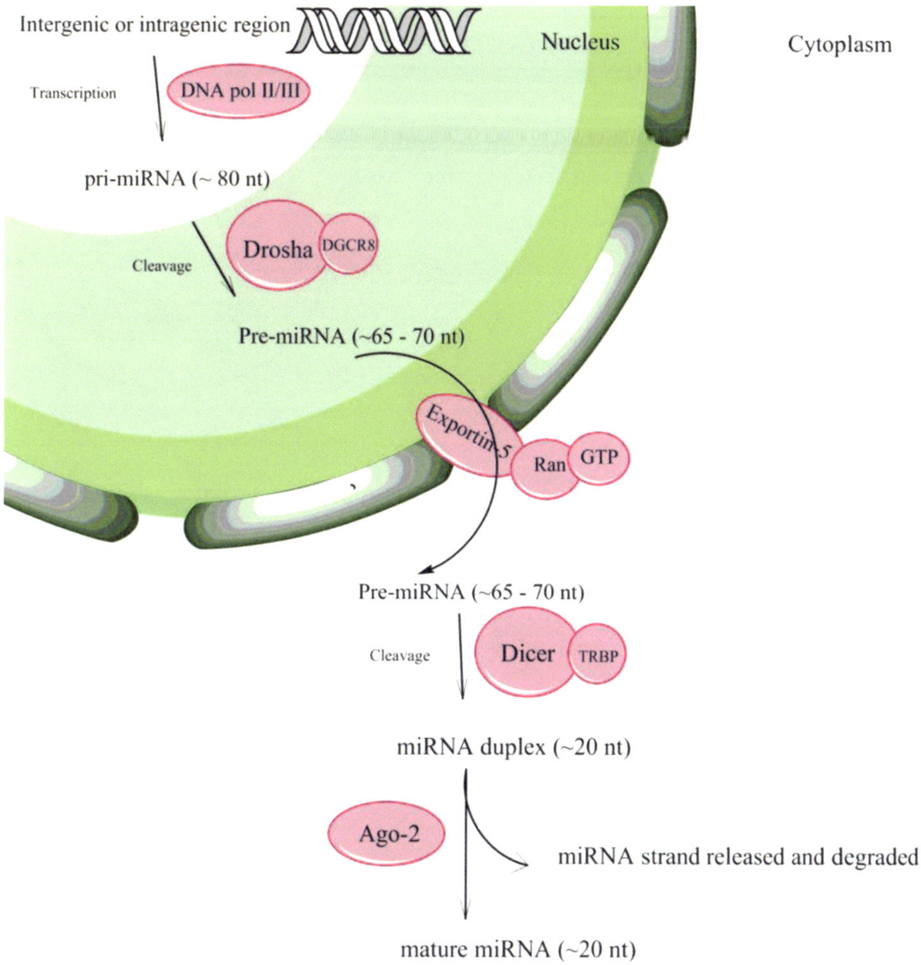

Figure 1.
Mechanism of miRNA's biosynthesis.

(DiGeorge syndrome critical region 8), then transported to cytoplasm through export factor Exportin-5.

b. Pri-miRNA is processed by called *Dicer-TRBP* (trans-activating region binding protein), a second RNase III endonuclease enzyme, to remove the terminal loop of pre-miRNA resulting in ~20 bp miRNA: miRNA* duplex.

iii. The *Dicer-TRBP* processed duplex is loaded onto Ago-2 (Argonaute) protein to form an miRNA induced silencing complex (miRISC). miRISC contains mature miRNA that regulates the gene expression, while another miRNA* will be released and degraded.

iv. Finally activated region (miRNA) of miRISC binds with 3′ UTR of targeted mRNA, ultimately leading to translational repression, deadenylation, or degradation of targeted mRNA [19].

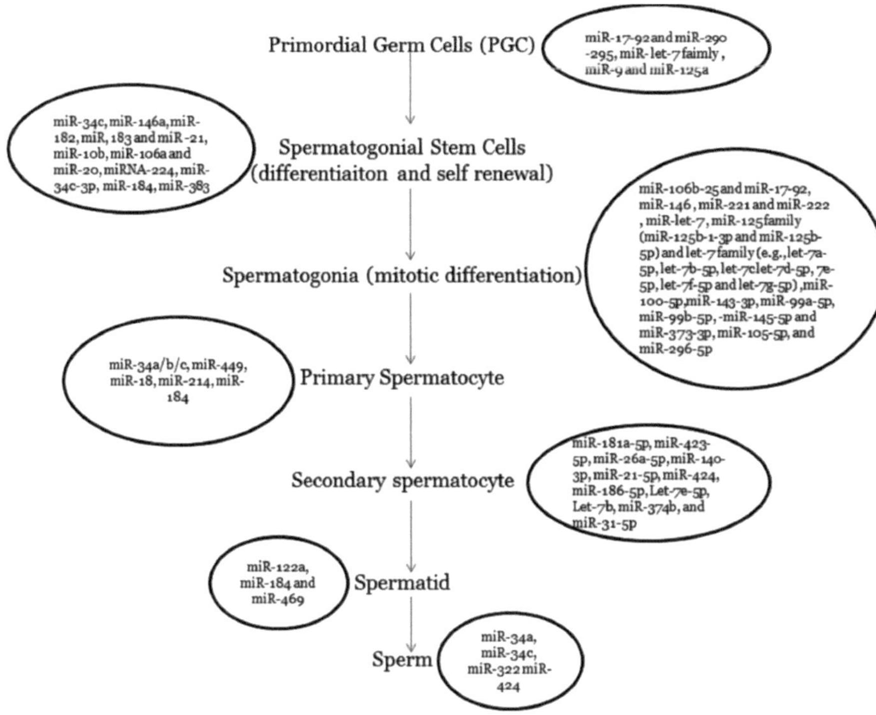

Figure 2.
miRNAs expressed during different stages of spermatogenesis in mammals.

4. miRNAs: regulators of biological processes

miRNAs play a vital role in the regulation of various biological phenomena including cellular differentiation, cell growth, programmed cell death, and embryonic development [20–22], whereas up- or downregulation may lead to serious abnormality. For instance, cardiovascular disease, cancer, diabetes, renal abnormality, schizophrenia, muscular dystrophy, and reproductive disorder especially related to sperm formation and its function have been linked with biosynthesis impairment, mutation, or improper regulation of miRNA [23–29]. miRNA is not solely responsible for the whole regulatory mechanism, but their activities are also dependent on other proteins or complexes depending upon the processor stage [30].

Mature human spermatozoa retain various miRNAs; moreover, variable expression of spermatozoal RNAs has been associated with male infertility [31]. miRNAs, present in primordial germ cells, spermatogonia, primary and secondary spermatocytes, spermatids, and mature spermatozoa, play an epigenetic role in the spermatogenesis and early development as well (**Figure 2**) [32].

5. miRNA as potential biomarker in male infertility

In order to confirm the male infertility, various methods have been adopted, but the most recent way is the use of biomarker. Biomarkers can be used to diagnose the disease before the appearance of physiological symptoms. miRNA is known as the most reliable biomarker due to various known properties.

5.1 Properties of biomarker

A biomarker molecule should be stable, target-specific, and sensitive to detection, noninvasive, and from an easily accessible source. In the field of medical science, protein molecules, which are easily found in serum plasma, have been used as a biomarker for the detection of pathological conditions and their prognosis. However, as a biomarker, protein molecules have some limitations such as reduced diagnostic value due to low sensitivity and specificity of their detection. On the other hand, miRNAs present in the extracellular or intracellular environment appear much earlier and detected at minute concentration, thus allowing early diagnosis. Expressions of miRNAs are often biological-stage-specific [33, 34]. Moreover, miRNA is observed as the homogeneous population of molecules, but protein molecules may become heterogeneous due to different posttranslational modifications.

miRNAs are more stable than mRNA but lesser stable than DNA. Extracellular miRNAs exist in microvesicles, exosomes, and lipoproteins or form a complex with Ago-2 protein, so protected from endogenous RNAse activity, which suggests their reliable use as a noninvasive biomarker for spermatogenic impairment [35–38]. Some miRNAs are stable at room temperature, sustain a repeated freeze-thaw cycle, and got stability under harsh conditions even found in degraded RNA preparations [39–41]. In a study, exosomal miRNAs were found to be stable at 4°C for 2 weeks, at −80°C for 2 months, and at −20°C for 5 year [42]. So their relative stability enhances their usage as biomarker molecules. miRNA (both extracellular and intracellular) can be isolated by using noninvasive procedures and detected with techniques in common routines such as RT-qPCR and miRNA microarray, which is more advantageous than conventional and invasive (e.g., prostate and testicular biopsy) diagnostic procedures [43–47]. Despite all these characteristics of miRNAs as a biomarker, the use of protein as a biomarker may not be completely replaced, but no doubt miRNAs can be labeled as a good candidate for complementary diagnosis tools.

Circulating (serum) miRNAs were firstly used as biomarkers for the detection of diffuse large B-cell lymphoma [48]. In another study, the downregulation of miR-34c, miR-122, and miR-181a was observed in the serum of patients suffering from oligo-asthenospermia [49]. Wang and his colleagues reported a decreased level of various miRNAs in azoospermic patients when compared with control [44]. Many other such published literature suggested that miRNAs are suitable biomarkers for diagnostic purposes [50, 51].

In mammals, sperm deliver genome and epigenome to the oocyte, which includes protein factors, methylation of DNA, and non-coding RNAs [52]. During mammalian spermatogenesis, mRNAs undergo posttranscriptional and posttranslational regulation in differentiating germ cells [53], so the regulatory role of miRNAs during the process of spermatogenesis can be observed clearly.

Many miRNAs as families or individual candidates are found to be very crucial in many systems of humans including the reproductive system. The role of some miRNA's family and individual miRNA candidates is summarized.

5.2 miRNA families

Let-7 **family** is a large family encoded by 12 different loci [54]. A well-known regulatory role of the let-7 family is gamete differentiation and embryonic implantation in humans [55, 56]. Different members of this family were identified in the testis, spermatozoa, and seminal plasma with differential expression [57–59].

miR-30-5p family (five members miR30a/b/c/d/e-5p), encoded by six loci located on chromosomes 1, 6, and 8 in humans. All miRNAs are observed in male reproductive tissue cells [60]. These miRNAs were expressed differentially in spermatozoa and seminal plasma of asthenozoospermic, oligozoospermic, and normozoospermic infertile men [39].

miR-345p/449-5p family with five miRNAs (miR-34a-5p, miR-34c-5p, miR-449a-5p, miR-449b-5p miR-449c-5p) has shown a very important regulatory role in mitosis [61]. These are highly expressed in male reproductive cells but variably expressed in pathologically infertile men especially nonobstructive azoospermic and obstructive azoospermic patients [62]. Their role was also investigated in the process of fertilization, cleavage division, and pre-implantation. These miRNAs are highly expressed in the sperm, as miR-34c-5p is the most abundant human sperm miRNA [52].

MiR-303-3p/370-3p/372-3p and 520-3p family each member of family miR-302-3p regulates over 450 target genes [63]. Members of this family were seen to be differentially expressed in the testis having histopathological impairments and in spermatozoa of patients with asthenozoospermia [62].

miR-99-5P/100-5P family is one of the most ancient families with three members (miR-99a/b/c) located in distinct chromosomal regions (ch 21, 19, and 11 respectively) in the human genome [64]. The member of this family shows differential expression in the testis of NOA patients [57].

miR-888 family (miR-888/ Mir-890, miR-891a/b, and miR-892a/b) is located on the X chromosome of primates only which has specific expression in epididymal tissues [65, 66]. Computational functional analyses predicted that the targets of the miR-888 family were related to morphogenesis of epididymis and sperm maturation [67].

5.3 Individual miRNA

hsa-miR-10b-5p, located on chromosome no 2(1q31.1), plays a pivotal role in gametogenesis as it is highly expressed in the testes. The expression level of hsa-miR-10B-5P, among others, was upregulated in round spermatids of NOA patients [57].

hsa-miR-27b-3p, present on chromosome 9 (9q22.32), was differentially expressed in the mature spermatozoa of infertile men. The expression of miR-27 has correlated with the expression of the CRISP2 (cysteine-rich secretory protein 2) gene, the highly expressed gene in the testis [59]. CGN1-CRISP2 complex has an important role in the development of the sperm tail (sperm motility) and predicts the regulatory role of miR27b-3p in spermatozoa development and motility potential [58].

miR-320a, located on chromosome 8, is highly expressed miRNA in epididymis and spermatozoa so has an important role in multiple reproductive processes [68]. Mmu-miR-320a (hsa-miR-320a) was exclusively expressed in murine Sertoli cells (SCs). The induction of apoptosis elicited miRNA expression was observed in meiotic spermatocytes and haploid spermatids. Forced expression of exogenous miR-320a in SCs may cause oligospermia and defection in sperm mobility, thus compromising the male fertility [69].

6. MicroRNAs: a key player in spermatogenesis

miRNAs play a vital role in the whole spermatogenic process, and their dysregulation ultimately leads to spermatogenic impairments [70]. To determine the role of miRNA, in male reproductive system, various models (mice) have been established

miRNA	Isolation of miRNA	Dysregulation	Cellular processes	Model organism	References
miR-19b and let-7a	Seminal plasma	Up-regulated	Failure in spermatogenesis	Human Oligozoospermia, non-obstructive and azoospermia	[79]
MiR-7-1-3p, miR-141 & miR-429	Seminal plasma	Up-regulated	Spermatogenesis impairment	Infertile men	[80]
hsa-miR-429	Semen	Up-regulated	Biomarker to access male infertility	Human Subfertile and non-obstructive azoospermia	[81]
hsa-miR-34b, hsa-miR-34c-5p & hsa-miR-122	Semen	Up-regulated	Biomarker to access male infertility	Human Subfertile and non-obstructive azoospermia	[81]
miR-34c-5p, miR-122, miR-146b-5p, miR-181a, miR-374b, miR-509-5p and miR-513-5p	Seminal plasma	Up-regulated in asthenozoospermia Down-regulated in azoospermia	Role in infertility	Infertile men (Asthenozoospermia and Azoospermia)	[39]
miR-27a	Semen	Upregulated	Low motility, abnormal Morphology	Infertile men Asthenoteratozoospermia and normozoospermia	[59]
miR-17-92 cluster (miR-17, miR-18a, and miR-20a)	Testes	Upregulated	Testicular atrophy, decreased sperm production	Mice	[82]
miR-17-92 (Mirc1) and miR-106b-25 (Mirc3) cluster	Testes	Knock-out	Reduced testes and mild spermetogenic defect	Mice	[83]
miR-146a			Role in differentiation of spermatogonia.	Mice	[84]
miR-221/222			Maintain the undifferentiated state of mammalian spermatogonia.		[85]
miR-135a	Spermatogonial stem cells	Downregulated	Downregulation of forkhead box protein O 1 (FOXO1) expression.	Rats	[86]

miRNA	Isolation of miRNA	Dysregulation	Cellular processes	Model organism	References
miR-449	Testis			Mice	[87]
MiR-518f	Seminal plasma	Downregulated	Effected sperm quality and testicular environment exposure of Bisphenol A	Human	[46]
miR- 23a/b- 3p	Semen	Upregulated	Oligoasthenozoospermia	Human	[88]

Table 1.
miRNAs, the cellular processes affected by their dysregulation.

by using the *Cre/Lox* system, which enables conditional manipulation of target genes, including knockout, insertion, replacement, activation, or modification of gene expression [44]. To understand the exact function of concerned miRNA *in vivo*, target deletion is the key step; however, in the absence of one miRNA, usually someone other has a compensatory role.

Double knockout of miR-34b/c and miR-449 in mice displayed severe disruption in spermatogenesis, dispensable fertilization, and pre-implantation development. Intracytoplasmic injection of miRNA-dKO sperm led to normal fertilization [52]. Deletion of miR34b/c and miR-449 in mice shows impaired spermatogenesis and spermatozoa maturation resulting in oligoasthenoteratozoospermia (OAT) [70]. Simultaneous inactivation of miR34b/c and miR449 in dKO mice leads to developmental defects and infertility [71, 72].

Salas-Huetos and his colleagues showed that 221 miRNAs were consistently detected in 10 healthy fertile men; among these most expressed, hsa-miR-191-5p was associated with sperm differentiation [73]. The first report on altered miRNA expression in patients with NOA showed that 154 miRNAs were differentially downregulated and 19 upregulated in NOA patients compared with fertile men [74]. Experimentally it is confirmed that specific genes are regulated by miRNAs involved in spermatogenesis. Decreased levels of estrogen-alpha (ERα) and a higher level of miR-100 and let-7b in oligospermia patients compared with fertile men indicated the regulatory role of miRNA over estrogen signaling [75–77]. Phosphatidylinositol-specific phospholipase C, X domain containing 3 (PLCXD3), expressed in spermatogenesis, was downregulated by miRNA34c-3p in severe oligozoospermic patients [78].

Conclusively, these results and some others (as shown in **Table 1**) confirm the regulatory role of miRNAs in male germ and somatic cells, and any change in their expression may lead to reproductive anomalies.

7. miRNAs: therapeutic advancements and infertility

In addition to the potential use of miRNAs as a biomarker, miRNAs have been considered therapeutic services against male infertility. miRNAs overexpression can be inhibited by anti-miR (laboratory designed molecule), or their downregulation might be supplemented with miRNAs mimics [89, 90]. A recent study showed that MRX34 (miRNA mimic of miR-34a) managed to suppress the tumor progression, and anti-miRs their inhibitory activity through binding to a miRNA, thus blocking it [91–94].

In RNA-based therapeutics strategies, the challenge of degradation of the oligonucleotide by RNases in serum or cellular compartments is averted using two distinct approaches, either by altering oligonucleotide or through encapsulations of RNAs for protection (by adding phosphorothioate-like groups or developing delivery vehicles [95].

After several preclinical studies involving miRNA therapeutics, only a small number of miRNAs have moved into clinical development [96]. This is because of the many challenges, including;

1. Difficulty in identifying the best miRNA candidates or miRNA targets for each disease type and the absence of efficient delivery systems in specific tissues. As described below, several novel delivery systems are currently being developed to develop miRNA therapeutics using a systematic approach.

2. miRNA and its target identification by using bioinformatics tools, in silico interaction, and *in vitro* experimentation (cell culture, etc.)

    a. Selection of miRNA chemistry such as 2'-methyl, locked nucleic acid (LNC), or phosphothionate.

    b. Optimization of the delivery system by viral particle encapsulation or through liposomes.

    c. *In vivo* testing by using a model organism so that target localization, the efficiency of delivery, and toxicity level can be reported.

    d. Clinical trial for dose optimization, determination of the mode of drug delivery, and toxicity analysis.

5. Another challenge is to provide stability, accuracy in *in vivo* targeting, avoid toxicity and thwarting off-target complex to a therapeutic miRNA [96].

6. To achieve the efficient therapeutic functioning, correct *in vivo* dose concentration has not been determined yet [97].

8. Conclusion

miRNAs play a vital role in developing an organism and regulating many biological processes in the living organism. This chapter summarized the role of miRNAs in male infertility. Many miRNAs are reported as regulators of many functions, including developing reproductive organs, spermatogenesis, spermiogenesis, sperm mobility, and fertilization. Despite using miRNAs as biomarkers, miRNAs are also investigated as more reliable therapeutic agents for various diseases such as cancer, diabetes, and infertility.

Conflict of interest

The authors declare no conflict of interest.

Author details

Mohsin Munawar*, Irfana Liaqat and Shaukat Ali
Government College University, Lahore, Pakistan

*Address all correspondence to: mohsinmunawar37yahoo.com

References

[1] Robay A, Abbasi S, Akil A, El-Bardisi H, Arafa M, Crystal RG, et al. A systematic review on the genetics of male infertility in the era of next-generation sequencing. Arab Journal of Urology. 2018;**16**(1):53-64

[2] Bracke A, Peeters K, Punjabi U, Hoogewijs D, Dewilde S. A search for molecular mechanisms underlying male idiopathic infertility. Reproductive Biomedicine Online. 2018;**36**(3):327-339

[3] Nieschlag E, Behre HM. Andrology: Male Reproductive Health and Dysfunction. Germany (Berlin): Springer Science & Business Media; 2001

[4] Manfo F, Nantia E, Mathur P. Effect of environmental contaminants on mammalian testis. Current Molecular Pharmacology. 2014;**7**(2):119-135

[5] Jodar M, Anton E. Small RNAs present in sand their role in reproduction. In: Reproductomics. United States: Academic Press; 2018. pp. 109-123

[6] Li S, Xu Z, Sheng J. tRNA-derived small RNA: A novel regulatory small non-coding RNA. Genes. 2018;**9**(5):246

[7] Trzybulska D, Vergadi E, Tsatsanis C. miRNA and other non-coding RNAs as promising diagnostic markers. Ejifcc. 2018;**29**(3):221

[8] Cai X, Hagedorn CH, Cullen BR. Human microRNAs are processed from capped, polyadenylated transcripts that can also function as mRNAs. RNA. 2004;**10**(12):1957-1966

[9] Selbach M, Schwanhäusser B, Thierfelder N, Fang Z, Khanin R, Rajewsky N. Widespread changes in protein synthesis induced by microRNAs. Nature. 2008;**455**(7209):58-63

[10] Sanger miRBase v.22.1; www.mirbase.org. [Accessed: May 08, 2022]

[11] Baskerville S, Bartel DP. Microarray profiling of microRNAs reveals frequent coexpression with neighboring miRNAs and host genes. RNA. 2005;**11**(3):241-247

[12] Vishnoi A, Rani S. MiRNA biogenesis and regulation of diseases: An overview. MicroRNA Profiling. 2017;**1**:270-282

[13] Friedman RC, Farh KK, Burge CB, Bartel DP. Most mammalian mRNAs are conserved targets of microRNAs. Genome Research. 2009;**19**(1):92-105

[14] Berezikov E, Cuppen E, Plasterk RH. Approaches to microRNA discovery. Nature Genetics. 2006;**38**(6):S2-S7

[15] Khawar MB, Mehmood R, Roohi N. MicroRNAs: Recent insights towards their role in male infertility and reproductive cancers. Bosnian Journal of Basic Medical Sciences. 2019;**19**(1):31

[16] Ambros V, Bartel B, Bartel DP, Burge CB, Carrington JC, Chen X, et al. A uniform system for microRNA annotation. RNA. 2003;**9**(3):277-279

[17] Budak H, Bulut R, Kantar M, Alptekin B. MicroRNA nomenclature and the need for a revised naming prescription. Briefings in Functional Genomics. 2016;**15**(1):65-71

[18] Bernstein E, Kim SY, Carmell MA, Murchison EP, Alcorn H, Li MZ, et al. Dicer is essential for mouse development. Nature Genetics. 2003;**35**(3):215-217

[19] Krol J, Loedige I, Filipowicz W. The widespread regulation of microRNA biogenesis, function and decay. Nature Reviews. Genetics. 2010;**11**(9):597-610

[20] Le Bot N. miRNAs and cell-cycle control in ESCs. Nature Cell Biology. 2012;**14**:658

[21] Cheng AM, Byrom MW, Shelton J, Ford LP. Antisense inhibition of human miRNAs and indications for an involvement of miRNA in cell growth and apoptosis. Nucleic Acids Research. 2005;**33**(4):1290-1297

[22] Dennis LM. MicroRNAs in Early Embryonic Development: Dissecting the Role of miR-290 through miR-295 in the Mouse. United States: Massachusetts Institute of Technology; 2008

[23] Latronico MV, Condorelli G. MicroRNAs and cardiac pathology. Nature Reviews. Cardiology. 2009;**6**(6):419-429

[24] Esquela-Kerscher A, Slack FJ. Oncomirs—microRNAs with a role in cancer. Nature Reviews. Cancer. 2006;**6**(4):259-269

[25] Hansen T, Olsen L, Lindow M, Jakobsen KD, Ullum H, Jonsson E, et al. Brain expressed microRNAs implicated in schizophrenia etiology. PLoS One. 2007;**2**(9):e873

[26] Li JY, Yong TY, Michael MZ, Gleadle JM. Review: The role of microRNAs in kidney disease. Nephrology (Carlton). 2010;**15**(6):599-608

[27] Sonkoly E, Wei T, Janson PC, Saaf A, Lundeberg L, Tengvall-Linder M, et al. MicroRNAs: Novel regulators involved in the pathogenesis of psoriasis. PloS One. 2007;**2**(7):e610

[28] Eisenberg I, Eran A, Nishino I, Moggio M, Lamperti C, Amato AA, et al. Distinctive patterns of microRNA expression in primary muscular disorders. Proceedings of the National Academy of Sciences of the United States of America. 2007;**104**(43):17016-17021

[29] Kantharidis P, Wang B, Carew RM, Lan HY. Diabetes complications: The microRNA perspective. Diabetes. 2011;**60**(7):1832-1837

[30] Kedde M, Agami R. Interplay between microRNAs and RNA-binding proteins determines developmental processes. Cell Cycle. 2008;**7**(7):899-903

[31] Sendler E, Johnson GD, Mao S, Goodrich RJ, Diamond MP, Hauser R, et al. Stability, delivery and functions of human sperm RNAs at fertilization. Nucleic Acids Research. 2013;**41**(7):4104-4117

[32] Pratt SL, Calcatera SM. Expression of microRNA in male reproductive tissues and their role in male fertility. Reproduction, Fertility, and Development. 2016;**29**(1):24-31

[33] Etheridge A, Lee I, Hood L, Galas D, Wang K. Extracellular microRNA: A new source of biomarkers. Mutation Research, Fundamental and Molecular Mechanisms of Mutagenesis. 2011;**717**(1-2):85-90

[34] Pal MK, Jaiswar SP, Dwivedi VN, Tripathi AK, Dwivedi A, Sankhwar P. MicroRNA: A new and promising potential biomarker for diagnosis and prognosis of ovarian cancer. Cancer Biology & Medicine. 2015;**12**(4):328

[35] Hunter MP, Ismail N, Zhang X, Aguda BD, Lee EJ, Yu L, et al. Detection of microRNA expression in human peripheral blood microvesicles. PLoS One. 2008;**3**(11):e3694

[36] Valadi H, Ekström K, Bossios A, Sjöstrand M, Lee JJ, Lötvall JO. Exosome-mediated transfer of mRNAs and microRNAs is a novel mechanism of genetic exchange between cells. Nature Cell Biology. 2007;**9**(6):654-659

[37] Sohel MH. Extracellular/circulating microRNAs: Release mechanisms, functions and challenges. Achievements in the Life Sciences. 2016;**10**(2):175-186

[38] Turchinovich A, Burwinkel B. Distinct AGO1 and AGO2 associated miRNA profiles in human cells and blood plasma. RNA Biology. 2012;**9**(8):1066-1075

[39] Wang C, Yang C, Chen X, Yao B, Yang C, Zhu C, et al. Altered profile of seminal plasma microRNAs in the molecular diagnosis of male infertility. Clinical Chemistry. 2011;**57**(12):1722-1731

[40] Glinge C, Clauss S, Boddum K, Jabbari R, Jabbari J, Risgaard B, et al. Stability of circulating blood-based microRNAs–pre-analytic methodological considerations. PLoS One. 2017;**12**(2):e0167969

[41] Jung M, Schaefer A, Steiner I, Kempkensteffen C, Stephan C, Erbersdobler A, et al. Robust microRNA stability in degraded RNA preparations from human tissue and cell samples. Clinical Chemistry. 2010;**56**(6):998-1006

[42] Ge Q, Zhou Y, Lu J, Bai Y, Xie X, Lu Z. miRNA in plasma exosome is stable under different storage conditions. Molecules. 2014;**19**(2):1568-1575

[43] Björkgren I, Petra S. The role of Dicer1 in the male reproductive tract. Asian journal of andrology 5. 2015;**17**(5):737

[44] Björkgren I, Gylling H, Turunen H, Huhtaniemi I, Strauss L, Poutanen M, et al. Imbalanced lipid homeostasis in the conditional Dicer1 knockout mouse epididymis causes instability of the sperm membrane. The FASEB Journal. 2015;**29**(2):433-442

[45] Li H, Huang S, Guo C, Guan H, Xiong C. Cell-free seminal mRNA and microRNA exist in different forms. PLoS One. 2012;7(4):e34566

[46] Barbu MG, Thompson DC, Suciu N, Voinea SC, Cretoiu D, Predescu DV. The roles of micrornas in male infertility. International Journal of Molecular Sciences. 2021;**22**(6):2910

[47] Khazaie Y, Esfahani MH. MicroRNA and male infertility: A potential for diagnosis. International Journal of Fertility & Sterility. 2014;**8**(2):113

[48] Lawrie CH, Gal S, Dunlop HM, Pushkaran B, Liggins AP, Pulford K, et al. Detection of elevated levels of tumour-associated microRNAs in serum of patients with diffuse large B-cell lymphoma. British Journal of Haematology. 2008;**141**(5):672-675

[49] Tian H, Li Z, Peng D, Bai X, Liang W. Expression difference of miR-10b and miR-135b between the fertile and infertile semen samples (p). Forensic Science International: Genetics Supplement Series. 2017;**6**:e257-e259

[50] Abu-Halima M, Backes C, Leidinger P, Keller A, Lubbad AM, Hammadeh M, et al. MicroRNA expression profiles in human testicular tissues of infertile men with different histopathologic patterns. Fertility and Sterility. 2014;**101**(1):78-86

[51] Trzybulska D, Bobjer J, Giwercman A, Tsatsanis C. Serum microRNAs in male subfertility—Biomarkers and a potential pathogenetic link to metabolic syndrome. Journal of Assisted Reproduction and Genetics. 2017;**34**(10):1277-1282

[52] Yuan S, Tang C, Zhang Y, Wu J, Bao J, Zheng H, et al. mir-34b/c and mir-449a/b/c are required for spermatogenesis, but

not for the first cleavage division in mice. Biol Open. 2015;**4**(2):212-223

[53] Braun RE. Post-transcriptional control of gene expression during spermatogenesis. Seminars in Cell & Developmental Biology. 1998;**9**(4):483-489

[54] Roush S, Slack FJ. The let-7 family of microRNAs. Trends in Cell Biology. 2008;**18**(10):505-516

[55] McIver SC, Roman SD, Nixon B, McLaughlin EA. miRNA and mammalian male germ cells. Human Reproduction Update. 2012;**18**(1):44-59

[56] Paul A, Sadek ST, Mahesan AM. The role of microRNAs in human embryo implantation: A review. Journal of Assisted Reproduction and Genetics. 2019;**36**(2):179-187

[57] Yao C, Yuan Q, Niu M, Fu H, Zhou F, Zhang W, et al. Distinct expression profiles and novel targets of MicroRNAs in human spermatogonia, pachytene spermatocytes, and round spermatids between OA patients and NOA patients. Molecular Therapy--Nucleic Acids. 2017;**9**:182-194

[58] Muñoz X, Mata A, Bassas L, Larriba S. Altered miRNA signature of developing germ-cells in infertile patients relates to the severity of spermatogenic failure and persists in spermatozoa. Scientific Reports. 2015;**5**(1):1-2

[59] Zhou JH, Zhou QZ, Yang JK, Lyu XM, Bian J, Guo WB, et al. MicroRNA-27a-mediated repression of cysteine-rich secretory protein 2 translation in asthenoteratozoospermic patients. Asian Journal of Andrology. 2017;**19**(5):591

[60] Ye L, Evans J, Gargett CE. Lim1/LIM1 is expressed in developing and adult mouse and human endometrium. Histochemistry and Cell Biology. 2012;**137**(4):527-536

[61] Fededa JP, Esk C, Mierzwa B, Stanyte R, Yuan S, Zheng H, et al. Micro RNA-34/449 controls mitotic spindle orientation during mammalian cortex development. The EMBO journal. 2016;**35**(22):2386-2398

[62] Noveski P, Popovska-Jankovic K, Kubelka-Sabit K, Filipovski V, Lazarevski S, Plaseski T, et al. Micro RNA expression profiles in testicular biopsies of patients with impaired spermatogenesis. Andrology. 2016;**4**(6):1020-1027

[63] Stenvang J, Petri A, Lindow M, Obad S, Kauppinen S. Inhibition of microRNA function by antimiR oligonucleotides. Silence. 2012;**3**(1):1-7

[64] Chen D, Chen Z, Jin Y, Dragas D, Zhang L, Adjei BS, et al. MicroRNA-99 family members suppress Homeobox A1 expression in epithelial cells. PLoS One. 2013;**8**(12):e80625

[65] Li J, Liu Y, Dong D, Zhang Z. Evolution of an X-linked primate-specific micro RNA cluster. Molecular Biology and Evolution. 2010;**27**(3):671-683

[66] Landgraf P, Rusu M, Sheridan R, Sewer A, Iovino N, Aravin A, et al. A mammalian microRNA expression atlas based on small RNA library sequencing. Cell. 2007;**129**(7):1401-1414

[67] Belleannée C. Extracellular microRNAs from the epididymis as potential mediators of cell-to-cell communication. Asian Journal of Andrology. 2015;**17**(5):730

[68] Feng R, Sang Q, Zhu Y, Fu W, Liu M, Xu Y, et al. MiRNA-320 in the human follicular fluid is associated with embryo quality in vivo and affects

mouse embryonic development in vitro. Scientific Reports. 2015;**5**(1):1-9

[69] Zhang LL, Ma J, Yang B, Zhao J, Yan BY, Zhang YQ, et al. Interference with lactate metabolism by mmu-miR-320-3p via negatively regulating GLUT3 signaling in mouse Sertoli cells. Cell Death & Disease. 2018;**9**(10):1-4

[70] Papaioannou MD, Nef S. microRNAs in the testis: Building up male fertility. Journal of Andrology. 2010;**31**(1):26-33

[71] Comazzetto S, Di Giacomo M, Rasmussen KD, Much C, Azzi C, Perlas E, et al. Oligoasthenoteratozoospermia and infertility in mice deficient for miR-34b/c and miR-449 loci. PLoS Genetics. 2014;**10**(10):e1004597

[72] Wu J, Bao J, Kim M, Yuan S, Tang C, Zheng H, et al. Two miRNA clusters, miR-34b/c and miR-449, are essential for normal brain development, motile ciliogenesis, and spermatogenesis. Proceedings of the National Academy of Sciences. 2014;**111**(28):E2851-E2857

[73] Salas-Huetos A, Blanco J, Vidal F, Mercader JM, Garrido N, Anton E. New insights into the expression profile and function of micro-ribonucleic acid in human spermatozoa. Fertility and Sterility. 2014;**102**(1):213-222

[74] Lian J, Zhang X, Tian H, Liang N, Wang Y, Liang C, et al. Altered microRNA expression in patients with non-obstructive azoospermia. Reproductive Biology and Endocrinology. 2009;**7**(1):1

[75] Safarinejad MR, Shafiei N, Safarinejad S. Association of polymorphisms in the estrogen receptors alpha, and beta (ESR1, ESR2) with the occurrence of male infertility and semen parameters. The Journal of Steroid Biochemistry and Molecular Biology. 2010;**122**(4):193-203

[76] Carreau S, Genissel C, Bilinska B, Levallet J. Sources of oestrogen in the testis and reproductive tract of the male. International Journal of Andrology. 1999;**22**(4):211-223

[77] Cheng C, Fu X, Alves P, Gerstein M. mRNA expression profiles show differential regulatory effects of microRNAs between estrogen receptor-positive and estrogen receptor-negative breast cancer. Genome Biology. 2009;**10**(9):1-7

[78] Abhari A, Zarghami N, Shahnazi V, Barzegar A, Farzadi L, Karami H, et al. Significance of microRNA targeted estrogen receptor in male fertility. Iranian Journal of Basic Medical Sciences. 2014;**17**(2):81

[79] Wu W, Hu Z, Qin Y, Dong J, Dai J, Lu C, et al. Seminal plasma microRNAs: Potential biomarkers for spermatogenesis status. Molecular Human Reproduction. 2012;**18**(10):489-497

[80] Wu W, Qin Y, Li Z, Dong J, Dai J, Lu C, et al. Genome-wide microRNA expression profiling in idiopathic non-obstructive azoospermia: Significant up-regulation of miR-141, miR-429 and miR-7-1-3p. Human Reproduction. 2013;**28**(7):1827-1836

[81] Abu-Halima M, Hammadeh M, Backes C, Fischer U, Leidinger P, Lubbad AM, et al. Panel of five microRNAs as potential biomarkers for the diagnosis and assessment of male infertility. Fertility and Sterility. 2014;**102**(4):989-997

[82] Xie R, Lin X, Du T, Xu K, Shen H, Wei F, et al. Targeted disruption of miR-17-92 impairs mouse spermatogenesis by activating mTOR signaling pathway. Medicine. 2016;**95**(7):345-367

[83] Tong MH, Mitchell DA, McGowan SD, Evanoff R, Griswold MD.

Two miRNA clusters, Mir-17-92 (Mirc1) and Mir-106b-25 (Mirc3), are involved in the regulation of spermatogonial differentiation in mice. Biology of Reproduction. 2012;**86**(3):72

[84] Huszar JM, Payne CJ. MicroRNA 146 (Mir146) modulates spermatogonial differentiation by retinoic acid in mice. Biology of Reproduction. 2013;**88**(1):15

[85] Yang QE, Racicot KE, Kaucher AV, Oatley MJ, Oatley JM. MicroRNAs 221 and 222 regulate the undifferentiated state in mammalian male germ cells. Development. 2013;**140**(2):280-290

[86] Moritoki Y, Hayashi Y, Mizuno K, Kamisawa H, Nishio H, Kurokawa S, et al. Expression profiling of microRNA in cryptorchid testes: miR-135a contributes to the maintenance of spermatogonial stem cells by regulating FoxO1. The Journal of Urology. 2014;**191**(4):1174-1180

[87] Bao J, Li D, Wang L, Wu J, Hu Y, Wang Z, et al. MicroRNA-449 and microRNA-34b/c function redundantly in murine testes by targeting E2F transcription factor-retinoblastoma protein (E2F-pRb) pathway. The Journal of Biological Chemistry. 2012;**287**(26):21686-21698

[88] Lee RC, Feinbaum RL, Ambros V. The *C. elegans* heterochronic gene lin-4 encodes small RNAs with antisense complementarity to lin-14. Cell. 1993;**75**(5):843-854

[89] He Z, Jiang J, Kokkinaki M, Tang L, Zeng W, Gallicano I, et al. MiRNA-20 and mirna-106a regulate spermatogonial stem cell renewal at the post-transcriptional level via targeting STAT3 and Ccnd1. Stem Cells. 2013;**31**(10):2205-2217

[90] Nedaeinia R, Sharifi M, Avan A, Kazemi M, Nabinejad A, Ferns GA, et al. Inhibition of microRNA-21 via locked nucleic acid-antimiR suppressed metastatic features of colorectal cancer cells through modulation of programmed cell death 4. Tumor Biology. 2017;**39**(3)

[91] Beg MS, Brenner AJ, Sachdev J, Borad M, Kang YK, Stoudemire J, et al. Phase I study of MRX34, a liposomal miR-34a mimic, administered twice weekly in patients with advanced solid tumors. Investigational New Drugs. 2017;**35**(2):180-188

[92] Bezan A, Gerger A, Pichler M. MicroRNAs in testicular cancer: Implications for pathogenesis, diagnosis, prognosis and therapy. Anticancer Research. 2014;**34**(6):2709-2713

[93] Costa AL, Lobo J, Jerónimo C, Henrique R. The epigenetics of testicular germ cell tumors: Looking for novel disease biomarkers. Epigenomics. 2017;**9**(2):155-169

[94] Gillis AJ, Stoop HJ, Hersmus R, Oosterhuis JW, Sun Y, Chen C, et al. High-throughput microRNAome analysis in human germ cell tumours. The Journal of Pathology: A Journal of the Pathological Society of Great Britain and Ireland. 2007;**213**(3):319-328

[95] Baumann V, Winkler J. miRNA-based therapies: Strategies and delivery platforms for oligonucleotide and non-oligonucleotide agents. Future Medicinal Chemistry. 2014;**6**(17):1967-1984

[96] Van Rooij E, Kauppinen S. Development of micro RNA therapeutics is coming of age. EMBO Molecular Medicine. 2014;**6**(7):851-864

[97] Am Hong C, Nam YS. Functional nanostructures for effective delivery of small interfering RNA therapeutics. Theranostics. 2014;**4**(12):1211

Chapter 10

The Role of Noncoding RNAs in the Response of Oil Palm Plants to Abiotic Stresses

Fernanda Ferreira Salgado, Priscila Grynberg and Manoel Teixeira Souza Junior

Abstract

The genus *Elaeis* comprises two species, *E. guineensis* Jacq. and *E. oleifera* (Kunth) Cortés, which are known as the African and the American oil palms, respectively. The African oil palm originated from West Africa and is the predominant species in commercial plantations. This oilseed crop is the number one source of consumed vegetable oil in the World. Several abiotic stressors affect the plant life cycle interfering with growth and productivity. Salinity and drought are abiotic stresses that affect plantations on all continents, resulting in the loss of billions of dollars annually. MicroRNAs (miRNAs) are small endogenous noncoding RNAs that impact almost all biological processes, affecting either the transcriptional or posttranscriptional regulation of gene expression. Here we describe the R&D initiatives on oil palm miRNAs, highlighting the current knowledge on miRNAs' involvement in oil palm response to abiotic stress and postulating possible miRNA-based strategies for the genetic improvement of oil palm salinity and drought stresses tolerance.

Keywords: abiotic stress, tolerance, transcription factor, transcriptome, noncoding RNA, oil palm, drought stress, salt stress

1. Introduction

Oil palm (*Elaeis guineensis* Jacq.) is known as the most productive oilseed crop in the World, bearing great economic importance due to its large-scale production and high efficiency of the extraction and refining processes to obtain palm oil and palm kernel oil [1, 2]. In 2021/2022, the World consumed approximately 82 million metric tons of palm oil and palm kernel oil, making this oilseed crop the number one source of consumed vegetable oil [3].

The oil palm industry faces criticism due to a series of unsustainable practices (deforestation and consequent biodiversity loss, increased greenhouse gas emissions, and environmental and aquatic pollution), finding itself under pressure to adopt new and innovative procedures that could help this sector reverse this negative public perception [4]. Darkwah and Ong-Abdullah [5] highlighted some of these procedures, such as choice for intensification over extensification, adoption of precision agriculture technologies, support for smallholder farmers, sustainability certification, and circular economy.

Oil palm plantations are in areas with tropical forests in the equatorial belt, as they need high rainfall throughout the year [6]. In Brazil, for instance, there is an extensive area with favorable conditions for cultivating oil palm outside the Amazon rainforest; however, those areas experience long periods of drought when oil palm does not meet the physiological water requirement to maintain productivity [7], and, consequently, need to be artificially irrigated with proper management to avoid soil salinization. Approximately 30% of the irrigated land area in the World is affected by salt [8], which, to a certain extent, shows a link between drought and salinity stresses.

Studies have shown that the progression of abiotic stresses is limiting global agricultural production, with no sign of reversal shortly [9–11], making it necessary to develop crops that are resilient to different abiotic stresses, such as drought and salinity, ensuring food security. Therefore, it is currently a challenge for plant scientists to develop crops resistant or tolerant to these conditions, capable of withstanding climatic instabilities and environmental stresses, especially combinations of these stresses. So, the research community aiming to develop knowledge and technology to allow oil palm breeding programs in Brazil and elsewhere to breed for superior genotypes must consider that.

Plants respond to environmental stimuli in a complex and highly coordinated manner at biochemical, physiological, and molecular levels [11–13]. When exposed to stress, rapid and effective reprogramming at the molecular level is required to adapt to unfavorable conditions [12, 14, 15]. This reprogramming regulates the expression of stress-responsive genes, especially at transcriptional and posttranscriptional levels [14, 16, 17].

micro RNAs (miRNAs) are posttranscriptional and translational regulators frequently correlated with plant stress tolerance and modulating stress response [15, 18, 19]. miRNAs have enormous potential for crop improvement, being the focus of studies by scientists in recent years [18, 20–22].

Therefore, the main objectives of this review are to describe the R&D initiatives known to date on oil palm (*Elaeis* spp.) miRNAs, to report on their biogenesis and mode of action, to summarize the current knowledge on miRNAs' involvement in oil palm response to abiotic stress, and to postulate possible miRNA-based strategies on the genetic improvement of oil palm's tolerance to abiotic stress.

2. miRNA biogenesis and mode of action

miRNAs are a class of endogenous, noncoding sRNAs transcribed from introns, exons, or intergenic regions [11]. They play a role in posttranscriptional RNA-mediated gene silencing and expression by complementary interaction with their mRNA target site [23, 24]. The biogenesis of plant miRNAs has been reported mainly in *Arabidopsis thaliana* (L.) *Heynh.* (**Figure 1**) [25].

Plant miRNAs range from 21 to 24 nucleotides in length [26]. Similar to protein-coding genes, miRNA genes (MIRs) are commonly transcribed by RNA polymerase II, forming a single-stranded precursor RNA called primary miRNAs (pri-miRNAs) that have imperfect self-complementary folding regions. Still in the nucleus, the 5′ m7G-cap and 3′ polyadenylation are added to promote better

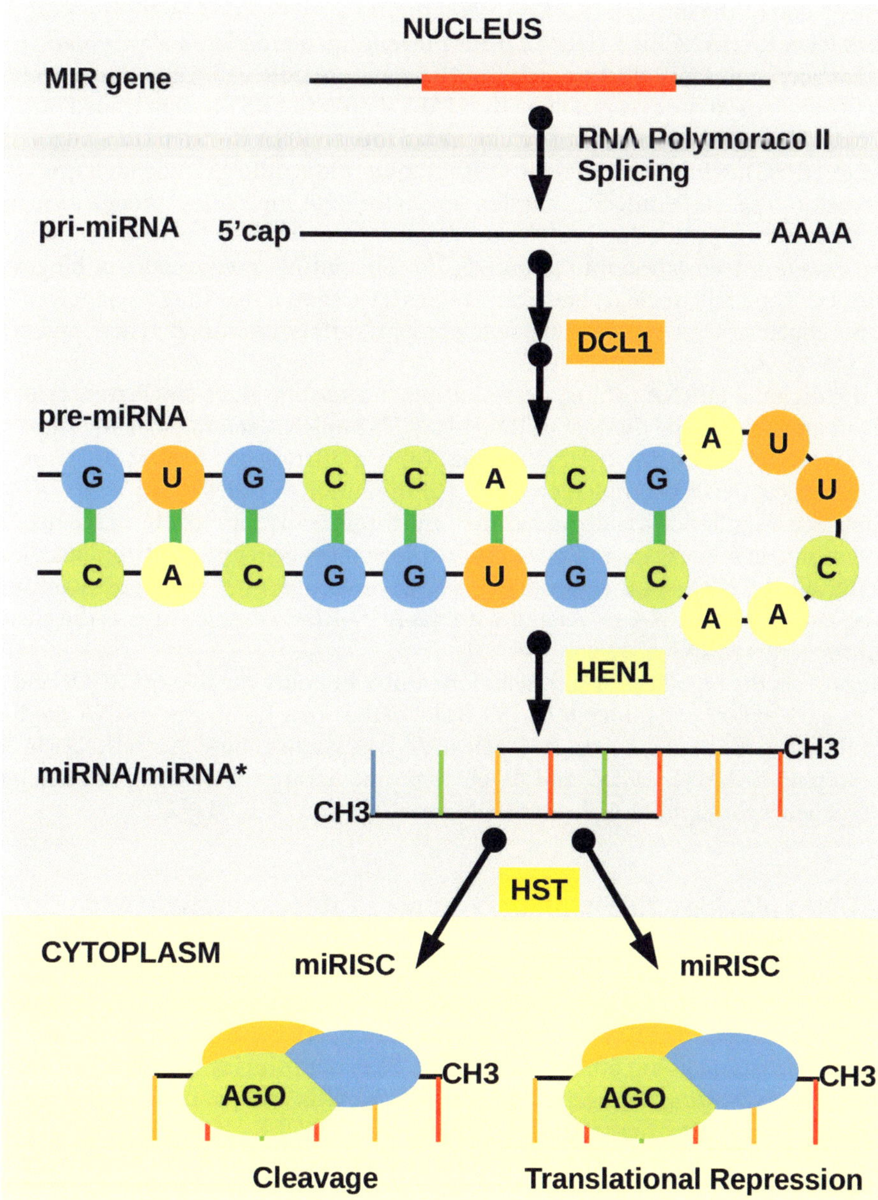

Figure 1.
Biogenesis of plant miRNAs. A miRNA gene is transcribed by RNA polymerase II, giving rise to a primary transcript (pri-miRNA), which is then capped and polyadenylated. DCL1 processes pri-miRNA, perhaps in two or more steps, and HEN1 methylate it to produce the miRNA/miRNA duplex. HST transports the duplex to the cytosol, and the miRNA strand gets incorporated into RISC. The nuclear export of miRNAs may occur before or after RISC assembly. According to the degree of complementarity with the target site, miRISC will either cleave the mRNA or inhibit its translation.*

stability. Then the pri-miRNAs are converted into miRNA precursor sequences (pre-miRNA) by the action of DICER-LIKE 1 (DCL1) along with other associated proteins [15, 27].

The 3′ end of the initial miRNA/miRNA* duplex is methylated by the nuclear protein HUA ENHANCER 1 (HEN1), thus preventing untemplated 3′ polymerization that accelerates miRNA turnover [28]. The mature miRNA is then transported from the nucleus to the cytoplasm by the HASTY protein (HST), then loaded onto AGONAUTE (AGO) proteins and incorporated into an RNA-induced silencing complex (RISC), while often the star miRNA molecules (miRNA *) do undergo degradation. The AGO/miRISC complex search for RNA molecules through sequence complementarity, promoting posttranscriptional gene silencing through endonucleolytic cleavage or translation inhibition [25, 29]. The miRNA mechanisms of biogenesis and function are still unclear; however, studies have shown that they are involved in several cellular processes, including development, differentiation, division, and cell death [11, 26, 30].

An individual miRNA can regulate multiple transcripts, and a single transcript can be acted upon by several distinct miRNAs [11]. The miRNA can regulate the expression of its target gene using three strategies: (a) degradation of a target transcript through almost perfect complementarity; (b) inhibition of translation; or (c) DNA methylation. Regulation via degradation of the target transcript results in the degradation of intron sequences, and these cleaved sequences generate dsRNA molecules with the aid of RDR2 and then produce I-siRNA molecules of 21 and 22 nucleotides. Subsequently, the I-siRNA associated with the AGO-RISC complex directs the cleavage of the target mRNA sequence [31, 32].

Regarding the regulation via translation inhibition, only the roles of AGO1 and AGO10 have so far been understood [33, 34]. On the other hand, the miRNA-mediated inhibition mechanism remains unclear. At last, studies show that miRNAs in *A. thaliana* bind to AGO4, AGO6, and AGO9 to promote transcriptional gene silencing of target genes through RNA-directed DNA methylation (RdDM) [27].

3. miRNAs playing a role in plant response to abiotic-drought and salinity-stress

Abiotic stress, such as deprivation or excess of water, high salinity, low or high temperature, heavy metals, and ultraviolet radiation, is a negative impact caused by nonliving factors on living organisms [35, 36]. They are primary stresses that arise in the plantations limiting seed germination, plant growth, and plant development; and, in some cases, resulting in the death of the plants.

Salinity and drought are two of the most prevalent abiotic stress worldwide, affecting plantations on all continents and resulting in the loss of billions of dollars annually. Plants have developed several mechanisms to combat drought stress, and several genes associated with the response of plants to this stress are known [12, 37]. One of these responses is the positive and/or negative regulation of several transcription factors (TF) related to numerous physiological and cellular functions [38].

The dehydration responsive elements (DREB) are TF related to the activation of genes responsive to drought stress tolerance, and its overexpression can result in tolerance to water deficit in plants. Similarly, the transcription factor MYB regulates negatively in plants during drought stress since it is related to stomata opening [11, 39]. However, the overexpression of other genes associated with drought stress in plants did not result in the expected drought tolerance, demonstrating the complexity of mechanisms responsible for plant tolerance to water stress [40].

Several research groups have identified and reported miRNAs responsive to water stress in several species, such as rice—*Oryza sativa* L. [41], soybean—*Glycine max* (L.) Merr. [42], barley—*Hordeum vulgare* L. [43], and Arabidopsis [44]. Those water stress-responsive miRNAs belong to three classes. The first class includes miRNAs targeting transcription factors that contribute to the gene regulation of the stress response, comprising miR156, miR159, miR165, miR169, miR171, miR172, miR319, and miR396 [21, 44, 45].

In the second class, the miRNAs are involved in the direct response to water stress, some of which are miR167, which is responsible for directing the auxin response factors ARF6 and ARF8 [46]; miR168, which targets the ARGONAUTE 1 (AGO1) mRNA [47]; and miR393 and miR394, which target F-box protein mRNAs that play roles in drought tolerance [45, 48, 49]. The last class contains miRNAs such as miR397 and miR408, which have hydrolase and oxidoreductase genes as their target gene [50, 51].

Zhou and colleagues [41] identified 30 miRNAs differentially expressed in rice under drought stress, 19 were new miRNAs. Regarding their expression, 14 were upregulated (miR159, miR169, miR171, miR319, miR395, miR474, miR845, miR851, miR854, miR896, miR901, miR903, miR1026, and miR1125) and 16 downregulated (miR156, miR159, miR170, miR171, miR172, miR319, miR396, miR397, miR408, miR529, miR896, miR1030, miR1035, miR1050, miR1088 and, miR1126). In soybean, upregulation of miRseq13, miR397ab, miR1513c, miR169-3p, and miR166-5p was observed in sensitive plants, while the same miRNAs were downregulated on tolerant crops [42].

When it comes to salinity stress, several genes are related to the plant's stress response, including those involved in ion channel activation, signal transduction, and modification regulated by plant growth factors, especially the morphological architecture of the root [52]. In *A. thaliana*, studies have shown increased expression of miRNAs miR156, miR158, miR159, miR165, miR167, miR168, miR169, miR171, miR319, miR393, miR394, miR396, and miR397 in response to salt stress, while miR398 was downregulated [21].

According to Ding and colleagues, when analyzing corn variants tolerant and sensitive to salt stress, members of the miR396, miR167, miR164, and miR156 families downregulated, while miRNAs miR474, miR395, miR168, and miR162 upregulated in the tolerant ones [18]. In radish (*Raphanus sativus*), 22 new and 49 already known miRNAs appeared under salt stress [53]. In young oil palm plants under saline stress, 27 new and 52 already known miRNAs appeared [15]. When analyzing the expression profile of these miRNAs, 72 of them showed negative differential expression and the remaining seven had no significant differential expression [15].

Recent studies allowed a better understanding of the mechanisms of action of miRNAs and their relationship in response to different abiotic stresses [38, 54, 55]. It is necessary to highlight that miRNAs are species-specific and present different expression levels when analyzed in distinct plant species or within a specific one under the same stress [15, 24].

4. miRNAs in oil palm (*Elaeis* spp.)

Despite many advancements in the prediction and characterization of miRNAs in plants, there are only a few studies where researchers report the identification and characterization of miRNAs in oil palm, either under abiotic stress conditions or not. Currently, there are 10 published studies reporting miRNAs identification and characterization in oil palm [15, 30, 56–63]. Considering the great economic importance of oil palm, the number of miRNA studies reported on this oilseed crop is relatively low (**Table 1**).

Nasaruddin and colleagues found five potential miRNA encoding sequences in oil palm by a combined homology and structural analysis approach, having roles in regulating the auxin response, floral development, and basal transcription [30]. Mehrpooyan, Othman, and Harikrishna [56] identified in oil palm six paralogs of miR172, a regulator of the APETALA2 (AP2)-like family transcription factors. Their results suggested that the expression of different miR172 precursor paralogs is tissue-specific and showed that each of the two mature miR172 isoforms had different expression patterns during floral development.

Low and colleagues identified 14 miRNAs in contigs assembled from sequences generated from the hypomethylated or gene-rich regions in the genomes of both species from the *Elaeis* genera [57]. Target prediction of these miRNAs identified just one putative target gene, similar to the Rab21-family small GTPase, a small GTP-binding protein of the Ras superfamily. Silva and colleagues identified 57 mature miRNAs in *E. guineensis* and 52 in *E oleifera*, respectively, revealing that majority of them are transcription factors involved in the plant development process [58].

According to Somyong et al. [59], miRNA159 is related to the determination of females in oil palm trees, which is directly related to the higher production of oil palm trees, since palm oil with high number of female inflorescence and of clusters is most favorable. Noting that no expression of EgmiR159a was found in male flowers in their study, confirming its role in female sexual differentiation (**Table 1**). Ho and colleagues identified 15 oil palm-specific miRNA candidates when investigating microRNA expression in female inflorescence at two stages of floral [60].

In Gao et al. [61], the micro RNA EgmiR179 regulates the biosynthesis of metabolites through the negative regulation of its target gene NDT1, increasing oil content in palm oil [61]. Zheng and colleagues identified 452 microRNAs (miRNAs), including 170 conserved miRNAs and 282 new miRNAs, when gaining insights into the oil palm regulatory mechanisms of lipid and fatty acid metabolism. They found 37 fatty acid synthesis-related genes as putative miRNA-target genes and indicated that 22 conserved miRNAs and 14 new ones might be involved in fatty acid metabolism pathways. Tregear et al. [63] reported finding 30 previously unreported oil palm miRNA genes in a molecular study of the process of sexual differentiation in the immature inflorescence of oil palm.

Our research group reported prospecting and characterizing miRNAs in oil palm plants under salinity stress (**Table 1**) [15]. That was the first step in a study prospecting and characterizing miRNAs in oil palm plants under salinity [64] or drought stress and looking for insights on commonalities—miRNAs and putative miRNA-target genes—on the molecular response of young oil palm plants to these two abiotic stresses.

We did find 81 miRNAs—52 known ones and 29 new ones (**Figure 2**)—and 139 differentially expressed putative miRNA-target genes [15, 64]. In Salgado et al. [15], miR166, miR169, miR319, miR396, miR529, and egu-miR24sds showed altered expression profiles in young oil palm plants subjected to salt stress, both targeting TF, indicating a miRNA-dependent posttransitional regulation during the plant's response to the environment.

All miRNAs identification and characterization studies done so far in oil palm allowed the identification of 55 miRNA families or groups of miRNAs that derive from a common ancestor (**Figure 3**).

Technology	Condition	miRNA	Species	Oil palm material	Publication
Small RNA-seq	Normal	miR159a	*E. guineensis*	Female flower	Somyong et al. [59]
3730 sequencing technology/ Blast	Normal	miR2911, miR2916, miR156j, miR2914, miR2910, miR319f, miR167g, miR319e, miR845a, miR845b	*E. guineensis* and *E. oleifera*	Leaf	Low et al. [57]
Blast	Normal	miR156, miR157, miR159, miR160, miR164, miR166, miR167, miR168, miR169, miR171, miR172, miR319, miR390, miR393, miR394, miR395, miR396, miR397, miR398, miR399, miR528, miR529, miR530, miR535, miR815, miR1428, miR1432, miR2118, miR2275, miR5148, miR5179, miR5532, miR5801	*E. guineensis* and *E. oleifera* and *Phoenix dactylifera*	Genome	da Silva et al. [58]
Blast	Normal	miR156, miR157, miR159, miR160, miR854	*E. guineensis*	Genome	Nasaruddin et al. [30]
RNA-seq	Normal	miR5179	*E. guineensis*	Fruit	Gao et al. [61]
Small RNA-seq	Salt stress	miR156, miR391, miR395a, miR536, miR156, miR160, miR166, miR167, miR169, miR171, miR172, miR395, miR396, miR399, miR528, miR156, miR159, miR166, miR319, miR393, miR535, miR156, miR162, miR169, miR529, miR530, miR168, miR319, miR159. egumiR01, egumiR02, egumiR03, egumiR04, egumiR05, egumiR06, egumiR07, egumiR08, egumiR09, egumiR10, egumiR11,egumiR12, egumiR13, egumiR14, egumiR15, egumiR16, egumiR17, egumiR18, egumiR19, egumiR20, egumiR21, egumiR22, egumiR23, egumiR24, egumiR25, egumiR26, egumiR27.	*E. guineensis*	Leaf	Salgado et al. [15]
Small RNA-seq	Normal	miR1432, miR160, miR163, miR166, miR168, miR172, miR1859, miR1873, miR2199, miR2654, miR396, miR4365, miR528, miR535, miR827, miR835, miR858, miR894, egumiR3, egumiR5, egumiR6, egumiR7, egumiR8, egumiR9, egumiR10, egumiR11, egumiR12, egumiR13, egumiR14, egumiR15.	*E. guineensis* *Tenera* hybrid palms (*Dura* × *Pisifera*)	Female Inflorescence	Ho et al. [60]

Technology	Condition	miRNA	Species	Oil palm material	Publication
Small RNA-seq	Normal	miR156, miR160, miR164, miR172, miR444, miR5179, miR528, miR167, egumiR259, egumiR223, egumiR218, egumiR255, egumiR43, egumiR132, egumiR172, egumiR113, egumiR273, egumiR158, egumiR275, egumiR138, egumiR59, egumiR201, egumiR209, egumiR116, egumiR129, egumiR211, egumiR7, egumiR210, egumiR274.	*E. guineensis*	Mesocarp	Zheng et al. [62]
Small RNA-seq	Normal	miR319, miRN1, miR168, miR482, miR2118, miR159, miR171, miR167, miR397, miR160, miR156, miR535, miR396, miR536, miR169, miR319, miR179, miR166, miR394, miR399, miR172, miR164, miRN4, miR390, miR393, miRN5, miRN6, miR162, miR827, miR398, miRN7, miR395, miRN8, miRN9, miRN10, miR408, miR528, miRN11.	*E. guineensis*	Immature Inflorescence	Tregear et al. [63]
Blast	Normal	miR172	*E. guineensis*	Inflorescence	Mehrpooyan et al. [56]

Table 1.
Summary of miRNA studies reported on oil palm.

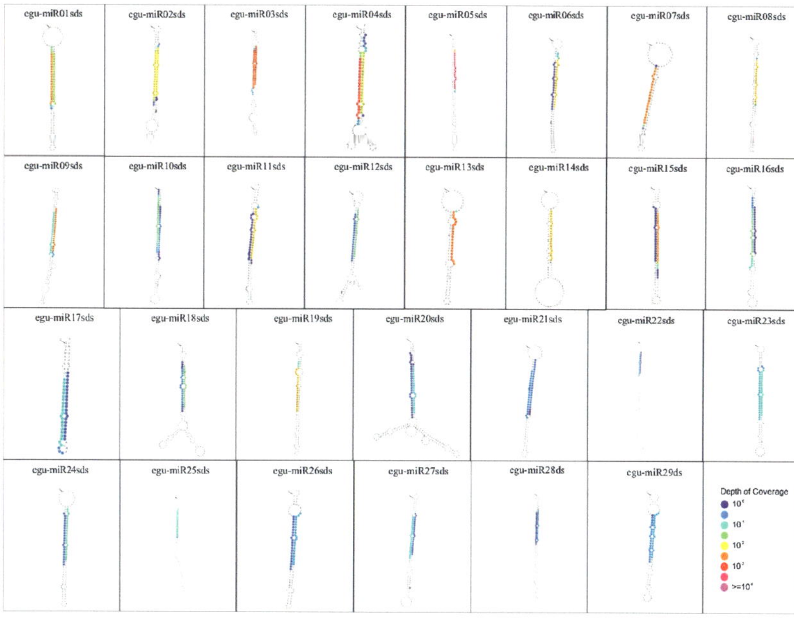

Figure 2.
Structure of the 29 new miRNAs identified in oil palm (Elaeis guineensis) plants exposed to abiotic stresses—salinity and drought (Source: [15, 64]).

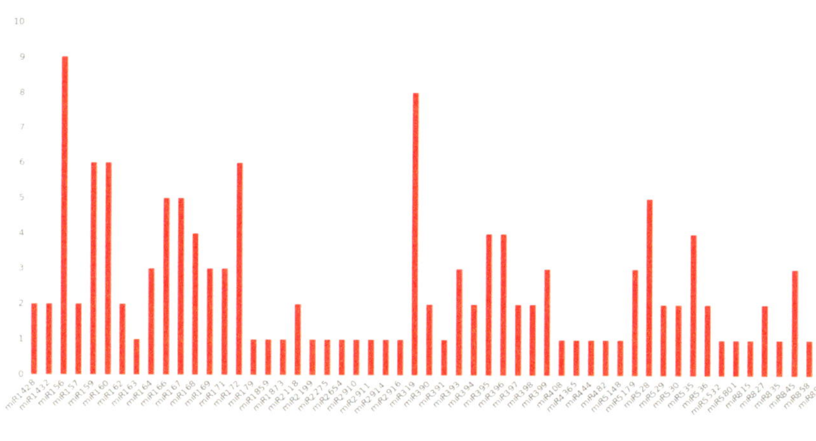

Figure 3.
Families of miRNAs found in oil palm, and the amount of members per family.

5. miRNA-based strategies to improve oil palm tolerance to abiotic stress

In the last decade, due to the recent advances in high-throughput sequencing techniques, vis-à-vis the empowerment of bioinformatics tools, much progress has been made in characterizing and understanding miRNAs mechanism of action, and predicting their target genes [65–68].

The possibility of the involvement of miRNAs in the regulation of genes directly related to the modulation of the impact of abiotic stress on plants has enabled researchers to take the next step by altering the expression levels of miRNAs, either by overexpression or knocking down strategies. This step attempts to gain further insights that could allow the development of distinct ways to generate superior genotypes harboring tolerance to those stresses, either by vertical or horizontal transfer of genes or even by genome editing [8].

According to Hajyzadeh et al. [69], the overexpression of miR408 in chickpea (*Cicer arietinum* L.) resulted in improved drought tolerance. Plants overexpressing the pre-miR408 from *A. thaliana* were without wilting and drying after 8 days of undergoing the drought treatment, unlike the control plants [69]. Arabidopsis plants overexpressing miR408 showed resilience to multi-stress environments—salinity and drought [70]. Through biochemical analysis and fluorescence imaging with measures of the photosystem efficiency, it was reported tolerance of the transformants compared to control ones [70].

Transgenic lines of creeping grass (*Agrostis stolonifer*a L.) overexpressing rice pre-miR393 showed a better tolerance response to saline stress (at 250 mM for 10 days), drought (15 days), and heat (40°C at day, 35°C at night, 13 days), confirming that miR393 is a potent candidate to confer resistance to multiple stresses [71]. According to Baek and colleagues, the overexpression of miR399f in Arabidopsis promoted greater tolerance to salinity and treatment with abscisic acid (ABA) [72]. Arabidopsis' putative miRNA-target genes—ABF3 and CSP41b—had low expression levels in transgenic plants, and these genes are related to stress due to their participation in ABA signaling [72].

Although the strategy of overexpression of miRNAs is dominant among the studies to obtain plants resistant to different stresses, the inhibition approach is also being promoted through the use of the short tandem target mimic (STTM) approach, causing loss of function [11]. Although there has been an increase in studies on the use of miRNAs to obtain plants resistant to multi-stress, there is still a long way to go.

According to Ferdous and colleagues, the overexpression of Hv-miR827 in barley (*H. vulgare* cv. "Golden Promise") influenced the grain weight and allowed the plants to recover after drought treatment, in addition to providing an improvement in the efficiency of the use of water [73]. Such behavior is also in transgenic Arabidopsis plants overexpressing the miRNA Ath-miR827 [74, 75].

miR319 is one of the oldest and most conserved miRNA families in plants, responsive to several stresses, including drought and salinity, based on high-throughput sequencing [76]. Studies have shown that its overexpression in transgenic creeping grass resulted in tolerance to salt and drought stresses; and it was linked to downregulation of at least four putative target genes of miR319 (AsPCF5, AsPCF6, AsPCF8, and AsTCP14) [77].

So far, no studies are known reporting on successfully horizontally transferring (or editing) miRNAs to or from oil palms aiming at achieving tolerance to abiotic stresses. Our research group prospected stress-responsive miRNAs and putative target genes that are good candidates for such endeavor [15, 64]. miRNAs and their putative target genes responsive to both stresses at once are the priority candidates for further studies.

Among putative target genes responsive to both stresses identified by our group in oil palm, there are some lncRNAs. Several studies have shown that lncRNAs play essential roles and different functions in the biological processes of plants. They can play a role as sRNA precursors to produce sRNAs, such as miRNAs and siRNAs. In response to different stresses, lncRNAs also play a role in the RNA-directed DNA methylation (RdDM) pathway [78–80].

6. Conclusions and future perspectives

Due to a series of unsustainable practices used by the oil palm industry, there is criticism pressuring it to adopt new and innovative procedures, including getting away from the tropical rain forests.

Predictably, primary stresses (abiotic and biotic) will arise once the industry establishes itself in those new areas for oil palm cultivation, forcing it to search for tools to deal in an economically sustainable way with them. Salinity and drought are on the top of such a list of primary abiotic stresses. Many studies report successful attempts to increase plants' tolerance to such stresses by altering the expression levels of miRNAs, either by overexpression or knocking down strategies. Despite the great economic importance of oil palm, we found only 10 published studies reporting miRNAs identification and characterization in this oilseed crop. When considering abiotic stresses, the scenario is even worst; only one published study so far. In this sense, it is clear that further studies are necessary on the role of miRNAs - and their putative target genes - in oil palm's response to abiotic stress. Besides that, as candidate genes become available from those studies, it will be necessary to validate their potential as tools to generate superior genotypes harboring tolerance to those stresses, either by vertical or horizontal transfer of genes or even by genome editing.

Acknowledgements

The author(s) disclosed receipt of the following financial support for the research, authorship, and/or publication of this article: The grant (01.13.0315.00 - DendêPalm Project) for this study was awarded by the Brazilian Innovation Agency—FINEP.

Conflict of interest

The authors declare no conflict of interest.

Author details

Fernanda Ferreira Salgado[1], Priscila Grynberg[2] and Manoel Teixeira Souza Junior[3]*

1 Universidade Federal de Lavras (UFLA), Lavras, MG, Brazil

2 Embrapa Recursos Genéticos e Biotecnologia, Brasília, DF, Brazil

3 Embrapa Agroenergia, Brasília, DF, Brazil

*Address all correspondence to: manoel.souza@embrapa.br

References

[1] Priscilla AS, Vanessa SC, Kátia CBR, Kelly SCD, Fábio ML, Roberto LC, et al. Drought tolerance in two oil palm hybrids as related to adjustments in carbon metabolism and vegetative growth. Acta Physiologiae Plantarum. 2017;**39**(58):1-12

[2] Le W, May L, Baoqing Y, Gen HY. Genes, pathways and networks responding to drought stress in oil palm roots. Scientific Reports. 2020;**10**(1):1-13. DOI: doi.org/10.1038/s41598-020-78297-z

[3] Statista. 2022. The Statistics Portal. Available from: www.statista.com/statistics/263937/vegetable-oils-global-consumption [Accessed: May 10, 2019]

[4] Matin Q, Kibrom TS, Hermanto S, Ingo G. Environmental, economic, and social consequences of the oil palm boom. Annual Review of Resource Economics. 2020;**12**:321-344. DOI: 10.1146/annurev-resource-110119-024922

[5] Dickson OD, Meilina OA. Sustainability of the oil palm industry. In: *Elaeis guineensis*. London: IntechOpen; 2021. DOI: 10.5772/intechopen.100156

[6] Furumo PR, Aide TM. Characterizing commercial oil palm expansion in Latin America: Land use change and trade. Environmental Research Letters. 2017;**12**(2):024008. DOI: 10.1088/1748-9326/aa5892

[7] Sérgio JC, Eduardo ALE, Taynar COT, Joedna S. Respostas fisiológicas de dendê submetidas ao estresse hídrico em condições do Cerrado. Revista Brasileira de Agropecuária Sustentável. 2018;**8**(4):92-99. https://doi.org/10.21206/rbas.v8i4.3055

[8] Vinay K, Tushar K, Varsha S, Shabir HW. Plant small RNAs: The essential epigenetic regulators of gene expression for salt-stress responses and tolerance. Plant Cell Reports. 2018;**37**(1):61-75. DOI: 10.1007/s00299-017-2210-4

[9] Petronia C, Maria GA, Giovanni P, Amodio F, Pasqualina W. Salinity Stress and Salt Tolerance. London, UK: Intech; 2012. p. 13. DOI: 10.1039/C7RA00172J%

[10] Khaled MH, Jonathan MF, David N, Alain L, Khaled M, Khaled MAA. Prospects for the study and improvement of abiotic stress tolerance in date palms in the post-genomics era. Frontiers in Plant Science. 2020;**11**(March):1-13. DOI: 10.3389/fpls.2020.00293

[11] Xu J et al. Exploring MiRNAs for developing climate-resilient crops: A perspective review. Science of the Total Environment. 2019;**653**:91-104. DOI: 10.1016/j.scitotenv.2018.10.340

[12] Banerjee S, Sirohi A, Ansari AA, Gill SS. Role of small RNAs in abiotic stress responses in plants. Plant Gene. 2017;**11**:180-189. DOI: 10.1016/j.plgene.2017.04.005

[13] Woodrow P et al. Ttd1a promoter is involved in DNA-protein binding by salt and light stresses. Molecular Biology Reports. 2011;**38**(6):3787-3794

[14] Djami-Tchatchou AT, Sanan-Mishra N, Ntushelo K, Dubery IA. Functional roles of microRNAs in agronomically important plants-potential as targets for crop improvement and protection. Frontiers in Plant Science. 2017;**8**(March)

[15] Salgado FF et al. Expression analysis of MiRNAs and their putative target genes confirm a preponderant role of transcription factors in the early response of oil palm plants to salinity stress. BMC Plant Biology. 2021;**21**(1):1-17. DOI: 10.1186/s12870-021-03296-9

[16] Sun G. MicroRNAs and their diverse functions in plants. Plant Molecular Biology. 2012;**80**(1):17-36

[17] Sunkar R. MicroRNAs with macro-effects on plant stress responses. Seminars in Cell and Developmental Biology. 2010;**21**(8):805-811. DOI: 10.1016/j.semcdb.2010.04.001

[18] Ding D et al. Differential expression of MiRNAs in response to salt stress in maize roots. Annals of Botany. 2009;**103**(1):29-38

[19] Sunkar R, Chinnusamy V, Zhu J, Zhu JK. Small RNAs as big players in plant abiotic stress responses and nutrient deprivation. Trends in Plant Science. 2007;**12**(7):301-309

[20] Denver JB, Ullah H. MiR393s regulate salt stress response pathway in arabidopsis thaliana through scaffold protein RACK1A mediated ABA signaling pathways. Plant Signaling and Behavior. 2019;**14**(6):1-7. DOI: 10.1080/15592324.2019.1600394

[21] Liu HH et al. Microarray-based analysis of stress-regulated MicroRNAs in arabidopsis thaliana. RNA. 2008;**14**(5):836-843

[22] Yu Y et al. Overexpression of soybean MiR169c confers increased drought stress sensitivity in transgenic arabidopsis thaliana. Plant Science. 2019;**285**(February):68-78. DOI: 10.1016/j.plantsci.2019.05.003

[23] Basso MF et al. MicroRNAs and new biotechnological tools for its modulation and improving stress tolerance in plants. Plant Biotechnology Journal. 2019;**17**(8):1482-1500

[24] Wang J et al. Non-coding RNAs and their roles in stress response in plants. Genomics, Proteomics and Bioinformatics. 2017a;**15**(5):301-312. DOI: 10.1016/j.gpb.2017.01.007

[25] Ding J, Zhou S, Guan J. Finding MicroRNA targets in plants: Current status and perspectives. Genomics, Proteomics and Bioinformatics. 2012;**10**(5):264-275. DOI: 10.1016/j.gpb.2012.09.003

[26] Sun X, Lin L, Sui N. Regulation mechanism of MicroRNA in plant response to abiotic stress and breeding. Molecular Biology Reports. 2019;**46**(1):1447-1457. DOI: 10.1007/s11033-018-4511-2

[27] Borges F, Martienssen RA. The expanding world of small RNAs in plants filipe. Nature reviews. Molecular Cell Biology. 2015;**16**(12):727-741

[28] Li J et al. Methylation protects MiRNAs and SiRNAs from a 3′-End Uridylation activity in arabidopsis. Current Biology. 2005;**15**(16):1501-1507

[29] Wang et al. Non-coding RNAs and their roles in stress response in plants Wang J et Al/MiRNA and LncRNA in plant stress response. Genomics, Proteomics and Bioinformatics. 2017b;**15**(5):301-312. DOI: 10.1016/j.gpb.2017.01.007

[30] Nasaruddin M, Nadirah, et al. Computational prediction of MicroRNAs from oil palm (Elaeis Guineensis Jacq.) expressed sequence tags. Asia-Pacific Journal of Molecular Biology and Biotechnology. 2007;**15**(3):107-113

[31] Arribas-Hernández L et al. The slicer activity of ARGONAUTE1 is

required specifically for the phasing, not production, of trans-acting short interfering RNAs in arabidopsis. Plant Cell. 2016;**28**(7):1563-1580

[32] Meng Y, Shao C, Ma X, Wang H. Introns targeted by plant MicroRNAs: A possible novel mechanism of gene regulation. Rice. 2013;**6**(1):1-10

[33] Li S et al. MicroRNAs inhibit the translation of target MRNAs on the endoplasmic reticulum in arabidopsis. Cell. 2013;**153**(3):562-574

[34] Shan Q et al. Multiplex and homologous recombination–mediated genome editing in arabidopsis and nicotiana benthamiana using guide RNA and Cas9. Nature Biotechnology. 2013;**31**(8):686-688

[35] Gull A, Lone AA, Wani NUI. Biotic and Abiotic Stresses in Plants. In: de Oliveira A, editor. Abiotic and Biotic Stress in Plants. London: IntechOpen; 2019. 6p. https://doi.org/10.5772/intechopen.85832

[36] Zhang H, Zhu J, Gong Z, et al. Abiotic stress responses in plants. Nature Reviews. Genetics. 2022;**23**:104-119. DOI: 10.1038/s41576-021-00413-0

[37] Shinozaki K, Yamaguchi-Shinozaki K. Gene networks involved in drought stress response and tolerance. Journal of Experimental Botany. 2007;**58**(2): 221-227

[38] Ayubov MS et al. Role of MicroRNAs and small RNAs in regulation of developmental processes and agronomic traits in gossypium species. Genomics. 2019;**111**(5):1018-1025. DOI: 10.1016/j.ygeno.2018.07.012

[39] Kumar R. Role of MicroRNAs in biotic and abiotic stress responses in crop plants. Applied Biochemistry and Biotechnology. 2014;**174**(1):93-115

[40] Ferdous J, Hussain SS, Shi BJ. Role of MicroRNAs in plant drought tolerance. Plant Biotechnology Journal. 2015;**13**(3):293-305

[41] Zhou L et al. Genome-wide identification and analysis of drought-responsive MicroRNAs in oryza sativa. Journal of Experimental Botany. 2010;**61**(15):4157-4168

[42] Kulcheski FR, de Oliveira LF, Molina LG, Almerão MP, Rodrigues FA, Marcolino J, et. al. Identification of novel soybean microRNAs involved in abiotic and biotic stresses. BMC genomics. 2011;**12**(307):1-17. https://doi.org/10.1186/1471-2164-12-307

[43] Deng P et al. Global identification of MicroRNAs and their targets in barley under salinity stress. PLoS One. 2015;**10**(9):1-20

[44] Sunkar R, Zhu J-K. Novel and stress-regulated MicroRNAs and other small RNAs from arabidopsis. 2004;**18**(August):957

[45] Jones-Rhoades MW, Bartel DP. Computational identification of plant MicroRNAs and their targets, including a stress-induced MiRNA. Molecular Cell. 2004;**14**(6):787-799

[46] Mahdavi-Darvari F, Noor NM, Ismanizan I. Epigenetic regulation and gene markers as signals of early somatic embryogenesis. Plant Cell, Tissue and Organ Culture. 2014;**120**(2):407-422. Available from: https://www.scopus.com/inward/record.uri?eid=2-s2.0-84921809786&doi=10.1007%2Fs11240-014-0615-0&partnerID=40&md5=9558f1d988ad53c4638fdf1142f417d2

[47] Vaucheret H, Vazquez F, Crété P, Bartel DP. The action of ARGONAUTE1 in the MiRNA pathway and its regulation by the MiRNA pathway are crucial

for plant development. Genes and Development. 2004;**18**(10):1187-1197

[48] Jain M et al. F-Box proteins in rice. Genome-wide analysis, classification, temporal and spatial gene expression during panicle and seed development, and regulation by light and abiotic stress. Plant Physiology. 2007;**143**(4): 1467-1483

[49] Navarro L, Dunoyer P, Jay F, Arnold B, Dharmasiri N, Estelle M, et al. A plant miRNA contributes to antibacterial resistance by repressing auxin signaling. Science. New York, N.Y. 2006;**312**(5772):436-439. https://doi.org/10.1126/science.1126088

[50] Apel K, Hirt H. Reactive oxygen species: Metabolism, oxidative stress, and signal transduction. Annual Review of Plant Biology. 2004;**55**:373-399

[51] Kimura M et al. Analysis of hydrogen peroxide–independent expression of the high-light–inducible ELIP2 gene with the aid of the ELIP2 promoter–luciferase fusion. Photochemistry and Photobiology. 2003;**77**(6):668

[52] Ku YS et al. Small RNAs in plant responses to abiotic stresses: Regulatory roles and study methods. International Journal of Molecular Sciences. 2015;**16**(10):24532-24554

[53] Sun X et al. Preparation and luminescence properties of Sr2EuxLa1-XAlO5 phosphor. Journal of Luminescence. 2015;**157**:197-200

[54] Kord H, Fakheri B, Ghabooli M, et al. Salinity-associated microRNAs and their potential roles in mediating salt tolerance in rice colonized by the endophytic root fungus Piriformospora indica. Funct Integr Genomics. 2019;**19**:659-672. https://doi.org/10.1007/s10142-019-00671-6

[55] Xu J, Chen Q, Liu P, Jia W, Chen Z, Xu Z. Integration of mRNA and miRNA Analysis Reveals the Molecular Mechanism Underlying Salt and Alkali Stress Tolerance in Tobacco. International journal of molecular sciences. 2019;**20**(10):1-18, 2391. https://doi.org/10.3390/ijms20102391

[56] Mehrpooyan F, Othman RY, Harikrishna JA. Tissue and temporal expression of MiR172 paralogs and the AP2-like target in oil palm (Elaeis Guineensis Jacq.). Tree Genetics and Genomes. 2012;**8**(6):1331-1343

[57] Low ET, Rosli R, Jayanthi N, Mohd-Amin AH, Azizi N, Chan KL, et al. Analyses of hypomethylated oil palm gene space. PloS one. 2014;**9**(1):1-15, e86728. https://doi.org/10.1371/journal.pone.0086728

[58] da Silva A, Cunha, et al. Computational identification and comparative analysis of MiRNA precursors in three palm species. Planta. 2016;**243**(5):1265-1277

[59] Somyong S et al. ACC oxidase and MiRNA 159a, and their involvement in fresh fruit bunch yield (FFB) via sex ratio determination in oil palm. Molecular Genetics and Genomics. 2016;**291**(3):1243-1257

[60] Huili H, Gudimella R, Ong-Abdullah M, Harikrishna JA. Expression of microRNAs during female inflorescence development in African oil palm (Elaeis guineensis Jacq.). Tree Genetics and Genomes. 2017;**35**(13):1-17. https://doi.org/10.1007/s11295-017-1120-5

[61] Gao LC et al. EgmiR5179 from the mesocarp of oil palm (Elaeis Guineensis Jacq.) regulates oil accumulation by targeting NAD transporter 1. Industrial Crops and Products. 2019;**137**(October 2018):126-136. DOI: 10.1016/j.indcrop.2019.05.013

[62] Zheng Y, Chen C, Liang Y, Sun R, Gao L, Liu T, et al. Genome-wide association analysis of the lipid and fatty acid metabolism regulatory network in the mesocarp of oil palm (*Elaeis guineensis* Jacq.) based on small noncoding RNA sequencing. Tree Physiology. 2019;**39**(3):356-371. DOI: doi.org/10.1093/treephys/tpy091

[63] Tregear JW, Richaud F, Collin M, Esbelin J, Parrinello H, Cochard B, et al. Micro-RNA-regulated *SQUAMOSA-PROMOTER BINDING PROTEIN-LIKE (SPL)* gene expression and cytokinin accumulation distinguish early-developing male and female inflorescences in oil palm (*Elaeis guineensis*). Plants (Basel, Switzerland). 2022;**11**(5):1-16, 685. https://doi.org/10.3390/plants11050685

[64] Salgado et al. The early response of oil palm (*Elaeis guineensis* Jacq.) plants to water deprivation: Expression analysis of miRNAs and their putative target genes, and similarities with the response to salinity stress. Unpublished

[65] Chuammitri P, Vannamahaxay S, Sornpet B, Pringproa K, Patchanee P. Detection and characterization of microRNA expression profiling and its target genes in response to canine parvovirus in Crandell Reese Feline Kidney cells. PeerJ. 2020;**8**:1-25, e8522. https://doi.org/10.7717/peerj.8522

[66] Khaksefidi, Reyhaneh Ebrahimi et al. 2015. "Differential expression of seven conserved MicroRNAs in response to abiotic stress and their regulatory network in helianthus annuus." Frontiers in Plant Science 6(September): 1-14.

[67] Zhang B, Wang Q. MicroRNA, a new target for engineering new crop cultivars. Bioengineered. 2016;**7**(1):7-10. DOI: 10.1080/21655979.2016.1141838

[68] Zhu QH, Wang MB. Molecular functions of long non-coding RNAs in plants. Genes. 2012;**3**(1):176-190

[69] Hajyzadeh M, Turktas M, Khawar KM, Unver T. MiR408 overexpression causes increased drought tolerance in chickpea. Gene. 2015;**555**(2):186-193. DOI: 10.1016/j.gene.2014.11.002

[70] Ma C, Burd S, Lers A. MiR408 is involved in abiotic stress responses in arabidopsis. Plant Journal. 2015;**84**(1):169-187

[71] Zhao J et al. Transgenic creeping bentgrass overexpressing osa-MiR393a exhibits altered plant development and improved multiple stress tolerance. Plant Biotechnology Journal. 2019;**17**(1):233-251

[72] Baek D et al. A role for arabidopsis MiR399f in salt, drought, and ABA signaling. Molecules and Cells. 2016;**39**(2):111-118

[73] Ferdous J et al. Drought-inducible expression of Hv-MiR827 enhances drought tolerance in transgenic barley. Functional and Integrative Genomics. 2017;**17**(2-3):279-292

[74] Aukerman M. Drought tolerant plants and related constructs and methods involving genes encooing MIR827. 2013;**1**(61)

[75] Aukerman M, Park W. Drought tolerant plants and related constructs and methods involving genes encoding MiR827. 2008;**1**(19). Available from: https://patents.google.com/patent/US20090165168A1/en

[76] Sunkar R, Zhu JK. Novel and stress-regulated MicroRNAs and other small RNAs from. Arabidopsis Plant Cell. 2004;**16**(August 2004):2019

[77] Man Z, Hong L. Role of microRNA319 in creeping bentgrass salinity and drought stress response. Plant Signaling and Behavior. 2014;**9**(4):e28700, DOI:10.4161/psb.28700

[78] Raj KJ, Swati M, Urmila B, Muhammad HR, Nat NVK. Genome wide identification and functional prediction of long non-coding RNAs responsive to sclerotinia sclerotiorum infection in brassica napus. PLoS One. 2016;**11**(7):1-19. DOI: 10.1371/journal.pone.0158784

[79] Matzke MA, Rebecca AM. RNA-directed DNA methylation: An epigenetic pathway of increasing complexity. Nature Reviews Genetics. 2014;**15**(6):394-408. DOI: 10.1038/nrg3683

[80] Wierzbicki AT. The role of long non-coding RNA in transcriptional gene silencing. Current Opinion in Plant Biology. 2012;**15**(5):517-522. DOI: 10.1016/j.pbi.2012.08.008

required specifically for the phasing, not production, of trans-acting short interfering RNAs in arabidopsis. Plant Cell. 2016;**28**(7):1563-1580

[32] Meng Y, Shao C, Ma X, Wang H. Introns targeted by plant MicroRNAs: A possible novel mechanism of gene regulation. Rice. 2013;**6**(1):1-10

[33] Li S et al. MicroRNAs inhibit the translation of target MRNAs on the endoplasmic reticulum in arabidopsis. Cell. 2013;**153**(3):562-574

[34] Shan Q et al. Multiplex and homologous recombination–mediated genome editing in arabidopsis and nicotiana benthamiana using guide RNA and Cas9. Nature Biotechnology. 2013;**31**(8):686-688

[35] Gull A, Lone AA, Wani NUI. Biotic and Abiotic Stresses in Plants. In: de Oliveira A, editor. Abiotic and Biotic Stress in Plants. London: IntechOpen; 2019. 6p. https://doi.org/10.5772/intechopen.85832

[36] Zhang H, Zhu J, Gong Z, et al. Abiotic stress responses in plants. Nature Reviews. Genetics. 2022;**23**:104-119. DOI: 10.1038/s41576-021-00413-0

[37] Shinozaki K, Yamaguchi-Shinozaki K. Gene networks involved in drought stress response and tolerance. Journal of Experimental Botany. 2007;**58**(2): 221-227

[38] Ayubov MS et al. Role of MicroRNAs and small RNAs in regulation of developmental processes and agronomic traits in gossypium species. Genomics. 2019;**111**(5):1018-1025. DOI: 10.1016/j.ygeno.2018.07.012

[39] Kumar R. Role of MicroRNAs in biotic and abiotic stress responses in crop plants. Applied Biochemistry and Biotechnology. 2014;**174**(1):93-115

[40] Ferdous J, Hussain SS, Shi BJ. Role of MicroRNAs in plant drought tolerance. Plant Biotechnology Journal. 2015;**13**(3):293-305

[41] Zhou L et al. Genome-wide identification and analysis of drought-responsive MicroRNAs in oryza sativa. Journal of Experimental Botany. 2010;**61**(15):4157-4168

[42] Kulcheski FR, de Oliveira LF, Molina LG, Almerão MP, Rodrigues FA, Marcolino J, et. al. Identification of novel soybean microRNAs involved in abiotic and biotic stresses. BMC genomics. 2011;**12**(307):1-17. https://doi.org/10.1186/1471-2164-12-307

[43] Deng P et al. Global identification of MicroRNAs and their targets in barley under salinity stress. PLoS One. 2015;**10**(9):1-20

[44] Sunkar R, Zhu J-K. Novel and stress-regulated MicroRNAs and other small RNAs from arabidopsis. 2004;**18**(August):957

[45] Jones-Rhoades MW, Bartel DP. Computational identification of plant MicroRNAs and their targets, including a stress-induced MiRNA. Molecular Cell. 2004;**14**(6):787-799

[46] Mahdavi-Darvari F, Noor NM, Ismanizan I. Epigenetic regulation and gene markers as signals of early somatic embryogenesis. Plant Cell, Tissue and Organ Culture. 2014;**120**(2):407-422. Available from: https://www.scopus.com/inward/record.uri?eid=2-s2.0-84921809786&doi=10.1007%2Fs11240-014-0615-0&partnerID=40&md5=9558f1d988ad53c4638fdf1142f417d2

[47] Vaucheret H, Vazquez F, Crété P, Bartel DP. The action of ARGONAUTE1 in the MiRNA pathway and its regulation by the MiRNA pathway are crucial

for plant development. Genes and Development. 2004;**18**(10):1187-1197

[48] Jain M et al. F-Box proteins in rice. Genome-wide analysis, classification, temporal and spatial gene expression during panicle and seed development, and regulation by light and abiotic stress. Plant Physiology. 2007;**143**(4): 1467-1483

[49] Navarro L, Dunoyer P, Jay F, Arnold B, Dharmasiri N, Estelle M, et al. A plant miRNA contributes to antibacterial resistance by repressing auxin signaling. Science. New York, N.Y. 2006;**312**(5772):436-439. https://doi.org/10.1126/science.1126088

[50] Apel K, Hirt H. Reactive oxygen species: Metabolism, oxidative stress, and signal transduction. Annual Review of Plant Biology. 2004;**55**:373-399

[51] Kimura M et al. Analysis of hydrogen peroxide–independent expression of the high-light–inducible ELIP2 gene with the aid of the ELIP2 promoter–luciferase fusion. Photochemistry and Photobiology. 2003;**77**(6):668

[52] Ku YS et al. Small RNAs in plant responses to abiotic stresses: Regulatory roles and study methods. International Journal of Molecular Sciences. 2015;**16**(10):24532-24554

[53] Sun X et al. Preparation and luminescence properties of Sr2EuxLa1-XAlO5 phosphor. Journal of Luminescence. 2015;**157**:197-200

[54] Kord H, Fakheri B, Ghabooli M, et al. Salinity-associated microRNAs and their potential roles in mediating salt tolerance in rice colonized by the endophytic root fungus Piriformospora indica. Funct Integr Genomics. 2019;**19**:659-672. https://doi.org/10.1007/s10142-019-00671-6

[55] Xu J, Chen Q, Liu P, Jia W, Chen Z, Xu Z. Integration of mRNA and miRNA Analysis Reveals the Molecular Mechanism Underlying Salt and Alkali Stress Tolerance in Tobacco. International journal of molecular sciences. 2019;**20**(10):1-18, 2391. https://doi.org/10.3390/ijms20102391

[56] Mehrpooyan F, Othman RY, Harikrishna JA. Tissue and temporal expression of MiR172 paralogs and the AP2-like target in oil palm (Elaeis Guineensis Jacq.). Tree Genetics and Genomes. 2012;**8**(6):1331-1343

[57] Low ET, Rosli R, Jayanthi N, Mohd-Amin AH, Azizi N, Chan KL, et al. Analyses of hypomethylated oil palm gene space. PloS one. 2014;**9**(1):1-15, e86728. https://doi.org/10.1371/journal.pone.0086728

[58] da Silva A, Cunha, et al. Computational identification and comparative analysis of MiRNA precursors in three palm species. Planta. 2016;**243**(5):1265-1277

[59] Somyong S et al. ACC oxidase and MiRNA 159a, and their involvement in fresh fruit bunch yield (FFB) via sex ratio determination in oil palm. Molecular Genetics and Genomics. 2016;**291**(3):1243-1257

[60] Huili H, Gudimella R, Ong-Abdullah M, Harikrishna JA. Expression of microRNAs during female inflorescence development in African oil palm (Elaeis guineensis Jacq.). Tree Genetics and Genomes. 2017;**35**(13):1-17. https://doi.org/10.1007/s11295-017-1120-5

[61] Gao LC et al. EgmiR5179 from the mesocarp of oil palm (Elaeis Guineensis Jacq.) regulates oil accumulation by targeting NAD transporter 1. Industrial Crops and Products. 2019;**137**(October 2018):126-136. DOI: 10.1016/j.indcrop.2019.05.013